Immunotherapy in Clinical Medicine

Guest Editors

NANCY MISRI KHARDORI, MD, PhD, FACP, FIDSA
ROMESH KHARDORI, MD, PhD, FACP, FACE

MEDICAL CLINICS OF NORTH AMERICA

www.medical.theclinics.com

May 2012 • Volume 96 • Number 3

SAUNDERS an imprint of ELSEVIER, Inc.

W.B. SAUNDERS COMPANY
A Division of Elsevier Inc.

1600 John F. Kennedy Boulevard ● Suite 1800 ● Philadelphia, Pennsylvania 19103-2899

http://www.theclinics.com

MEDICAL CLINICS OF NORTH AMERICA Volume 96, Number 3
May 2012 ISSN 0025-7125, ISBN-13: 978-1-4557-5064-1

Editor: Pamela Hetherington
Developmental Editor: Teia Stone

Medical Clinics of North America (ISSN 0025-7125) is published bimonthly by Elsevier Inc., 360 Park Avenue South, New York, NY 10010-1710. Months of issue are January, March, May, July, September, and November. Periodicals postage paid at New York, NY, and additional mailing offices. Subscription prices are USD 232 per year for US individuals, USD 424 per year for US institutions, USD 117 per year for US students, USD 295 per year for Canadian individuals, USD 551 per year for Canadian institutions, USD 184 per year for Canadian students, USD 358 per year for international individuals, USD 551 per year for international institutions and USD 184 per year for international students. To receive student/resident rate, orders must be accompanied by name of affiliated institution, date of term, and the *signature* of program/residency coordinator on institution letterhead. Orders will be billed at individual rate until proof of status is received. Foreign air speed delivery is included in all *Clinics* subscription prices. All prices are subject to change without notice. **POSTMASTER:** Send address changes to *Medical Clinics of North America*, Elsevier Health Sciences Division, Subscription Customer Service, 3251 Riverport Lane, Maryland Heights, MO 63043. **Customer Service: Telephone: 1-800-654-2452** (U.S. and Canada); **1-314-447-8871** (outside U.S. and Canada). **Fax: 1-314-447-8029. E-mail: journalscustomerservice-usa@elsevier.com** (for print support); **journalsonlinesupport-usa@ elsevier.com** (for online support).

Reprints. For copies of 100 or more of articles in this publication, please contact the Commercial Reprints Department, Elsevier Inc., 360 Park Avenue South, New York, NY 10010-1710. Tel.: 212-633-3812; Fax: 212-462-1935; E-mail: reprints@elsevier.com.

Medical Clinics of North America is also published in Spanish by McGraw-Hill Interamericana Editores S. A., P.O. Box 5-237, 06500 Mexico, D.F., Mexico.

Medical Clinics of North America is covered in *MEDLINE/PubMed (Index Medicus), Current Contents, ASCA, Excerpta Medica, Science Citation Index, and ISI/BIOMED.*

Printed in the United States of America.

GOAL STATEMENT

The goal of *Medical Clinics of North America* is to keep practicing physicians up to date with current clinical practice by providing timely articles reviewing the state of the art in patient care.

ACCREDITATION

The *Medical Clinics of North America* is planned and implemented in accordance with the Essential Areas and Policies of the Accreditation Council for Continuing Medical Education (ACCME) through the joint sponsorship of the University of Virginia School of Medicine and Elsevier. The University of Virginia School of Medicine is accredited by the ACCME to provide continuing medical education for physicians.

The University of Virginia School of Medicine designates this enduring material activity for a maximum of 15 *AMA PRA Category 1 Credit*(s)™ for each issue, 90 credits per year. Physicians should only claim credit commensurate with the extent of their participation in the activity.

The American Medical Association has determined that physicians not licensed in the US who participate in this CME enduring material activity are eligible for a maximum of 15 *AMA PRA Category 1 Credit*(s)™ for each issue, 90 credits per year.

Credit can be earned by reading the text material, taking the CME examination online at http://www.theclinics.com/home/cme, and completing the evaluation. After taking the test, you will be required to review any and all incorrect answers. Following completion of the test and evaluation, your credit will be awarded and you may print your certificate.

FACULTY DISCLOSURE/CONFLICT OF INTEREST

The University of Virginia School of Medicine, as an ACCME accredited provider, endorses and strives to comply with the Accreditation Council for Continuing Medical Education (ACCME) Standards of Commercial Support, Commonwealth of Virginia statutes, University of Virginia policies and procedures, and associated federal and private regulations and guidelines on the need for disclosure and monitoring of proprietary and financial interests that may affect the scientific integrity and balance of content delivered in continuing medical education activities under our auspices.

The University of Virginia School of Medicine requires that all CME activities accredited through this institution be developed independently and be scientifically rigorous, balanced and objective in the presentation/discussion of its content, theories and practices.

All authors/editors participating in an accredited CME activity are expected to disclose to the readers relevant financial relationships with commercial entities occurring within the past 12 months (such as grants or research support, employee, consultant, stock holder, member of speakers bureau, etc.). The University of Virginia School of Medicine will employ appropriate mechanisms to resolve potential conflicts of interest to maintain the standards of fair and balanced education to the reader. Questions about specific strategies can be directed to the Office of Continuing Medical Education, University of Virginia School of Medicine, Charlottesville, Virginia.

The faculty and staff of the University of Virginia Office of Continuing Medical Education have no financial affiliations to disclose.

The authors/editors listed below have identified no professional or financial affiliations for themselves or their spouse/partner:

Jatinder P. Ahluwalia, MD; Emilie Beke, MD; André Delannoy, MD, PhD; Timothy Devos, MD, PhD; Daan Dierickx, MD; Robyn S. Fallen, BHSc; Carmel Fratianni, MD; Pamela Hetherington (Acquisitions Editor); Michael Gonzales, MD; Smita Gupta, MD; Nancy Misri Khardori, MD, PhD, FIDSA (Guest Editor); Ajay Kher, MBBS; Hermenio C. Lima, MD, PhD; Chaitanya Mamillapali, MBBS, MRCP; Anne V. Miller, MD; Jignesh Modi, MD; Sriya K.M. Ranatunga, MD, MPH; Lokesh Shanini, MD; Sushma Singh, MD; Vidya Sundareshan, MD; Collin R. Terpstra, MD; Andrew Wolf, MD (Test Author).

The authors/editors listed below identified the following professional or financial affiliations for themselves or their spouse/partner:

Donna Graves, MD is on the Speakers' Bureau for TEVA Pharmaceutricals, Bayer Healthcare, and Novartis.
Vivek Kak, MD is on the Speakers' Bureau for Cubist Pharmaceutical and Forest Pharmaceutical.
Romesh Khardori, MD, PhD (Guest Editor) receives research support from Eli Lilly.
Vijay Kher, MD, DM is an industry funded research/investigator, and is on the Speakers' Bureau and Advisory Board for Novartis India, and Roche, India; is on the Advisory Board for Torrent Pharmaceuticals; and is an industry funded research/investigator and is on the Speakers' Bureau for Pancea Biotec.
Steven Vernino, MD, PhD has a licensing contract with Athena Diagnostics, is on the Advisory Board for Myasthenia Gravis Foundation, receives research support from Chelsea Therapeutics, and is on the editorial board for Archives of Neurology.
Philip Wood, D.Phil., FRCP, FRCPath is on the Advisory Board for Baxter, CSL Behring, Octapharma, and Shire.

Disclosure of Discussion of Non-FDA Approved Uses for Pharmaceutical Products and/or Medical Devices

The University of Virginia School of Medicine, as an ACCME provider, requires that all faculty presenters identify and disclose any off-label uses for pharmaceutical and medical device products. The University of Virginia School of Medicine recommends that each physician fully review all the available data on new products or procedures prior to clinical use.

TO ENROLL

To enroll in the Medical Clinics of North America Continuing Medical Education program, call customer service at 1-800-654-2452 or visit us online at http://www.theclinics.com/home/cme. The CME program is available to subscribers for an additional fee of USD 228.

MEDICAL CLINICS OF NORTH AMERICA

FORTHCOMING ISSUES

July 2012
COPD
Stephen I. Rennard, MD, and
Bartolome R. Celli, MD, *Guest Editors*

September 2012
Heart Failure
Prakash Deedwania, MD, *Guest Editor*

RECENT ISSUES

March 2012
Thyroid Disorders and Diseases
Kenneth D. Burman, MD, *Guest Editor*

January 2012
Coronary Risk Factors Update
Valentin Fuster, MD, PhD, and
Jagat Narula, MD, PhD,
Guest Editors

November 2011
Pulmonary Diseases
Ali I. Musani, MD, *Guest Editor*

RELATED INTEREST

Immunology and Allergy Clinics, February 2012 (Volume 32, Issue 1)
Food Allergy
Anna Nowak-Węgrzyn, MD, *Guest Editor*

DOWNLOAD
Free App!

Review Articles
THE CLINICS

NOW AVAILABLE FOR YOUR iPhone and iPad

Contributors

GUEST EDITORS

NANCY MISRI KHARDORI, MD, PhD, FACP, FIDSA
Professor of Medicine and Microbiology and Molecular Cell Biology, Division of Infectious Diseases, Department of Internal Medicine and Microbiology and Molecular Cell Biology, Eastern Virginia Medical School, Norfolk, Virginia

ROMESH KHARDORI, MD, PhD, FACP, FACE
Professor of Medicine and Endocrinology; Director, Endocrinology Fellowship Training Program, Division of Endocrinology and Metabolism, Department of Internal Medicine, Strelitz Center for Diabetes and Endocrine Disorders, Eastern Virginia Medical School, Norfolk, Virginia

AUTHORS

JATINDER P. AHLUWALIA, MD
Staff Physician, Gastroenterology Clinic of Acadiana and Lafayette General Medical Center, Lafayette; Clinical Associate Professor of Medicine, Gastroenterology and Hepatology, Department of Medicine, Tulane University, New Orleans, Louisiana

EMILIE BEKE, MD
Department of Internal Medicine, University Hospitals Leuven, Leuven, Belgium

ANDRÉ DELANNOY, MD, PhD
Hôpital de Jolimont, Haine-Saint-Paul and Cliniques Universitaires St Luc, Brussels, Haine-Saint-Paul, Belgium

TIMOTHY DEVOS, MD, PhD
Department of Hematology, University Hospitals Leuven, Leuven, Belgium

DAAN DIERICKX, MD
Department of Hematology, University Hospitals Leuven, Leuven, Belgium

ROBYN S. FALLEN, BHSc
Michael G. DeGroote School of Medicine, Waterloo Regional Campus, McMaster University, Kitchener, Ontario, Canada

CARMEL FRATIANNI, MD, FACE
Division of Endocrinology and Metabolism, Department of Internal Medicine, Southern Illinois University School of Medicine, Springfield, Illinois

MICHAEL GONZALES, MD
Division of Endocrinology and Metabolism, Department of Internal Medicine, Strelitz Center for Diabetes and Endocrine Disorders, Eastern Virginia Medical School, Norfolk, Virginia

DONNA GRAVES, MD
Assistant Professor, Department of Neurology and Neurotherapeutics, UT Southwestern Medical Center, Dallas, Texas

SMITA GUPTA, MD
Diabetes and Endocrinology Consultants, Indianapolis, Indiana

VIVEK KAK, MD
Allegiance Health, Jackson, Michigan

NANCY MISRI KHARDORI, MD, PhD, FACP, FIDSA
Professor of Medicine and Microbiology and Molecular Cell Biology, Division of Infectious Diseases, Departments of Internal Medicine, and Microbiology and Molecular Cell Biology, Eastern Virginia Medical School, Norfolk, Virginia

ROMESH KHARDORI, MD, PhD, FACP, FACE
Professor of Medicine and Endocrinology; Director, Endocrinology Fellowship Training Program, Division of Endocrinology and Metabolism, Department of Internal Medicine, Strelitz Center for Diabetes and Endocrine Disorders, Eastern Virginia Medical School, Norfolk, Virginia

AJAY KHER, MBBS
The Transplant Institute, Beth Israel Deaconess Medical Center, Boston, Massachusetts

VIJAY KHER, MD, DM
Division of Nephrology and Renal Transplant Medicine, Kidney and Urology Institute, Medanta–The Medicity, Gurgaon, India

HERMENIO C. LIMA, MD, PhD
Associate Clinical Professor, Division of Dermatology, Department of Medicine, Michael G. DeGroote School of Medicine, McMaster University, Kitchener, Ontario, Canada

CHAITANYA MAMILLAPALI, MBBS, MRCP
Division of Endocrinology and Metabolism, Department of Internal Medicine, Southern Illinois University School of Medicine, Springfield, Illinois

ANNE V. MILLER, MD
Assistant Professor, Division of Rheumatology, Department of Internal Medicine, Southern Illinois University School of Medicine, Springfield, Illinois

JIGNESH MODI, MD
Division of Infectious Diseases, Department of Internal Medicine, Southern Illinois University School of Medicine, Springfield, Illinois

SRIYA K.M. RANATUNGA, MD, MPH
Associate Professor, Division of Rheumatology, Department of Internal Medicine, Southern Illinois University School of Medicine, Springfield, Illinois

LOKESH SHAHANI, MD
Department of Medicine, Southern Illinois University School of Medicine, Springfield, Illinois

SUSHMA SINGH, MD
Division of Infectious Diseases, Department of Internal Medicine, Eastern Virginia Medical School, Norfolk, Virginia

VIDYA SUNDARESHAN, MD
Division of Infectious Diseases, Department of Internal Medicine, Southern Illinois University School of Medicine, Springfield, Illinois

COLLIN R. TERPSTRA, MD
Division of Allergy, Department of Medicine, Michael G. DeGroote School of Medicine, McMaster University, Hamilton, Ontario, Canada

STEVEN VERNINO, MD, PhD
Professor, Department of Neurology and Neurotherapeutics, UT Southwestern Medical Center, Dallas, Texas

PHILIP WOOD, D.Phil., FRCP, FRCPath
Department of Clinical Immunology, St James's University Hospital, Leeds, Yorkshire, United Kingdom

Contents

> In humans, the immune system is a complex organ system involving cells and soluble mediators whose function is, essentially, protection. However, disequilibrium in this intricate system leads to disease in itself. To modulate these responses, immunotherapy is now the primary or adjunct treatment of many diseases. In addition, immunologic tests now diagnose several diseases.

> The 2 most commonly encountered primary immunodeficiency syndromes in adult practice are antibody deficiency disorders and hereditary angioedema. Immunologic therapy for these disorders has significantly improved patient management. Therapy with immunoglobulin leads to improvement in overall quality of life. With increasing survival rates and decreasing levels of life-threatening infections in patients with primary antibody deficiencies, disease complications are more commonly encountered. Treatment of these complications with monoclonal antibody therapy seems promising and is likely to increase in the future. More recently, several additional agents have become available, including novel drugs targeted at different elements of the disease process.

> The development of an infection involves interplay between the host's immune system and the virulence of the infecting microorganism. The traditional treatment of an infection involves antimicrobial chemotherapy to kill the organism. The use of immunotherapies in infections includes treatment options that modulate the immune response and can lead to control of infections. These therapies are expected to become more important therapeutic options with the increase in infections due to multidrug-resistant organisms and the increasing number of immunocompromised patients.

> Over the past several decades, rheumatology has directed its focus to understanding and countering the immune dysregulation underlying autoimmune diseases with rheumatologic manifestations. Older therapies, effective though poorly understood, are being scrutinized anew and are

yielding the immune-modulating mechanisms behind their efficacy. New therapies, the "biologics," are drugs tailored to address specific immune defects and imbalances. This article discusses the current standard and biologic immunotherapies of the rheumatic diseases, correlating our current understanding of their mechanisms with dysfunctions believed to be present in the major autoimmune syndromes, especially rheumatoid arthritis and systemic lupus erythematosus.

Therapy for autoimmune demyelinating disorders has evolved rapidly over the past 10 years to include traditional immunosuppressants as well as novel biologicals. Antibody-mediated neuromuscular disorders are treated with therapies that acutely modulate pathogenic antibodies or chronically inhibit the humoral immune response. In other inflammatory autoimmune disorders of the peripheral and central nervous system, corticosteroids, often combined with conventional immunosuppression, and immunomodulatory treatments are used. Because autoimmune neurologic disorders are so diverse, evidence from randomized controlled trials is limited for most of the immunotherapies used in neurology. This review provides an overview of the immunotherapies currently used for neurologic disorders.

Inflammatory bowel disease affects an increasing number of patients worldwide and is associated with significant morbidity. The dysregulation of the immune system with increased expression of proinflammatory cytokines and increased mucosal expression of vascular adhesion molecules play an important role in its pathogenesis. Strategies targeting TNF-alpha and alpha4-integrin have led to the development of novel therapies for treatment of patients with IBD. This article discusses the efficacy of immunologic agents currently approved for treating Crohn disease and ulcerative colitis and reviews the risks and challenges associated with their use.

Immunotherapy has been used for the treatment of renal diseases for a long time, and there has been significant progress in such treatment. This review focuses on the use of immunotherapy for the treatment of glomerular diseases. The use of immunosuppression in the treatment of minimal change disease, membranous nephropathy, primary focal segmental glomerulosclerosis, lupus nephritis, immunoglobulin-A nephropathy, antineutrophil cytoplasmic antibody–associated disease, and anti–glomerular basement membrane disease is discussed.

Treatment modalities and therapeutic response experience support the use of immunotherapy in the treatment of many diseases in all fields of medicine. The aim of this article is to conduct and present a review of literature on the use of immunotherapy in the treatment of skin diseases analyzing scientific literature available up to January 2012. Studies that presented evidence-based data were selected. The article discusses how blocking or reverting the effect of a specific immunologic disequilibrium can treat dermatoses and intends to transfer a large amount of immunotherapy knowledge into a historical perspective for physicians naive to immunotherapy practices.

In this article, the evidence on the clinical use of monoclonal antibodies in the treatment of immune-mediated hematologic disorders is described. Insights into pathogenic mechanisms have revealed a major role of both B and T cells. Controlled trials have shown conflicting results, necessitating further research regarding pathogenesis, mechanism of action, and resistance. Although the use of more potent and specific monoclonal antibody therapy, mainly targeting costimulation signals, may improve response rates and long-term outcome, its use should be carefully balanced against potential side effects.

Type 1 diabetes is an autoimmune disease that gradually destructs insulin-producing beta cells. Over the years, clinicians' knowledge regarding the immunopathogenesis of this disease has greatly increased. Immunotherapies that can change the course of immune-mediated destruction and preserve and possibly regenerate the pancreatic beta cells seem to be promising in preclinical trials but so far have been unsuccessful in human studies. This article reviews the important immune interventions for type 1 diabetes that have been tried so far targeting the different stages of disease development and provides an insight into what the future might hold.

In Graves ophthalmopathy, immunotherapy is offering an opportunity of reducing bad outcomes that lead to disfigurement and impairment of vision. These therapies are not perfect; however, we now have a chance to achieve better outcomes. In asthma, immune therapy using passive immunity targeting key proinflammatory cytokine/chemokines and medications of their effects has opened an avenue of research into a safe and durable therapy. Omalizumab appears to be safe and effective in clinical use. In regional pain syndrome, immune mechanisms may be involved in sustaining long-standing pain, and IVIG may moderate pain sensitivity by reducing immune activation.

Preface
Immunotherapy in Clinical
Medicine

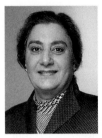 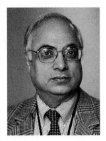

Nancy Misri Khardori, MD, PhD, FIDSA   Romesh Khardori, MD, PhD
Guest Editors

Active Immunotherapy in the form of pre-exposure primary and secondary (booster) vaccination has made the most significant impact on the current state of human health and longevity by preventing childhood and adult infectious diseases. The current availability of a vaccine (HPV vaccine) that prevents a number of cancers by inducing an immune response to a virus has opened up the field of preventive cancer vaccines. Passive immunotherapy using preformed antibodies and modulation of cytokine cascade by agonists and antagonists has added to the therapeutic armamentarium for diseases involving many organ systems. A brief overview of the history and current status of immunotherapy is presented in the first article. The next 10 articles review in detail the current status of immunological therapies in various diseases. The major focus of these articles is on clinically available immunotherapies. However, all the authors have included information on investigational and evolving immunotherapies. Such therapies for potentially fatal acute infectious disease caused by resistant pathogens are the need of the hour considering that no novel antimicrobial agents are in the pipeline. Even if such novel agents did become available, microbes developing resistance to antimicrobial agents are by now an expectation rather than news. It seems that understanding and utilizing physiology will be the most lasting intervention against pathology of human disease. That being the case, broadening and deepening of basic science curricula during medical school and graduate training should be a priority for educators and policy-makers. Simply teaching about a list of currently prevalent diseases in a superficial manner is likely feeding them today without concern for tomorrow. We find one of Osler's quotes most appropriate in this context: "We are easily misled by our experience and not only are the reactions (of patients) themselves variable, but we, the doctors, are so fallible, ever beset with the common and fatal facility of reaching conclusions from superficial observations, and constantly misled by the ease with which our mind fall into the ruts of one or two experiences."

Med Clin N Am 96 (2012) xiii–xiv
doi:10.1016/j.mcna.2012.04.005
0025-7125/12/$ – see front matter © 2012 Elsevier Inc. All rights reserved.

medical.theclinics.com

It is clear that this issue of *Medical Clinics of North America* was made possible by the high quality of the diligent and meticulous work of the contributing authors. For this we owe them our appreciation and gratitude. We owe special thanks to Sandra Finch of the Department of Internal Medicine at Eastern Virginia Medical School for the assistance she provided in bringing this issue to fruition.

Nancy Misri Khardori, MD, PhD, FIDSA
Division of Infectious Diseases
Department of Internal Medicine
and Microbiology and Molecular Cell Biology
Eastern Virginia Medical School
700 West Olney Road
Norfolk, VA 23507, USA

Romesh Khardori, MD, PhD
Division of Endocrinology and Metabolism
Department of Internal Medicine
Strelitz Center for Diabetes and Endocrine Disorders
Eastern Virginia Medical School
855 West Brambleton Avenue
Norfolk, VA 23510, USA

E-mail addresses:
nkhardori@gmail.com (N.M. Khardori)
rkhardori@gmail.com (R. Khardori)

Erratum

With regard to the article "LDL Cholesterol: The Lower the Better," by Seth S. Martin, Roger S. Blumenthal, and Michael Miller, which appeared in *Medical Clinics of North America,* Jan. 2012 96(1):13–26, the publisher would like to clarify that **Table 1** on page 22 and **Table 2** on page 23 have incorrect titles. The correct title for **Table 1** is "Risk factors for the development of myopathy" and the correct title for **Table 2** is "Major safety and efficacy outcomes across strata of achieved LDL-C (percentage of subjects)."

Table 1
Risk factors for the development of myopathy

Concomitant Medications	Other Conditions
Fibrate	Advanced age (especially >80 years)
Nicotinic acid (rarely)	Women > Men especially at older age
Cyclosporine	Small body frame, frailty
Antifungal azoles	Multisystem disease
Macrolide antibitors	Multiple medications
HIV protease inhibitors	Perioperative period
Nafazadone	Alcohol abuse
Verapamil, Amiodarone	Grapefruit juice (>1 quart/day)

Abbreviation: HIV, human immunodeficiency virus.
From Wiviott SD, Cannon CP, Morrow DA, et al. PROVE IT-TIMI 22 Investigators. Can low-density lipoprotein be too low? The safety and efficacy of achieving very low low-density lipoprotein with intensive statin therapy: a PROVE IT-TIMI 22 substudy. J Am Coll Cardiol 2005;46:1414; with permission.

doi:10.1016/j.mcna.2012.05.007
0025-7125/12/$ – see front matter
medical.theclinics.com

Table 2
Major safety and efficacy outcomes across strata of achieved LDL cholesterol (percent of subjects)

| | Achieved LDL Cholesterol (mg/dL) | | | | |
| | >80–100 | >60–80 | >40–60 | <40 | |
Safety Measure	n = 256	n = 576	n = 631	n = 193	p Trend
Muscle side effects[a]					
Myalgia	6.4	4.3	6.2	5.7	0.75
Myositis	0.4	0.6	0.6	0	0.64
CK >3× ULN	2.3	0.7	1.9	1.0	0.18
CK >10× ULN	0	0	0.3	0	0.45
Rhabdomyolysis	0	0	0	0	1.0
Liver side effects					
ALT >3× ULN	3.2	3.0	3.2	2.6	0.98
Study drug discontinued because of LFT	2.0	2.6	2.4	1.6	0.83
Other					
Hemorrhagic stroke	0.4	0.2	0	0	0.12
Retinal AE	0.4	0.9	1.0	0	0.48
Suicide/trauma death	0	0	0	0	1.0
Study drug discontinued because of any AE	10.2	9.4	9.7	9.8	0.99
Major efficacy measures					
Death	1.1	1.4	1.3	0.5	0.59
CHD death	0.5	0.5	0.6	0.0	0.06
Myocardial infraction	1.0	0.7	0.5	0.6	0.009
Any stroke	0.8	0.9	0.6	1.6	0.32
Primary composite[a]	26.1	22.2	20.4	20.4	0.10

Abbreviations: AE, adverse event; ALT, alanine aminotransferase; CHD, coronary heart disease; CK, creatine kinase; LFT, liver function test; LDL-C, low-density lipoprotein cholesterol; ULN, upper limit of normal.

[a] Primary composite: percent of subjects with any of the following: death, myocardial infarction, stroke, unstable angina requiring rehospitalization, and revascularization. Myalgia: muscle symptoms without CK elevation. Myositis: muscle symptoms with CK elevation. Rhabdomyolysis: muscle symptoms with CK >10 × ULN and evidence of renal dysfunction.

Adapted from Pasternak RC, Smith SC Jr, Bairey-Merz CN, et al. American College of Cardiology; American Heart Association; National Heart, Lung and Blood Institute. ACC/AHA/NHLBI Clinical Advisory on the Use and Safety of Statins. Circulation 2002;106:1027; with permission.

Immunotherapy in Clinical Medicine: Historical Perspective and Current Status

Lokesh Shahani, MD[a], Sushma Singh, MD[b],
Nancy Misri Khardori, MD, PhD, FIDSA[b],*

KEYWORDS

- Immunotherapy • Vaccination • Immunoglobulins • Cytokines

Key Points

- The use of immunotherapy crosses disciplines and involves several diseases.
- Active immunotherapy in the form of vaccines remains the single most significant intervention in decreasing childhood mortality.
- The use of immunotherapy for the modulation of immune responses in noninfectious diseases is now the standard of care.

INTRODUCTION

Immunotherapy is broadly defined as the prevention and/or treatment of diseases by inducing, enhancing, or suppressing immune response, and has been recently reviewed in the context of biological disease modifiers.[1]

The concept of inducing protection against diseases dates back to the eighteenth century, before the germ theory of disease was scientifically proved. When microbiological methods to cultivate various organisms became available, methods to render these organisms nonpathogenic while maintaining immunogenicity made it possible to control and/or eradicate several acute and potentially fatal childhood infectious diseases. This active immunoprotection by routinely used vaccines has made the most significant contribution to the current status of human health and longevity.

---

[a] Department of Medicine, Southern Illinois University School of Medicine, 801 North Rutledge, PO Box 9636, Springfield, IL 62794, USA
[b] Division of Infectious Diseases, Department of Internal Medicine and Microbiology and Molecular Cell Biology, Eastern Virginia Medical School, 700 West Olney Road, Norfolk, VA 23507, USA
* Corresponding author.
E-mail address: KhardoriNM@evms.edu

Med Clin N Am 96 (2012) 421–431
doi:10.1016/j.mcna.2012.04.001   medical.theclinics.com
0025-7125/12/$ – see front matter © 2012 Published by Elsevier Inc.

Passive immunotherapy, in the form of serum from recovering patients, was used even before the availability of antimicrobial therapy in the mid 1940s and was further improved by the use of antitoxins raised in animals. In 1944, the fractionation of human immunoglobulin for the treatment of measles overcame the problem of serum sickness and introduced the concept of pooled immunoglobulin therapy. Molecular technology has now offered development and the use of defined monoclonal antibodies against factors involved in the pathogenesis of diseases.

Immunotherapy has become an integral part of clinical practice. Articles that follow in this issue discuss the use of immunotherapy in various organ system disorders.

ACTIVE IMMUNOTHERAPY: VACCINATION

Active immunotherapy has been in use over the past 2 centuries to prevent the morbidity and mortality associated with various infectious diseases. Smallpox, a disease of the past, was a major killer in the eighteenth century. In 1796, Edward Jenner discovered that deliberate infection with the cowpox virus caused mild disease and, thereby, resulted in subsequent immunity to the smallpox virus infection. This discovery was a pioneering work in immunotherapy and also one of the greatest revolutions in medical therapy.[2,3] Vaccination (Latin: *vacca*, cow) was so named because the first vaccine was derived from a virus affecting cows. Using the same concept, effective vaccines in the form of either killed or attenuated pathogens have been developed for several infectious diseases (**Table 1**).

Louis Pasteur and coworkers first adopted the concept of physical attenuation of pathogenic organisms for the purpose of immunization in the early twentieth century. The concept came from an observation Pasteur made in 1881. A culture of *Pasteurella multocida* lying on his bench over the summer break failed to cause disease when injected into chickens. These chickens did not develop disease after a challenge with a newly made culture either. This finding led Pasteur[4] to the conclusion that the chickens were immune to the disease because of the previous exposure to aged and, probably, damaged culture. The physical attenuation of the organisms led to the discovery of vaccines against anthrax and rabies. Pasteur exposed *Bacillus anthracis* to oxygen before using it for vaccinating animals. He produced the first vaccine for rabies by growing the virus in rabbits and then weakening it by drying the affected nerve tissue.

In 1907, Calmette and colleagues[5] used passage in artificial media to attenuate *Mycobacterium bovis*, and in 1937, Theiler and Smith[6] used passage in mice and chick embryos to attenuate yellow fever virus before its use in human vaccines. In the middle of the twentieth century it was discovered that passage through cell culture was also a means of attenuation, probably by fortuitous selection of mutants better adapted to replication in vitro than in the living host. This technique allowed the selection of mutants by isolation of single clones and incubation at temperatures below the normal temperature of the host. Thus, the period between 1950 and 1980 saw the development of numerous attenuated virus vaccines, including those for poliomyelitis, measles, rubella, mumps, and varicella.[7] The ability to mix RNA segments from attenuated strains with RNA-encoding protective antigens from circulating wild strains led to the discovery of the influenza virus and rotavirus vaccines.

The use of completely inactivated vaccines started in the nineteenth century and was initially directed against typhoid and cholera.[7] More recently, the Salk poliomyelitis and hepatitis A vaccines contained whole inactivated viruses.[7] The recognition of extracellular bacterial toxins resulted in Ramon developing immunogenic but nontoxic toxoids for diphtheria and tetanus.[7] Later it became possible to separate

Table 1
Vaccines for infectious diseases available in the United States

Name of Causative Organism	Disease Prevented	Type of Vaccine
Bacillus anthracis	Anthrax	Acellular protein derived from B anthracis V770-NP1-R
Bordetella pertussis	Pertussis	Acellular component of B pertussis
Clostridium tetani	Tetanus	Inactivated toxin
Corynebacterium diphtheriae	Diphtheria	Inactivated toxin
Haemophilus influenzae type b	Invasive H influenzae infections	Conjugated polysaccharide
Hepatitis A virus	Hepatitis A	Inactivated whole virus
Hepatitis B virus	Hepatitis B	Recombinant containing hepatitis B surface antigen
Human papillomavirus	Anogenital warts, genital cancers	Recombinant quadrivalent vaccine
Influenza virus	Seasonal and pandemic influenza	Inactivated virus and live cold-adapted virus
Japanese encephalitis virus	Japanese encephalitis	Inactivated cell culture–derived and live attenuated vaccines
Measles virus	Measles	Live attenuated vaccine
Mumps virus	Mumps	Live attenuated vaccine
Mycobacterium tuberculosis	Tuberculosis	Live attenuated vaccine
Neisseria meningitidis	Meningococcal meningitis, meningococcemia	Capsular polysaccharide and tetravalent conjugate vaccines
Poliomyelitis virus	Poliomyelitis	Oral, live, attenuated vaccine and inactivated (killed) virus vaccine
Rabies virus	Rabies	Killed virus vaccine
Rotavirus	Rotavirus-related gastroenteritis	Oral, live, attenuated vaccine
Rubella virus	Rubella, congenital rubella syndrome	Live attenuated vaccine
Salmonella typhi	Typhoid fever	Oral, live, attenuated vaccine and parenteral capsular polysaccharide
Streptococcus pneumoniae	Invasive pneumococcal infections	Capsular polysaccharide and conjugate vaccines
Varicella-zoster virus	Chicken pox, herpes zoster	Live attenuated virus vaccine
Variola virus	Smallpox	Live attenuated virus vaccine
Yellow fever virus	Yellow fever	Live attenuated virus vaccine

and use subunits of organisms in the form of extracts of infected tissues (used in rabies vaccine), capsular polysaccharides (used in typhoid Vi and pneumococcal vaccines), and proteins (used in acellular pertussis vaccine).[7] Late in the twentieth century, the concept of conjugation of proteins to polysaccharides was used to develop polysaccharide vaccines with better efficacy and memory response.[8]

Genetic engineering has led to the construction of inactivated antigens and attenuation of organisms through directed mutation. The first success of genetic engineering was a hepatitis B vaccine manufactured in a yeast recombinant carrying the gene for hepatitis B virus surface protein.[9]

PASSIVE IMMUNOTHERAPY

The first use of passive immunization dates back to the Christmas night of 1891, in Berlin, when injecting diphtheria antitoxin cured a young boy who had diphtheria.[10,11] Passive immunization was discovered by Emil Behring and Shibasaburo Kitasato at the Robert Koch Institute of Hygiene in Berlin. Their work demonstrating that serum obtained from an animal injected with diphtheria toxin could be used to neutralize a fatal dose of toxin in another animal was published in 1890.[12] The commercial production of antidiphtheria serum led to its use in other parts of Europe in the summer of 1894 with favorable results.[13] By the early twentieth century, serum therapy was being used to treat bacterial infections, such as those caused by *Streptococcus pneumoniae* and *Neisseria meningitidis*.[14] Side effects, such as serum sickness and lack of neutralization property, for different serotypes of *S pneumoniae* combined with the discovery of penicillin and the dawn of the antibiotic era limited the use of serum therapy.[14]

IMMUNOGLOBULINS

In 1944, the production of human immunoglobulins for the treatment of measles overcame the problem of serum sickness and introduced the concept of pooled human immunoglobulins, which are used to date.[15] Serum therapy with hyperimmune immunoglobulins continues to be used for the prophylaxis or treatment of various bacterial and viral diseases. This therapy is routinely used for the prophylaxis of viral diseases, such as those caused by cytomegalovirus, respiratory syncytial virus (RSV), and hepatitis B virus. Antibodies against toxins are used for the treatment and prophylaxis of bacterial diseases, such as tetanus, botulism, and diphtheria.[16] Antivenoms used for stings and snakebites are therapeutic counterparts of noninfectious diseases.[17]

Intravenous immunoglobulin (IVIG), a preparation of human polyclonal antibodies pooled from several healthy donors, has been used for a variety of conditions. The goals of treatment with IVIG are (1) replacement therapy in humoral immunodeficiency disorder, (2) protection of the recipient against infection, and (3) suppression of inflammatory and immune-mediated processes. IVIG was initially used for the treatment of autoimmune and inflammatory diseases followed by the prophylaxis and treatment of infectious diseases. IVIG has been used in the treatment of sepsis, whereby it reduces the pathology by targeting and suppressing inflammation.[18–21] Limited evidence exists for the use of IVIG in the treatment of bacterial infections for which toxin production is the major mediator of pathogenesis, for example, toxin-producing organisms, such as *Staphylococcus aureus*, streptococci, and clostridia (**Box 1**).

Anti-D immunoglobulin is prepared from pooled source plasma selected for high titers of antibodies to Rh(D)-positive erythrocytes. This immunoglobulin has made a tremendous impact on Rh(D) alloimmunization during pregnancies, with routine postpartum administration of a single dose of the immunoglobulin and routine antenatal administration in the third trimester.[22]

MONOCLONAL ANTIBODIES

In 1975, Georges Köhler and César Milstein of the Medical Research Council Laboratory of Molecular Biology in Cambridge described a method of obtaining antigen-specific antibodies in large amounts.[23] It was possible to produce high-affinity specific monoclonal antibodies using this hybridoma technology. Muromonab, a murine-derived

---

Box 1
The US Food and Drug Administration–approved uses of immunoglobulin

- Idiopathic thrombocytopenic purpura

- Primary immunodeficiency states

- Secondary immunodeficiency in chronic lymphocytic leukemia

- Pediatric human immunodeficiency virus infection

- Kawasaki syndrome

- Prevention of graft-versus-host disease and infection in adult hematopoietic cell transplantation

- Chronic inflammatory demyelinating polyneuropathy

Data from Bussel JB, Giulino L, Lee S, et al. Update on therapeutic monoclonal antibodies. Curr Probl Pediatr Adolesc Health Care 2007;37:118.

---

monoclonal antibody used to prevent organ allograft rejection, was the first therapeutic antibody approved for clinical use in 1986.[17] This was followed by the development of humanized chimeric monoclonal antibodies, daclizumab and basiliximab, both targeting interleukin 2 (IL-2) and used for the prevention of organ rejection.[17]

In 1997, the first cancer therapeutic antibody, rituximab, was approved for targeting CD20 in patients with low-grade non-Hodgkin lymphoma and showed a response rate of 57% in patients receiving 8 weekly treatments.[24] This was rapidly followed by the development of a humanized antibody known as trastuzumab, which was produced by complementarity-determining region grafting and is used for the treatment of HER2/neu-positive breast cancer. The blockade of tumor necrosis factor α (TNF-α) has been the focus of immunotherapy for the treatment of autoimmune disorders, such as rheumatoid arthritis and inflammatory bowel disease. The 2 approved agents that target TNF-α include infliximab, a chimeric monoclonal antibody targeted against TNF-α, and etanercept, a p75 TNF receptor dimer linked to the Fc portion of IgG1.[2]

Palivizumab, a human monoclonal antibody, is the only currently approved antibody for the treatment of infectious diseases. This antibody was developed as a prophylactic treatment against the RSV. In acute infections, the neutralizing therapeutic antibodies may help suppress viral replication and give the host immune system time to develop an effective response for viral clearance.[17] Furthermore, the activation of natural killer cells through antibody-dependent cellular cytotoxicity leads to killing of infected cells.[17]

The cytotoxicity of monoclonal antibodies is increased by linking them to a toxin or a radionuclide, which is then targeted to the tumor cell by the antibody. The first immunotoxin-armed antibody was gemtuzumab ozogamicin, which links a CD33-specific antibody to calicheamicin and is used in the treatment of myelogenous leukemia.[2] These oncotoxins manifest toxicity to the normal tissue and hence have a narrow therapeutic window. Radiolabeled monoclonal antibodies have been developed to overcome this barrier. CD20, which has an expression limited to B cells, is a major target used in the therapy for B-cell leukemia and lymphoma. Rituximab and its version armed with yttrium Y 90 (ibritumomab tiuxetan) have been approved for the treatment of non-Hodgkin lymphoma.[2,25] Similarly, bevacizumab is an antiangiogenic antibody that binds to and inhibits the vascular endothelial growth factor (VEGF). The addition of this agent to standard chemotherapy for the treatment of metastatic colorectal cancer was found to significantly increase median survival in comparison with chemotherapy alone.[26]

Ranibizumab is a recombinant humanized monoclonal antibody fragment (Fab), which binds to and inhibits human VEGF-A. Ranibizumab inhibits VEGF from binding to its receptors and thereby suppresses neovascularization and slows vision loss. This agent is used in the treatment of some forms of age-related macular degeneration. Similarly, abciximab is a Fab of a chimeric human-murine monoclonal antibody, which binds to platelet IIb/IIIa receptors, resulting in steric hindrance and thus inhibition of platelet aggregation. Clinical uses of abciximab include unstable angina and clot prevention in various coronary stenting procedures.[27,28]

CANCER IMMUNOTHERAPY

The initial hint that the immune system might respond to cancer was observed in the eighteenth century when it was noted that infections causing fever in patients with cancer were occasionally associated with cancer remission.[22] In 1893, William Coley, a New York surgeon, started investigating this phenomenon in detail. He observed that a patient with cancer had complete remission of cancer after 2 episodes of erysipelas caused by *Streptococcus pyogenes.* Coley subsequently injected streptococcal cultures into patients with cancer and observed tumor regression in some patients.[29] The bacterial preparation was named Coley's toxin, and around 900 patients with cancer were treated with this preparation. Most of the patients treated had inoperable sarcoma, and a 10% response rate was observed.[22] This treatment did not last long because of the high temperature caused by the bacterial products and the low response rate; however, this was the beginning in tumor immunology.[30]

This was followed by the observation of tuberculosis (TB) and its possible antitumor effect in the twentieth century. In 1929, Raymond Pearl[31] reported an autopsy study from the Johns Hopkins Hospital in Baltimore showing a lower frequency of cancer in patients with TB. Pearl observed that surviving patients had a higher incidence of active or healed TB than patients who had died of cancer. Conversely, he observed a lower incidence of cancer in patients dying of TB than in similarly matched control subjects. The immunotherapeutic properties of the BCG vaccine were first studied in the 1950s when Old and colleagues[32] demonstrated that mice infected with bacille Calmette-Guérin (BCG) showed resistance to transplantable tumors. This study was followed by that of Zbar and colleagues[33] in the 1970s, which demonstrated the tumor inhibitory properties of BCG mediated by the delayed hypersensitivity reaction against tumor cells. Based on further extensive animal studies and clinical trials, intravesicular BCG has now emerged as the most effective local therapy for superficial bladder cancer.[34]

The immunologic theories of Burnet and Fenner[35] have had a major impact on the understanding of cancer immunotherapy. The investigators' initial theory of acquired immunologic tolerance proposed that lymphocytes able to respond to self-tissues were depleted early in life during the development of the immune system and also supported the view that it is impossible for immunotherapy to rearm the immune system such that it recognizes and fights cancerous self-tissues. Burnet's[36] cancer immunosurveillance theory supports the current belief that tumors can be recognized by the lymphocytes and eliminated by the immune system. Furthermore, some tumor cells evade immune elimination to become successful. Both the innate and adaptive immune systems are involved in tumor recognition and clearance, and tumor elimination involves the same immunologic mechanism used to combat pathogens.[30]

The recognition of cancer-associated antigens by the tumor-bearing host and the mounting of an immune response against these antigens is the basis of the study of cancer vaccines. The immunoglobulin idiotype is an antigenic target present in B-cell lymphomas and could function as a tumor-specific antigen, which can be used in vaccines to target lymphomas.[37] This concept was first practiced by using both an idiotype granulocyte-macrophage colony-stimulating factor (GM-CSF) fusion protein and a naked DNA immunization to develop a therapeutic vaccine for B-cell lymphoma.[38]

Efforts to enhance vaccination have focused on the function of antigen-presenting cells, such as dendritic cells, and activation of T cells. Interferon-γ can be used to generate mature dendritic cells for vaccines in which a long-memory CD8+ response is desired.[2] The concept of the use of GM-CSF to induce dendritic cell differentiation has been adopted recently.[2,39] Furthermore, immunotherapies have been enhanced by modification of the antigenic peptide by epitope engineering, which involves altering the antigen to increase its affinity for major histocompatibility complex (MHC) molecules.[2]

Cytokines are proteins that regulate the immune system and participate in intercellular communication. Several agents have been approved for clinical use in immunotherapy. Interferons comprise a group of related proteins whose effects include antiviral activity, growth regulatory properties, inhibition of angiogenesis, regulation of cell differentiation, enhancement of MHC antigen expression, and a wide variety of immunomodulatory activities. Interferon-α has been used in the treatment of hairy cell leukemia, malignant melanoma, follicular lymphoma, AIDS-related Kaposi sarcoma, and hepatitis B and C. Interferon-β is used in the treatment of multiple sclerosis and interferon-γ in the treatment of chronic granulomatous disease and osteoporosis.[2] Genes encoding these cytokines have been used in vaccine preparation to elicit a broad T-cell response. GM-CSF has been used, as mentioned earlier, to elicit a T-cell response. Furthermore, the gene encoding the interleukins has also been incorporated to elicit a T-cell response. For example, IL-2 is used for the treatment of metastatic renal cancer and malignant melanoma.[40]

ALLERGEN-SPECIFIC IMMUNOTHERAPY

Allergen-specific immunotherapy (ASIT) is the process of administering slowly increasing doses of specifically relevant allergens for the treatment of IgE-mediated allergic diseases.[41] This kind of immunotherapy dates back to the BC era, when King Mithridates VI (132–63 BC) used increasing doses of snake venom to immunize himself against the toxin.[42] ASIT originated in the early twentieth century. In 1902, Dunbar[43] tried to adopt the concept of protective immunity in the treatment of hay fever by developing a hyperimmune serum in animals vaccinated with pollen extract to cure hay fever. The first successful trial of ASIT dates back to the work of Leonard Noon and John Freeman, who postulated that the toxin component of the pollen was responsible for generating the symptom constellation of hay fever and that a pollen antitoxin would be protective. A protocol of subcutaneous injections of pollen extracts with increasing doses was developed according to a defined schedule for patients with hay fever. The trial of 84 patients treated with the ASIT regimen showed that ASIT was effective in patients with allergy and that it seemed to confer an acquired immunity lasting for at least 1 year after cessation of treatment.[44] Controlled clinical trials demonstrating the effectiveness of ASIT were conducted in the 1950s.[45]

For decades, whole-body extracts of bees and wasps were used for protection against insect venom anaphylaxis. Loveless and Cann,[46] who were studying beekeepers, recognized that these individuals underwent active immunization every day through contact with the bees. The investigators were able to transfer immunity from the beekeeper's serum and highlighted the concept of blocking antibodies. In 1979, the landmark study led by Larry Lichtenstein at the Johns Hopkins University in Baltimore showed that venom-specific immunotherapy was clinically superior to therapy on whole-body extract.[47]

The major breakthrough in ASIT occurred in 1998 when the World Health Organization released their guideline supporting the safety, efficacy, and standardization of

ASIT.[48] ASIT has grown with the identification of different allergens and different routes and techniques of administration, and it has now become a gold standard for the treatment of IgE-mediated allergic diseases involving several allergens.

DIAGNOSTIC IMMUNOLOGY

Diagnostic immunology is a growing and significant field of immunology. Georges Widal, a French investigator, was the first to identify the appearance of antibodies after an acute infection. This concept gave rise to the Widal test for diagnosis of typhoid fever, which adhered to the principle that the presence of antibodies signified a recent infection. Serologic diagnosis provided clinically important information when the identification of the causative agent was not possible. Wassermann, Neisser, Bruck, and Schucht used a liver suspension from a patient with syphilis (which served as an antigen) in a complement fixation reaction that simplified the diagnosis of syphilis.[49]

Soon after the isolation of the tubercle bacillus, Robert Koch realized that patients with TB might develop a reaction to an extract of the microorganism. This observation evolved into a skin test in which old tuberculin or the purified protein derivative is injected into the skin, where it produces a delayed hypersensitivity response, signifying recent or past contact with tubercle bacillus. Delayed-type hypersensitivity reactions are still useful for the epidemiology of diseases, such as TB and histoplasmosis, in which cell-mediated responses are more significant than antibody responses.[49]

Gruber and Durham showed that antiserum could agglutinate the corresponding bacterial cells in the test tube. This finding led to the use of antibodies as highly specific laboratory reagents. The ability of known antibodies to neutralize viruses is a major tool in the identification of viral agents isolated from patients. The application of antibodies as specific reagents has far exceeded their use in the diagnosis of infectious diseases. Immunoassays are applied in all components of the modern diagnostic laboratory. The most sensitive assays for hormones, such as those used in pregnancy tests, depend on potent antibodies.[49]

The knowledge that antibodies are formed against self-tissue antigens gave rise to diagnostic immunology for autoimmune diseases, which in turn led to the identification of antinuclear antibodies, which is now the standard for diagnosis of autoimmune disorders.[49] At present, immunologic methods are being routinely used for diagnostic and prognostic markers of malignant disease.

SUMMARY

Historically, the concept of immunotherapy started with the observation that patients who had suffered from and survived certain types of illness were subsequently protected and that it was possible to transfer this protection passively to other patients who had the disease or did not have it yet. These diseases were subsequently proved to be of microbial origin. A host reacting to microbes as foreign objects and mounting a defensive response could be explained rather easily. With an understanding of the immunology of autoimmune disorders, cancer immunology, transplant immunology, and allergic disorders, the global concept of immunogen, to which the host immune system reacts, evolved. This has made immunotherapy possible in many diseases, as reviewed in the articles elsewhere in this issue.

REFERENCES

1. Khardori NM. Biologic response modifiers in infectious disease. Infect Dis Clin North Am 2011;25(4):723–31.

2. Waldmann TA. Immunotherapy: past, present and future. Nat Med 2003;9(3): 269–77.
3. Plotkin SA. Vaccines: the fourth century. Clin Vaccine Immunol 2009;16(12):1709–19.
4. Geison GL. The Private Science of Louis Pasteur. Princeton (NJ): Princeton University Press; 1995.
5. Calmette A, Guerin C, Breton M. Contribution a l'etude de la tuberculose experimental du cobaye (infection et essais de vaccination par la voie digestive). Ann Inst Pasteur (Paris) 1907;21:401–16 [in French].
6. Theiler M, Smith HH. The use of yellow fever virus modified by in vitro cultivation for human immunization. J Exp Med 1937;65:787–800.
7. Plotkin SA. Vaccines: past, present and future. Nat Med 2005;11(Suppl 4):S5–11.
8. Moingeon P. Cancer vaccines. Vaccine 2001;9:1305–26.
9. McAleer WJ, Buynak EB, Maigetter RZ, et al. Human hepatitis B vaccine from recombinant yeast. Nature 1984;307:178–80.
10. Singer C, Underwood EA. A short history of medicine. 2nd edition. Oxford (UK): Oxford University Press; 1962.
11. Llewelyn MB, Hawkins RE, Russell SJ. Discovery of antibodies. BMJ 1992 21; 305(6864):1269–72.
12. Behring EA, Kitasato S. Uber das Zustandekommen der Diphtherie-Immunitat und der Tetanus-Immunitat bei Thieren. Dtsch Med Wochenschr 1890;49: 1113–4 [in German].
13. Chothia C, Lesk AM, Tramontano A, et al. Conformations of immunoglobulin hypervariable regions. Nature 1989;342:842–83.
14. Casadevall A, Scharff MD. Serum therapy revisited: animal models of infection and development of passive antibody therapy. Antimicrob Agents Chemother 1994;38:1695–702.
15. Stokes J Jr, Maris EP, Gellis SS. The use of concentrated normal human serum gamma globulin (human immune serum globulin) in the prophylaxis and treatment of measles. J Clin Invest 1944;23:531.
16. Keller MA, Stiehm ER. Passive immunity in prevention and treatment of infectious diseases. Clin Microbiol Rev 2000;13:602–14.
17. Chan CE, Chan AH, Hanson BJ, et al. The use of antibodies in the treatment of infectious diseases. Singapore Med J 2009;50(7):663–73.
18. Werdan K. Intravenous immunoglobulin for prophylaxis and therapy of sepsis. Curr Opin Crit Care 2001;7:354–61.
19. Sriskandan S, Ferguson M, Elliot V, et al. Human intravenous immunoglobulin for experimental streptococcal toxic shock: bacterial clearance and modulation of inflammation. J Antimicrob Chemother 2006;58:117–24.
20. Vernachio JH, Bayer AS, Ames B, et al. Human immunoglobulin G recognizing fibrinogen-binding surface proteins is protective against both *Staphylococcus aureus* and *Staphylococcus epidermidis* infections in vivo. Antimicrob Agents Chemother 2006;50:511–8.
21. Abougergi MS, Kwon JH. Intravenous immunoglobulin for the treatment of *Clostridium difficile* infection: a review. Dig Dis Sci 2011;56:19–26.
22. Wiemann B, Starnes CO. Coley's toxins, tumor necrosis factor and cancer research: a historical perspective. Pharmacol Ther 1994;64:529–64.
23. Kohler G, Milstein C. Continuous cultures of fused cells secreting antibody of predefined specificity. Nature 1975;256:495–7.
24. McLaughlin P, Grillo-López AJ, Link BK, et al. Rituximab chimeric anti-CD20 monoclonal antibody therapy for relapsed indolent lymphoma: half of patients respond to a four-dose treatment program. J Clin Oncol 1998;16:2825–33.

25. Witzig TE, Gordon LI, Cabanillas F, et al. Randomized controlled trial of yttrium-90-labeled ibritumomab tiuxetan radioimmunotherapy versus rituximab for patients with relapsed or refractory low-grade, follicular, or transformed B-cell non-Hodgkin's lymphoma. J Clin Oncol 2002;20:2453–63.
26. Giantonio BJ, Catalano PJ, Meropol NJ, et al. Bevacizumab in combination with oxaliplatin, fluorouracil, and leucovorin (FOLFOX4) for previously treated metastatic colorectal cancer: results from the Eastern Cooperative Oncology Group Study E3200. J Clin Oncol 2007;25:1539.
27. Bussel JB, Giulino L, Lee S, et al. Update on therapeutic monoclonal antibodies. Curr Probl Pediatr Adolesc Health Care 2007;37:118.
28. Knezevic-Maramica I, Kruskall MS. Intravenous immune globulins: an update for clinicians. Transfusion 2003;43:1460–80.
29. Coley WB. The treatment of malignant tumors by repeated inoculations of erysipelas. With a report of ten original cases. Am J Med Sci 1893;105:487–511.
30. Parish CR. Cancer immunotherapy: the past, the present and the future. Immunol Cell Biol 2003;81:106–13.
31. Pearl R. Cancer and tuberculosis. Am J Hyg 1929;9:97.
32. Old LJ, Clarke DA, Benacerraf B. Effect of bacillus Calmette-Guerin infection on transplanted tumours in the mouse. Nature 1959;184:291.
33. Zbar B, Bernstein ID, Rapp HJ. Suppression of tumor growth at the site of infection with living Bacillus Calmette-Guérin. J Natl Cancer Inst 1971;46:831.
34. Bassi P. BCG (bacillus of Calmette Guerin) therapy of high-risk superficial bladder cancer. Surg Oncol 2002;11:77–83.
35. Burnet FM, Fenner F, editors. The production of antibodies. London: Macmillan; 1949.
36. Burnet FM. Immunological aspects of malignant disease. Lancet 1967;1:1171–4.
37. Lynch RG, Graff RJ, Sirisinha S, et al. Myeloma proteins as tumor-specific transplantation antigens. Proc Natl Acad Sci U S A 1972;69:1540–4.
38. Bendandi M, Gocke CD, Kobrin CB, et al. Complete molecular remissions induced by patient-specific vaccination plus granulocyte-monocyte colony-stimulating factor against lymphoma. Nat Med 1999;5:1171–7.
39. Pardoll DM. Spinning molecular immunology into successful immunotherapy. Nat Rev Immunol 2002;2:227–38.
40. Rosenberg SA, Yang JC, Topalian SL, et al. Treatment of 283 consecutive patients with metastatic melanoma or renal cell cancer using high-dose bolus interleukin-2. JAMA 1994;271:907–13.
41. Ring J. Allergy in practice. Berlin, Heidelberg (Germany), New York (NY): Springer; 2005.
42. Schadewaldt H. Geschichte der allergie, vol. 1–4. 1st edition. München-Deisenhofen: Dustri-Verlag; 1979–1983.
43. Dunbar WP. The present state of our knowledge of hay-fever. J Hyg 1902;13:105.
44. Freeman J. Vaccination against hay fever. Report of results during the last three years. Lancet 1914;1:1178.
45. Frankland AW. High and low dosage pollen extract treatment in summer hay fever and asthma. Acta Allergol 1955;9:183–7.
46. Loveless MH, Cann JR. Distribution of allergic and blocking activity in human serum proteins fractionated by electrophoresis convection. Science 1953;117:105–8.
47. Hunt KJ, Valentine MD, Sobotka AK, et al. A controlled trial of immunotherapy in insect hypersensitivity. N Engl J Med 1978;299:157–61.

48. Bousquet J, Lockey R, Malling HJ, et al, WHO panel members. Allergen immunotherapy: therapeutic vaccines for allergic diseases. A WHO position paper.
J Allergy Clin Immunol 1998;102:558–62.
49. Rose NR. Genesis and evolution of diagnostic and clinical immunology. Clin
Vaccine Immunol 1999;6(3):289–90.

Immunotherapy for Primary Immunodeficiency Diseases

Philip Wood, D.Phil., FRCP, FRCPath

KEYWORDS

- Antibody deficiency • Immunoglobulin therapy
- Common variable immunodeficiency • Hereditary angioedema
- C1 inhibitor

Key Points

- The primary immunodeficiencies are a rare group of disorders in which the fundamental defect is an inability to maintain effective immune response to invading pathogen.

- The two conditions most commonly seen in adult primary immunodeficiency practice are the primary antibody deficiencies and Hereditary Angioedema.

- Immunoglobulin replacement therapy is most commonly indicated in defects of antibody production.

- Replacement therapy with immunoglobulin in primary antibody deficiencies increases life expectancy and reduces infection frequency and severity.

- Treatment of disease-associated complications of primary antibody deficiencies with monoclonal antibody therapy appears promising and is likely to increase in the future.

- Therapy for Hereditary angioedema has historically been focussed on plasma-derived C1 inhibitor. More recently a number of additional agents have become available for therapy, including novel drugs targeted at different elements of the disease process.

INTRODUCTION

The primary immunodeficiencies are a rare group of disorders for which the fundamental defect is an inability to maintain effective immune response to invading pathogens. These disorders can be categorized into several different groups.

1. Combined immunodeficiencies, in which defects of both cellular and humoral immunity result most commonly from single gene defects in genes encoding proteins critical for lymphocyte development. These disorders usually present in early childhood and are usually fatal without hematopoietic stem cell transplantation.

Department of Clinical Immunology, St James's University Hospital, Beckett Wing, Leeds, Yorkshire LS9 7TF, UK
E-mail address: philipwood1@nhs.net

Med Clin N Am 96 (2012) 433–454
doi:10.1016/j.mcna.2012.04.010
0025-7125/12/$ – see front matter © 2012 Elsevier Inc. All rights reserved.

2. Antibody deficiencies, which result from a variety of single gene defects and most commonly more complex polygenic disorders, whereby failure of an effective immunoglobulin response to infection places the individual at significant risk of life-threatening infection, most commonly with encapsulating bacteria such as *Streptococcus pneumoniae* or *Haemophilus influenzae.*
3. Complement deficiencies, in which the genetically defined inability to produce of the complement components places the individual at risk from a variety of infections and potentially inflammatory complications. In addition, genetic deficiency of C1 inhibitor (hereditary angioedema [HAE]) leads to potentially life-threatening attacks of angioedema precipitated by infection, trauma, and other triggers.
4. Phagocytic disorders, most notably chronic granulomatous disease, which usually result from an X-linked or autosomal recessive inheritance, and whereby susceptibility to infection with catalase-negative bacteria, most typically *Staphylococcus aureus,* resulting in abscesses and granuloma formation, are the hallmark.
5. Defects in innate immunity, at present most commonly those involving the Toll-like receptor pathways, where the lack of an effective inflammatory response both increases susceptibility to infection from bacterial and fungal pathogens, and results in tissue damage as a consequence of recurrent infection.

Immunoglobulin replacement therapy is most commonly indicated in defects of antibody production, but is often used in the context of severe combined immunodeficiency, both before and after stem cell transplant, whereby poor B-cell engraftment may require a long-term immunoglobulin support. Some defects in innate immunity, in particular the hyper–immunoglobulin E (IgE) syndrome, can develop a degree of antibody deficiency, which may require immunoglobulin replacement therapy.

This article focuses on the 2 conditions most commonly seen in adult primary immunodeficiency practice, the primary antibody deficiencies and HAE. These conditions and their management are reviewed, with particular attention to the use of plasma-derived and more recent therapies that have become available. The history of plasma fractionation and immunoglobulin replacement therapy as well as current practices and products available are addressed, focusing on the therapeutic benefit and risk of treatment. The primary antibody deficiencies are focused upon, as these are the most common of the primary immunodeficiencies and those for which immunoglobulin replacement therapy is most widely indicated. In addition, the evidence of efficacy of immunoglobulin replacement therapy is most clearly demonstrated in this group of disorders. The therapies for HAE are reviewed, looking at the recent significant expansion in therapeutic options available.

CLINICAL PRESENTATION

The primary antibody deficiencies are a group of disorders whereby the fundamental defect is an inability to produce an effective antibody response to infection (**Table 1**). Some of these disorders result from single genetic mutations encoding proteins that play a critical role in B-lymphocyte development, including X-linked agammaglobulinemia (XLA), defects in molecules critically involved in signaling from the pre–B-cell receptor,[1] and molecules involved in later processes of class switching and somatic hypermutation.[2] More complex polygenic disorders, including the most common antibody deficiency, common variable immune deficiency (CVID), result in a more varied clinical phenotype for which the common theme is an inadequate immunoglobulin response to infection.

The International Union of Immunological Societies has developed diagnostic criteria for a wide range of primary immunodeficiencies, including the commoner primary

Table 1
Primary antibody deficiencies

Disease	B Cells	Immunoglobulins	Inheritance	Gene Defect	Mechanism
Early Defects					
Abnormalities in pre–B-cell receptor complex	Absent/low	All reduced	AR	CD79a IGHM μ heavy chain λ5 surrogate light chain *BLNK*	B-cell differentiation failure
XLA	Absent/low	All reduced	X-linked	Btk	B-cell differentiation failure
Later Defects					
B-cell intrinsic immunoglobulin class switch recombination (Ig-CSR) deficiencies	Normal	Normal/raised IgM Low IgG and IgA	AR AR AR	CD40 AID UNG	T-cell cooperation failure
CVID-like syndromes	≥1%	Low IgG and IgA with normal/raised IgM	None	Homozygous defects (eg, ICOS, TACI) Heterozygosity/polymorphism (eg, TACI)	B-cell function failure

Abbreviations: AR, autosomal recessive; CVID, common variable immune deficiency; XLA, X-linked agammaglobulinemia.

antibody deficiencies.[3] Infections with encapsulated bacteria such as *Haemophilus influenzae* and *Streptococcus pneumoniae* are the most common presenting features,[4,5] with recurrent pneumonia, sinusitis, otitis media, and acute bronchitis the most common infective histories obtained from patients presenting with primary antibody deficiency. Often infections respond to standard treatment, only to recur once therapy has finished. Bronchiectasis and chronic sinusitis remain common complications before diagnosis and treatment.[6]

In addition to these infective presentations, the underlying dysregulation of the immune system, thought to be inherent in CVID, is illustrated by the observation that patients can present with systemic or organ-specific autoimmunity[4,5,7]; this is most commonly hematologic. Other organ-specific autoimmunity, for example, pernicious anemia secondary to autoantibodies directed against intrinsic factor, is also common and can be the presenting feature of the condition.

A subgroup of patients with CVID can present with or develop during the course of their disease a granulomatous syndrome affecting the liver, spleen, lungs, and gastrointestinal tract. These conditions can often appear similar to other granulomatous ones such as Crohn disease or sarcoidosis, and can lead to diagnostic confusion and delay in appropriate therapy.

HISTORY OF IMMUNOGLOBULIN REPLACEMENT THERAPY

Following the report by Colonel Ogden Bruton in 1953 of what was subsequently identified as XLA,[8] treated with replacement plasma, early attempts to replace absent immunoglobulin progressed from the use of fresh frozen plasma to relatively impure preparations of immunoglobulin, given intramuscularly.

The processes of cold-ethanol and pH fractionation to extract immunoglobulin from plasma was developed in the 1940s, with preparations containing 70% to 80% monomeric immunoglobulin G (IgG) and substantial amounts of immunoglobulins A (IgA) and M (IgM). Such preparations proved useful in reducing infections in patients with XLA when given intramuscularly, but produced life-threatening anaphylactic reactions when given intravenously. Enzymatic modifications of IgG resulted in more monomeric preparations but with significant loss of function, including complement-binding activity. The identification of processes that could result in the preparation of intact IgG at high purity, involving low pH and trace pepsin concentrations, precipitation by polyethylene glycol (PEG), or purification using diethylaminoethanol-exchange chromatography, paved the way for the development of stable products that could be administered intravenously, and many patients with primary antibody deficiencies were moved onto these newer preparations.

MODERN MANUFACTURING PROCESSES

The quality of plasma collected directly affects the final quality of the plasma product produced (intravenous [IVIg] and subcutaneous [SCIg] immunoglobulin preparations and C1-inhibitor concentrate). Strict quality assurance measures in place throughout the process ensure high levels of reliability and consistency. Collection centers are subject to oversight by national and international regulatory authorities, and should comply with good manufacturing practice. Plasma donors have a documented medical history and should be exempt from risk factors for plasma-borne infectious agents. On collection, most plasma for IVIg is frozen to $-25°$ to $-30°C$ within 24 hours, and kept in this state for several months. Individual donations are screened for human immunodeficiency virus (HIV)-1 and -2 and hepatitis C virus (HCV) antibodies, as well as hepatitis B surface antigen (HBsAg). Many manufacturers now screen mini-pools of donations for genomic viral markers of HIV, hepatitis A, B, and C, and parvovirus B19. The manufacturing pool should then be screened negative for HCV nucleic acid test (NAT), HIV antibodies, and HBsAg, often now with additional screening for hepatitis A RNA and parvovirus B19 DNA.

In most processes plasma is then subjected to controlled thawing to 2° to 3°C, known as cryoprecipitation, with the cryoprecipitate removed leaving a "cryo-poor" fraction containing the immunoglobulin, after removal of fibrinogen by ethanol precipitation at neutral pH. Subsequent processes may involve ion-exchange chromatography, the use of caprylic acid, incubation at low pH, and the use of nanofiltration to ensure the highest purity and maximal yield. Key steps are summarized in **Box 1**. Previously end products were produced in lyophilized form, but this resulted in a risk of aggregate formation on reconstitution, and the discovery that IgG remains stable in liquid form at pH 4.25 and that patients could tolerate such preparations has resulted in a move to liquid preparations at low pH with the addition of stabilizers such as polyols, sugars and, increasingly, amino acids such as proline or isoleucine. For several years, IVIg products were provided at 5% concentration, requiring several hours of infusion time and with the disadvantage of comparatively high total volumes. The latter issue could be of relevance in elderly or frail patients with cardiorespiratory disease or renal impairment. More recently, manufacturers have moved to more concentrated products for intravenous use, typically 10%, resulting in faster infusion times and smaller overall volume product.[9–12]

Early SCIg products were developed using products originally designed for intramuscular use, typically at 16% concentration. More recently, CSL-Behring has developed a 20% product (Hizentra) for use subcutaneously. Again the smaller volumes and higher concentration bring the potential benefit of larger dose of and faster infusion times. It is likely that manufacturers will move toward generally higher concentrations of products to improve the potential for higher dosing and more rapid infusion times, which will improve treatment quality for patients.

TREATMENT PROTOCOLS

Once a diagnosis has been made, this should be fully explained to both patient and family. The implications of this lifelong diagnosis and potential complications should be outlined at an early stage. Therapeutic options should then be discussed with the patient and appropriate written information given to allow the patient to make an informed choice.

Many patients receive immunoglobulin therapy via the intravenous route, most commonly given in the hospital or clinic setting, but in some countries in the home setting after appropriate training. Replacement dosing has historically been in the

---

Box 1
Key steps in plasma fractionation

1. Donor selection

2. Plasma collection

3. Freezing and quarantine

4. Viral screening (HIV, hepatitis A virus [HAV], hepatitis B virus [HBV], HCV, parvovirus B19)

5. Cryoprecipitation and cold-ethanol fractionation

6. Additional viral removal steps (eg, detergent treatment, nanofiltration, caprylate)

7. Final product

range of 200 to 600 mg/kg, given at an interval of 2 to 4 weeks. Routine cannulation is all that is required, and infusions generally last a few hours, depending on the manufacturer's guidelines for infusion rates.

HOME THERAPY

Patients and their carers can be trained to undertake therapy at home.[13,14] Once patients are stabilized and can tolerate therapy, usually with IVIg, they should be offered the option of home therapy. Formal psychological evaluations are not routinely performed but discussions with the patient and carers are held, after written information has been given, before accepting a patient and carer into the training program. Willingness to undertake the training and a stable home environment are the key factors to successful home therapy. Many centers in the United Kingdom have experience and expertise in training patients to self-administer IVIg at home. Hospital-based training involves the achievement of competence in aseptic technique, intravenous cannulation, preparation of the delivery system, and management of adverse reactions. When patients and carers are considered to be ready to undertake home infusions, a formal agreement is made between the patient and carer, the medical and nursing teams, and the general practitioner that home treatment can commence. The nursing team makes a home visit for the first infusion to confirm competence in the home setting. Many patients in the United Kingdom and other European countries successfully undertake this form of treatment.

Training for home SCIg therapy is technically much more straightforward than for IVIg therapy. The insertion of a butterfly needle or equivalent using standard aseptic techniques can be readily shown to patients or carers for children, and the use of low-volume battery-operated pump devices allows infusions of up to 20 mL at a single site to be delivered in times around 1 hour. Larger children and adults usually need to infuse at 2 sites, on either the anterior abdomen or thigh. There is some evidence that a rapid push technique is acceptable to patients.[15]

EFFICACY OF IMMUNOGLOBULIN THERAPY
Survival Rates

There are numerous randomized controlled trials (RCTs) examining the effectiveness of immunoglobulin treatment, but no placebo-controlled trial data. The UK Medical Research Council reported 201 case histories of immune-deficient patients treated with low doses (0.1 g/kg/mo) of intramuscular immunoglobulin (IMIg), with a 10-year survival of 37%.[16] By contrast, Cunningham-Rundles and Bodian[5] reported 248 patients with CVIDs, the vast majority of whom received IVIg (0.4 g/kg/mo) throughout the period of observation: these patients had a 10-year survival of 78%. Liu and colleagues[17] concluded from these data that mortality was markedly higher in those treated with low-dose immunoglobulin. More recent European data show a further increase in survival rates.[18] However, factors in addition to increased immunoglobulin dose such as improved diagnosis and management of complications are likely to have made a significant contribution to the increased survival seen in those patients treated with IVIg.

Infection Rates

Replacement immunoglobulin therapy reduces the rate of bacterial infections, days of antibiotic usage and days of fever, hospital admissions, and incidence of pneumonia (**Table 2**).[19–22] Patients receiving higher-dose therapy have significantly fewer total episodes of infections per patient, and the duration of infections is significantly shorter

Table 2	
Clinical benefits of immunoglobulin replacement therapy in primary antibody deficiency	
Issue	**Grade of Evidence**
Increased life expectancy	2++
Reduction in the rate of bacterial infection	2++
Greater morbidity from diagnostic and treatment delay	2++
Reduction in infections with increased dose	1++
Improved quality of life with replacement therapy	2++

compared with low-dose therapy.[23] Previous studies comparing IMIg (at 0.08–0.1 g/kg/mo) with IVIg (at 0.4 g/kg/mo) also showed that higher doses of immunoglobulin reduce the rates of bacterial infections.[24]

Low levels of IgG (<6 g/L) immediately before therapy (termed trough levels) are associated with moderate lung damage (bronchiectasis)[25] Significantly higher rates of pneumonia (per patient-year) were found in patients with trough IgG levels less than 5 g/L ($P = .06$).[25] There was also an increased risk of chronic lung disease and sinusitis with time in patients with low IgG levels.[6] Data from Rolfman and colleagues[19] showed that an IgG trough level greater than 9 g/L reduced validated infection rates from more than 10% to 5.6%. It has been shown that there is a significant correlation between prevention of pneumonia and IgG trough levels ($P = .012$).[20] More recently, a large multicenter study demonstrated that IVIg therapy should be aimed at maintaining a trough level above 4 g/L to maintain the reduced incidence of pneumonia after therapy, and that patients with CVID who have low IgA (<0.07 g/L), low IgM, and bronchiectasis at presentation have a higher risk of pneumonia despite therapy.[26] A crossover study comparing IVIg with SCIg therapy demonstrated equivalent efficacy in terms of infection frequency,[27] and this has been demonstrated more recently in other studies.[28,29] However, dosing when changing patients from intravenous to subcutaneous treatment should be adjusted on an individual basis to achieve similar levels of IgG.[30]

These data support the contention that higher doses of immunoglobulin and higher trough levels are associated with fewer infections. However, this does not translate into ideal dosage or trough IgG levels for all patients, as the level at which infections are prevented varies widely between patients. Recent data suggest that clinical measures in individual patients may be more important than aiming for a specific trough IgG level,[31] although a meta-analysis concluded that progressively higher trough IgG levels (achieved by increased dosing) correlated with a reduced incidence of pneumonia during therapy.[32]

It is also unclear as to whether a starting dose adjusted for body weight is an appropriate approach for all patients. There was no relationship between annual dose and trough IgG level, regardless of infusion frequency, or adjustment for weight or body mass index.[33] Whether increased doses are associated with an improved outcome has yet to be established. Despite this lack of clear evidence, surveys suggest many clinicians use dosing to achieve appropriate trough levels,[34] and guidelines attempting to standardize treatment dosing and frequency have been produced by several different countries, often as part of demand-management strategies.[35,36]

RISKS OF IMMUNOGLOBULIN THERAPY

The risks of immunoglobulin therapy fall into 3 main categories: immediate reaction, delayed reaction, and pathogen transmission.

Immediate Reactions

Immediate reactions occurring during infusions can be severe, including anaphylaxis. Patients experience a clinical syndrome similar to type I hypersensitivity reactions, with urticaria, angioedema, bronchospasm and, potentially, cardiovascular collapse. The etiology of such reactions remains unclear, and although there have been reports of antibodies potentially directed against IgA found in the infusion product, the overall contribution of these to adverse reactions remains unclear.[37] As already noted, manufacturers attempt to keep the IgA content of their products as low as possible to minimize this risk. Of probable greater risk is the presence of untreated bacterial or low-grade viral infection, and the incidence of potentially severe side effects when the patient is acutely infected remains high. For this reason clinical units commonly operate a policy of ensuring that the patient is apyrexial for a 48-hour period before any infusion.

Delayed Reactions

Patients can also experience delayed reactions to immunoglobulin products, occurring several hours after infusion, and most commonly involving headache, backache, and occasional rigors. Again the precise etiology of these reactions remains unclear, although both immune complex formation and reactivity to components used in the manufacturing process that appear in the final product may be implicated in such reactions. The osmotic activity of the IVIg preparations, particularly in those older products where carbohydrates motives are used as stabilizers, may cause a degree of fluid shift into the intravascular space during infusion. This shift may be exacerbated if the patient is relatively dehydrated, and may contribute to the headache and other delayed side effects seen. It is likely that residual infections, particularly in patients who have end-organ damage such as bronchiectasis or sinusitis, may be important in the nature of these reactions.

It is clear that patients tolerate different products to differing extents,[38] and if reactions persist, the brand of IVIg should be changed. In general, however, there is acceptance that the patient should be maintained on the same product if at all possible, to reduce the potential risk of infection transmission, although there is no direct evidence to support this practice. Adverse reactions to SCIg appear to be generally much less common, more likely as a consequence of the route of administration, with subcutaneous therapy being delivered into a relatively inert space in comparison with the intravenous route, rather than inherent differences between intravenous and subcutaneous products.

Pathogen Transmission

There is an inevitable risk from pooled donated plasma of the transmission of plasma-borne infectious agents. IVIg produced by cold-ethanol fractionation has been regarded as inherently safer than those products prepared from cryoprecipitate fractions such as Factor VIII. However, transmission of HCV has been reported previously, although viral transmission has not been reported since the last outbreak of HCV nearly 20 years ago.[39,40] These outbreaks resulted in a high level of vigilance regarding donor and plasma selection, and a review of manufacturing processes to assess their impact on viral reduction or inactivation. Cold-ethanol fractionation and incubation at low pH both contribute to significant reduction in viral concentrations in experimental conditions, although not being regarded as sufficient. Additional measures including pasteurization, solvent detergent treatment, the use of caprylic acid treatment, and nanofiltration have all been demonstrated to significantly remove viral particles during the manufacturing processes. Manufacturers currently use a multistage approach with all of these methods often used in combination.

The other major long-term risk, albeit at this stage theoretical, is the transmission of prions in plasma. The epidemic of bovine spongiform encephalopathy (SSE) in the United Kingdom and a small number of other countries in the 1990s, and the reported link between SSE and a novel form of Creutzfeldt-Jakob disease (new variant CJD) led to major concerns about the safety of plasma donated from individuals resident in those countries affected by SSE, in particular the United Kingdom. As a result of these concerns, a ban was placed on the use of UK-derived plasma for the manufacturers of immunoglobulin and other plasma-derived products. This ban remains in place and is likely to do so for the foreseeable future. Manufacturers' own assessments indicate that significant removal of prion particles (4–5 log reduction) occurs during the fractionation process, filtration steps, and precipitation procedures, suggesting that the risk transmission from immunoglobulin products is likely to be extremely low. However, case reports of transmission of new variant CJD by blood transfusion indicate that the theoretical risk remains, and it is critical that during the consenting process, patients, their families, and carers are made fully aware of the long-term potential risk from treatment. These risks clearly must be balanced against the evidence of benefit from therapy.

CONSEQUENCES OF DELAYED THERAPY

Data from the United Kingdom in the later 1980s and early 1990s indicated that patients with primary antibody deficiencies experienced a median diagnostic delay of 3.5 years.[41,42] More recent data suggest that this may have declined to a median of 1 year.[43] In the United Kingdom, this reduction in delay may have been attributable to the publication of previous reports including the UK Consensus[44] and the distribution of national guidelines in 1995. However, the delay in diagnosis depends on the type of antibody deficiency.[43]

Diagnostic delay results in treatment delay and morbidity following further infections. An episode of pneumonia before treatment results in a 10-fold increase in risk of pneumonia after therapy.[21] Inadequate replacement therapy with immunoglobulin places the patient at greater risk of recurrent respiratory tract infections, chronic bronchitis, and rhinosinusitis.[4,5] Infectious diarrhea occurs with increased frequency in untreated patients with both CVID and XLA.[45] Central nervous system infections have been reported as both a presenting feature and complication of primary antibody deficiency, particularly prediagnosis or during suboptimal therapy.[25] Such infectious episodes are significantly reduced with adequate immunoglobulin replacement therapy.

In addition to acute infection, end-organ damage can result from delayed diagnosis and therapy. End-stage lung disease with the development of respiratory insufficiency remained the most common cause of morbidity in large cohort studies from the 1990s,[4,5] although there is a lack of more recent data. Patients may also suffer from autoimmune hematologic disorders. In the largest case series of CVID reported (326 patients),[46] 11% had a history of autoimmune hematologic disease.

Rheumatologic complications of primary antibody deficiencies are primarily those caused by acute or chronic infection that resolve on appropriate antibiotic therapy and are prevented by the institution of immunoglobulin therapy.[47] Skin infections may be fungal, bacterial, or viral.[48] Patients on immunoglobulin therapy remain at risk of several organ-specific and systemic complications, including inflammatory bowel disease, neurodegeneration, and malignancy (reviewed in Ref.[49]). Estimates of the overall increased risk of malignancy vary from 1.8-fold to 13-foid, with the risk linked to the primary antibody deficiency rather than the genetic background of the individual.[50] The occurrence of these and other complications emphasizes the need for regular clinical review by appropriately trained specialists and further investigation as required.

CURRENT AVAILABILITY

There are several plasma fractionation companies manufacturing both intravenous and subcutaneous products. Current availability in the United Kingdom is shown in **Table 3**. Most manufacturers provide both intravenous and subcutaneous products derived from the same plasma donation pool and, as outlined earlier, the current trend is toward higher concentration of product, with the benefits of reduced volume and infusion time.

It is clear that patients with primary immunodeficiencies tolerate certain products more than others. This difference may partly be due to the IgA content of products and the presence of anti-IgA antibodies in the patient, although the data on this issue remain unclear, and in any event manufacturers all ensure that the IgA content of their products is as low as possible. However, the issue of variable tolerability underlies the consensus best-practice approach of ensuring that patients have access to a range of products, and this is endorsed by national professional societies (eg, The United Kingdom Primary Immunodeficiency Network; http://www.ukpin.org.uk/. In addition, it is desirable to ensure continuity of product in an individual patient unless clinically a change of product is required. Patients should not have their product changed purely on the grounds of cost or convenience.

QUALITY-OF-LIFE ISSUES

There is only one study that has directly compared health-related quality of life before and after immunoglobulin therapy.[51] This study of 25 patients with CVID or XLA used analysis of medical records, data registers, and 3 questionnaires (a study-specific

Table 3 Currently available intravenous and subcutaneous immunoglobulin products (United Kingdom)		
Product	**Manufacturer**	**Concentration (% v/v)**
Intravenous		
Kiovig	Baxter	10
Vigam	BPL	5
Gammaplex	BPL	5
Intratect	Biotest	10
Privigen	CSL-Behring	10
Flebogamma diff 5%	Grifols	5
Flebogamma diff 10%	Grifols	10
Octagam 5%	Octapharma	5
Octagam 10%	Octapharma	10
Subcutaneous		
Subcuvia	Baxter	16
Subgam	BPL	16
Vivaglobin	CSL-Behring	16
Hizentra	CSL-Behring	20

questionnaire in addition to the Sickness Impact Profile)[52] to assess the overall quality of life before and 18 months after initiation of SCIg therapy. After 18 months of SCIg therapy, patients reported significant improvements across all areas of health-related function to levels comparable with healthy individuals. In addition, the patient group reported reduced fear of infections and decreased anxiety for their future health. It is reasonable to conclude that initiation of therapy with immunoglobulin was a major factor in the improvements seen, although other factors relating to diagnosis and support from health professionals are likely also to have been contributory. Other studies support the overall concept that patients prefer home-based therapy and report improved quality of life when transferring from hospital-based IVIg therapy.[29,53]

Other studies have assessed the quality of life of individuals already receiving immunoglobulin replacement therapy.[54] Eighty-three percent of a cohort of adult XLA patients rated their health as good, very good, or excellent. The responses indicated that the adult males with XLA had equivalent quality of life to the general male population, other than in their perception of their own health. In this study, XLA patients had a better quality of life in every parameter when compared with individuals with diabetes. Although direct comparison is not possible, more historical data on XLA patients indicates significant morbidity and poor survival rates in adult life, particularly from the era before IVIg,[55] indicating that earlier diagnosis and prompt initiation of adequate immunoglobulin replacement therapy improves overall quality of life. This proposal is supported by recent data from Iran.[56]

By contrast, a study comparing patients with CVID receiving IVIg with patients suffering from diabetes mellitus or congestive cardiac failure found that patients with CVID had significantly worse health-related quality of life than patients with either of these other conditions, unrelated to socioeconomic or disease-related factors.[57] However, this does not indicate that initiation of immunoglobulin replacement therapy fails to improve overall life quality. Overall, studies looking at quality-of-life issues in primary antibody deficiencies suggest that replacement therapy with immunoglobulin given by either the intravenous or subcutaneous route is a contributory factor in the improvement of life quality. There are no studies assessing how diagnostic or treatment delay affects this, although pretreatment data provide some indication as to the overall poor quality of life suffered by individuals with either undiagnosed or untreated primary antibody deficiencies. It could be inferred that because increased dose reduces overall infection burden, this would improve quality of life further, but this has not been demonstrated directly.

THE ECONOMIC BENEFITS OF DIAGNOSIS AND APPROPRIATE THERAPY

There are a few studies assessing the cost-effectiveness of immunoglobulin therapy, but none comparing no therapy with replacement therapy. All studies are limited by the costs of immunoglobulin at the time of the study. However, an early study compared the potential cost-effectiveness of changing from IMIg to IVIg.[58] Because IMIg therapy has often been used as a surrogate marker for no effective therapy, this study represents an attempt to compare therapy with no therapy. Twenty-three children with a variety of primary antibody deficiency states were assessed in the 2 years before and the 3 years following the change from IMIg to IVIg. The number of days with antibiotics, number of absences from school, number of days in bed or hospital, and the number of days with infection or fever were assessed at 3-week intervals. The change from IMIg to IVIg produced a 90% decrease in the number of hospital bed days. Based on 1990 Italian costs (in lira; 1000 lira = $1) the relative costs of antibiotic therapy, hospitalization, and immunoglobulin drug costs per month for a 20-kg child were L953,000 for IMIg, reduced to L826,000 for IVIg. Given that the quoted figures for drug costs were L160,000 for IMIg and L468,000 for IVIg, this illustrates the significant overall cost saving of adequate therapy with IVIg. Other studies have compared the estimated relative overall treatment costs of IVIg with SCIg. Such studies are limited by the relative drug costs, which in the case of the study of Gardulf and colleagues[59] in 1995 were based on an approximate cost of $14,000 per annum for IVIg against $4650 for SCIg. Perhaps not surprisingly, this study reported a lower overall cost for home SCIg therapy compared with hospital-based IVIg therapy. A more recent study[60] compared the costs to the German health insurance system of providing level or SCIg from 18 centers in Germany. Costs were taken from the standard tariffs for drugs and health services in the German health care system in 2003. For adults the overall costs per annum were €31.027 for IVIg and €14,893 for SCIg. Within these costs the drug costs were €30,456 and €13,874, respectively. Because these data are derived from a unit cost of €86.40 for IVIg and €38.54 for SCIg, at price equivalence there is effectively no cost difference between the two therapy routes. Smaller but similar costs applied to children in the study.

Cost-Effectiveness of Immunoglobulin Replacement Therapy

As part of a cost-effectiveness review on immunoglobulin therapy, Liu and colleagues[17] developed a Markov model to assess the cost-effectiveness of immunoglobulin therapy. This model used derived mortality data based on survival estimates from current immunoglobulin replacement regimes (mainly IVIg) compared with historical data (mainly IMIg), although the investigators acknowledged that such a comparison was difficult due to the lack of placebo-controlled RCT data. Nevertheless, a conversion of the costs used by Hogy and colleagues[60] into United Kingdom costs resulted in estimated costs per annum of £18,600 for hospital-based IVIg therapy and £11,580 for home-based IVIg therapy. Costs of SCIg therapy (exclusively based at home) were £11,760, reflecting the similar unit costs of SCIg and IVIg in the United Kingdom. Taking these data assumptions into account the economic model predicted a base case incremental cost-effectiveness ratio (ICER) per quality-assessed life year of approximately £30,000. The ICER for immunoglobulin therapy in primary immunodeficiency compares favorably to the use of prophylactic therapy in hemophilia.[61]

IMMUNOTHERAPY FOR AUTOIMMUNE AND GRANULOMATOUS COMPLICATIONS IN PRIMARY ANTIBODY DEFICIENCY

It is well recognized that patients with CVID disorders can develop a variety of autoimmune and granulomatous complications of their disease, and a significant percentage have such complications at presentation.[49] Management of these conditions has been, and continues to be, a significant clinical challenge, although the availability of several biologic agents, in particular the anti-CD20 monoclonal antibody rituximab and the anti–tumor necrosis factor (TNF) agents infliximab and etanercept, has increased the therapeutic options available for the treatment of these serious and potentially life-threatening complications.

Hematologic Autoimmunity

Immune thrombocytopenic purpura and autoimmune hemolytic anemia develop in a significant proportion of patients with CVID.[46] Based on previous evidence of efficacy for the use of rituximab in these conditions occurring outside the context of primary immunodeficiency, rituximab has been used to treat such complications in patients with CVID. Successful treatment of autoimmune hemolytic anemia has been reported in children,[62] and several case reports demonstrated efficacy in immune thrombocytopenic purpura.[63–65] A retrospective report of 33 patients from several centers (immune thrombocytic purpura [n = 22 cases], autoimmune hemolytic anemia [n = 5], or both [n = 7]) showed an overall initial response rate to rituximab was 85% including 74% complete responses with relapse in 10 of the initial responders after a mean follow-up of 39 months (±30).[66] Severe infections occurred after rituximab in 8 adults (24%), although 4 were not on immunoglobulin replacement therapy, raising doubts about the diagnosis of CVID. Dosing regimens have varied in published studies, but evidence suggests that sustained benefit can be achieved, although the underlying immune dysregulation resulting in these complications remains an ongoing problem.

Granulomatous Disease

Granulomatous disease of the lungs, liver, spleen, and other organs is another significant disabling and potentially life-threatening complication of CVID. Therapeutic options remain limited but there have been reports of benefit from the use of anti-TNF agents, in particular infliximab,[67–69] following the success of this agent in diseases with presumed similar immunopathology such as Crohn disease. With both of these agents, reservations remain about the further compromise of effective immunity in individuals for whom the immune system is already partially ineffective although, in the case of rituximab, the fact that CVID patients are receiving replacement immunoglobulin therapy alleviates any concerns about increased B-cell dysfunction occurring as a consequence of treatment.

IMMUNOTHERAPY IN HAE

HAE is an autosomal dominant disorder caused by mutations in the gene for C1 inhibitor. C1 inhibitor, a member of the Serpin family, is critical in the regulation of both the complement pathway and the contact pathway. Evidence indicates that lack of inhibition of the contact pathway leads to unregulated activity of kininigen, leading to the uncontrolled production of bradykinin. Bradykinin seems to be the major mediator of the angioedema suffered by patients with this disorder.[70] Clinically patients present with recurrent bouts of evolving angioedema most commonly involving limbs, gastrointestinal tract, and upper airway, resulting in significant pain and, in the case of airway involvement, potential life-threatening angioedema episodes. In contrast to histaminergic angioedema, the clinical evolution of angioedema occurs more slowly, reaching a peak after several hours, but with much longer persistence. Attacks can be life-threatening, and prompt therapy is desirable to reverse angioedema and relieve pain.

Early attempts at therapy for this disorder used plasma products.[71,72] Such agents contain amounts of C1 inhibitor sufficient to prevent progression of angioedema, but carry the concerns that other complement components present in plasma may paradoxically fuel further episodes. It is not clear how clinically relevant this might be but, at the very least, it is likely that the available C1 inhibitor may be consumed in complement cascade blockade rather than prevention of further bradykinin production.

Plasma-Derived C1 Inhibitor Concentrate

Production of C1 inhibitor from plasma is broadly similar to the processes already described for the production of immunoglobulin. Donated plasma is screened for the presence of HBsAg, and antibodies to HIV-1 and -2 and HCV. In addition, plasma is tested by for genomic material of HCV, HBV, HAV, HIV-1, and parvovirus B19. Manufacturing pools are tested for HBsAg and anti–HIV-1/-2. Only manufacturing nonreactive for HCV RNA, HBV DNA, HAV RNA, HIV-1 RNA, and high titers of parvovirus B19 are released. Viral reduction steps in the manufacturing process include pasteurization (10 hours at 60°C) and hydrophobic interaction columns. The ability to produce pasteurized C1 inhibitor derived from plasma has, until recently, been the mainstay of therapy for acute attacks for this disorder, although its availability has been limited mainly to the United Kingdom and European countries often on an unlicensed basis, and controlled trial evidence of efficacy has been available only comparatively recently.[73] Nevertheless, pasteurized C1 inhibitor concentrate used at a dose of 20 units per kg of body weight is an effective therapy for acute angioedema in this condition and remains the recommended first-line therapy for acute angioedema in this disorder, according to recently published international consensus guidelines.

Icatibant

More recently the bradykinin antagonist icatibant has become available for the treatment of acute angioedema attacks in HAE. This small peptide binds to the bradykinin B2 receptor with a high binding affinity (1000-fold higher for the B2 receptor than for the inducible B1 receptor)[74] and confers several potential advantages over plasma-derived C1 inhibitor, not least the fact that being a non–plasma-derived product it does not carry the potential risks of infection transmission. In addition, the bioavailability of icatibant appears to be equivalent whether given subcutaneously or intravenously, allowing rapid subcutaneous administration. This rapidity has practical advantages in the hospital setting, where intravenous cannulation is not required, and more recently evidence has become available that self-administration in the nonhospital setting during an attack is both effective and well tolerated by patients. The ability of patients to self-administer at home in the early stages of an attack of acute angioedema has potential health resource implications, and its recent licensing for self-administration in the United Kingdom and Europe has allowed the development of home therapy programs, similar in scope to those described for SCIg therapy. After initial pilot studies,[75,76] 2 RCTs compared icatibant for the treatment of cutaneous or abdominal attacks in the For Angioedema Subcutaneous Treatment (FAST) studies.[77] In FAST-1, 56 patients were randomized to receive icatibant at a dose of 30 mg or placebo, with the icatibant group demonstrating reduction in the median time to clinically significant relief of symptoms, although this did not attain statistical significance. This finding was attributed to the early allowable use of rescue medication inherent in the study design. In the FAST-2 study, the efficacy of icatibant was compared with tranexamic acid, with the primary end point being reached in 2 hours with icatibant compared with 12 hours with tranexamic acid ($P<.001$) in a group of 74 patients. No significant side effects were reported. In these initial studies no patients with laryngeal angioedema were included, but the later FAST-3 study demonstrated the efficacy of icatibant in the control of mild to moderate laryngeal angioedema.[78]

Nanofiltered Plasma-Derived C1 Inhibitor

The use of nanofiltration as an additional viral removal step has been applied to the manufacture of plasma-derived C1 inhibitor concentrate. Cinryze is a nanofiltered plasma-derived C1 inhibitor that has shown efficacy in controlled trials. Intriguingly the nanofiltered product has an extended half-life, allowing the drug to be used as prophylactic therapy. Two randomized trials to evaluate nanofiltered C1 inhibitor concentrate in the management of HAE have been published.[79] The first compared nanofiltered C1 inhibitor concentrate with placebo for treatment of an acute attack of angioedema in 68 subjects (35 in the C1 inhibitor group and 33 in the placebo group). Participants were given 1 or 2 intravenous injections of the study drug (1000 units each). The median time to the onset of unequivocal relief from an attack (used as the primary end point) was 2 hours in the subjects treated with C1 inhibitor concentrate but more than 4 hours in those given placebo ($P = .02$). The second study was a crossover trial involving 22 subjects comparing prophylactic twice-weekly injections of nanofiltered C1 inhibitor concentrate (1000 units) with placebo during 2 12-week periods. The primary end point was the number of attacks of angioedema per period. In the second study, the number of attacks per 12-week period was 6.26 with C1 inhibitor concentrate given as prophylaxis, compared with 12.73 with placebo ($P<.001$); the subjects who received the C1 inhibitor concentrate also had significant reductions in both the severity and the duration of attacks, in the need for open-label rescue therapy, and in the total number of days with swelling. The addition of a nanofiltration step in the manufacture of Cetor (Sanquin, the Netherlands) has been shown not to affect pharmacokinetic parameters or efficacy in a randomized, double-blind, controlled crossover study looking at use in both acute attacks and prophylaxis, with no adverse events and no induction of anti-C1 antibodies.[80]

Recombinant Human C1 Inhibitor (Ruconest)

Ruconest (rhuC1INH) is another new C1 inhibitor concentrate product, secreted in the milk of transgenic rabbits, and has been licensed for treatment of acute attacks of HAE. The glycosylation pattern of the recombinant product differs from plasma-derived C1 inhibitor, resulting in a shorter half-life but equipotency. Initial safety studies in asymptomatic HAE patients demonstrated good tolerability[81] and in placebo-controlled studies rhuC1INH at 100 (n = 29) and 50 (n = 12) U/kg body weight resulted in a significant reduction for the primary end-point time (beginning of relief of symptoms) compared with saline (n = 29). Failure of treatment occurred in 59% (17/29) of the saline group compared with 0% (0/12) of the 50-U/kg group and 10% (3/29) of the 100-U/kg group. No postexposure antibody responses against rhuC1INH or host-related impurities were observed. Open-label extensions of these trials are in progress, but evidence suggests that the recombinant product remains equally effective with repeated use. A minor but significant issue with the recombinant product concerns the reactivity in patients allergic to rabbit epithelium. During safety studies an individual with previously undisclosed rabbit allergy developed anaphylaxis after administration of recombinant C1 inhibitor, and patients should therefore be screened by skin-prick testing or serum IgE testing to rabbit epithelium before prescription.[82] There is, as yet, no evidence that patients develop IgE antibodies to rabbit epithelium or C1 inhibitor following administration of the recombinant product.

Ecallantide

Ecallantide is a recombinantly produced small protein based on one of the domains of the human tissue factor pathway inhibitor, and is a potent and selective inhibitor of plasma kallikrein. As indicated earlier, kallikrein is the enzyme that acts on high molecular weight kininigen to generate bradykinin,[83] the compound responsible for formation of angioedema. Two double-blind, placebo-controlled studies have demonstrated the efficacy of this compound in controlling acute attacks of angioedema. In the first study[84] 72 patients were given 30 mg of either ecallantide or placebo, with a primary end point of a treatment outcome score (range -100 [worsening] to $+100$ [improvement]) 4 hours after drug administration. There was a significant difference in the scores between treatment and placebo groups, with more rapid improvement in symptoms in the drug group. A similar study in 96 patients

Table 4		
Current availability of therapies for C1-inhibitor deficiency (hereditary angioedema)		
Product	**Manufacturer**	**Licensed Uses**
Berinert (pdC1INH)	CSL-Behring	Acute attacks (self-administration)
Cinryze (npdC1INH)	ViroPharma	Acute attacks (prophylaxis)
Ruconest (rhuC1INH)	Pharming	Acute attacks
Firazyr (Icatibant)	Shire	Acute attacks (self-administration)
Kalbitor (Ecallantide)	Dyax	Acute attacks

demonstrated similar results,[85] and in a majority of cases a single dose is sufficient, although subsequent dosing may be necessary. Current data suggest that ecallantide may have a significant adverse event rate regarding anaphylaxis; 5% of patients may experience hypersensitivity reactions, with anaphylaxis possibly occurring in 2%. At present ecallantide is approved in the United States for the treatment of acute attacks, but is not yet approved in Europe.

Self-Administration of Therapies for HAE

There is now increasing interest in the use of some of the aforementioned agents for self-administration by patients with HAE suffering an acute episode of angioedema. Icatibant is licensed for self-administration with the subcutaneous route, making the training process for patients and carers considerably more simple. Self-administration of plasma-derived C1 inhibitor for the treatment of acute attacks has been reported,[86] and in a small study (n = 9) was shown to improve quality of life as assessed by the Dermatology Quality of Life Index and SF-36 questionnaires.[87] C1 inhibitor (Berinert) has recently been given approval by the US Food and Drug Administration for self-administration outside the hospital setting. Prophylactic use of plasma-derived C1 inhibitor seems to be tolerated,[88] and cinryze has been demonstrated to be effective as prophylaxis.[79,89] A recent International Working Group meeting has published evidence-based recommendations for the therapeutic management of angioedema caused by hereditary C1 inhibitor deficiency, and has produced a set of recommended consensus treatment approaches for this disorder.[90] Currently available therapies for HAE and their indications are listed in **Table 4**.

SUMMARY

Primary immunodeficiency diseases are rare and can present at any age. The most commonly encountered diseases in adults, primary antibody deficiencies and HAE, can be effectively managed by immunotherapeutic interventions. The ability to fractionate donated plasma to produce stable immunoglobulin for intravenous and subcutaneous use has dramatically improved overall survival and quality of life in patients with primary antibody deficiencies. With increased survival in primary antibody deficiencies has come the development of complications of disease not directly related to recurrent infection. The use of biologics in the form of monoclonal antibody therapies is becoming established as the treatment of choice for such problems as autoimmune hematologic disorders and granulomatous diseases.

In a similar way, fractionation of plasma to produce C1 inhibitor concentrate has allowed effective therapy for acute angioedema episodes in patients with HAE. More recently, several significant additions to the therapy for HAE have become available, with the potential to alleviate some of the concerns over potential pathogen transmission from plasma-derived products, offering choice to patients and the ability to self-administer therapy, thus allowing greater patient control over their disease. Significant challenges remain in the treatment of HAE, including timing and appropriateness of self-administration, and in these straightened economic circumstances concerns over long-term funding for these agents.

Nevertheless, increased understanding of the pathogenesis of these disorders combined with technological and genetic manufacturing advances has expanded the immunotherapy available for primary immunodeficiency disorders, a trend that is certain to continue.

REFERENCES

1. Conley ME, Broides A, Hernandez-Trujillo V, et al. Genetic analysis of patients with defects in early B-cell development. Immunol Rev 2005;203:216–34.
2. Kracker S, Gardes P, Durandy A. Inherited defects of immunoglobulin class switch recombination. Adv Exp Med Biol 2010;685:166–74.
3. Notarangelo LD, Fischer A, Geha RS, et al. Primary immunodeficiencies: 2009 update. J Allergy Clin Immunol 2009;124(6):1161–78.
4. Hermaszewski RA, Webster AD. Primary hypogammaglobulinaemia: a survey of clinical manifestations and complications. Q J Med 1993;86(1):31–42.
5. Cunningham-Rundles C, Bodian C. Common variable immunodeficiency: clinical and immunological features of 248 patients. Clin Immunol 1999;92(1):34–48.
6. Kainulainen L, Varpula M, Liippo K, et al. Pulmonary abnormalities in patients with primary hypogammaglobulinemia. J Allergy Clin Immunol 1999;104(5):1031–6.
7. Michel M, Chanet V, Galicier L, et al. Autoimmune thrombocytopenic purpura and common variable immunodeficiency: analysis of 21 cases and review of the literature. Medicine (Baltimore) 2004;83(4):254–63.
8. Bruton OC. Agammaglobulinemia (congenital absence of gamma globulin); report of a case [passim]. Med Ann Dist Columbia 1953;22(12):648–50.
9. Church JA, Leibl H, Stein MR, et al. Efficacy, safety and tolerability of a new 10% liquid intravenous immune globulin [IGIV 10%] in patients with primary immunodeficiency. J Clin Immunol 2006;26(4):388–95.
10. Shah SR. A newer immunoglobulin Intravenous (IGIV) Gammagard liquid 10%: evaluation of efficacy, safety, tolerability and impact on patient care. Expert Opin Biol Ther 2008;8(6):799–804.
11. Stein MR, Nelson RP, Church JA, et al. Safety and efficacy of Privigen, a novel 10% liquid immunoglobulin preparation for intravenous use, in patients with primary immunodeficiencies. J Clin Immunol 2009;29(1):137–44.
12. Berger M, Pinciaro PJ, Althaus A, et al. Efficacy, pharmacokinetics, safety, and tolerability of Flebogamma 10% DIF, a high-purity human intravenous immunoglobulin, in primary immunodeficiency. J Clin Immunol 2010;30(2):321–9.
13. Gardulf A, Hammarstrom L, Smith CI. Home treatment of hypogammaglobulinaemia with subcutaneous gammaglobulin by rapid infusion. Lancet 1991;338(8760):162–6.
14. Chapel H, Brennan V, Delson E. Immunoglobulin replacement therapy by self-infusion at home. Clin Exp Immunol 1988;73(1):160–2.
15. Shapiro R. Subcutaneous immunoglobulin therapy by rapid push is preferred to infusion by pump: a retrospective analysis. J Clin Immunol 2010;30(2):301–7.
16. UK Medical Research Council. Hypogammaglobulinaemia in the United Kingdom. Special Report Series. London (HMSO): UK Medical Research Council; 1971. p. 310.

17. Liu Z, Albon E, Hyde C. The effectiveness and cost-effectiveness of immunoglob-ulin replacement therapy for primary immunodeficiency and chronic lymphocytic leukaemia: a systematic review and economic evaluation. Birmingham: West Midlands Health Technology Assessment Group, Dept of Public Health & Epide-miology, University of Birmingham; 2006. p. 54.
18. Chapel H, Lucas M, Lee M, et al. Common variable Immunodeficiency disorders: division into distinct clinical phenotypes. Blood 2008;112(2):277–86.
19. Roitman CM, Schroeder H, Berger M, et al. Comparison of the efficacy of IGIV-C, 10% (caprylate/chromatography) and IGIVSD, 10% as replacement therapy in primary immune deficiency. A randomized double-blind trial. Int Immunopharma-col 2003;3(9):1325–33.
20. Aghamohammadi A, Moin M, Farhoudi A, et al. Efficacy of intravenous immuno-globulin on the prevention of pneumonia in patients with agammaglobulinemia. FEMS Immunol Med Microbiol 2004;40(2):113–8.
21. Busse PJ, Razvi S, Cunningham-Rundles C. Efficacy of intravenous immunoglob-ulin in the prevention of pneumonia in patients with common variable immunode-ficiency. J Allergy Clin Immunol 2002;109(6):1001–4.
22. de Gracia J, Vendrell M, Alvarez A, et al. Immunoglobulin therapy to control lung damage in patients with common variable immunodeficiency. Int Immunophar-macol 2004;4(6):745–53.
23. Eijkhout HW, van Der Meer JW, Kallenberg CG, et al. The effect of two different dosages of intravenous immunoglobulin on the incidence of recurrent infections in patients with primary hypogammaglobulinemia. A randomized, double-blind, multicenter crossover trial. Ann Intern Med 2001;135(3):165–74.
24. Cunningham-Rundles C, Siegal FP, Smithwick EM, et al. Efficacy of intravenous immunoglobulin in primary humoral immunodeficiency disease. Ann Intern Med 1984;101(4):435–9.
25. Plebani A, Soresina A, Rondell R, et al. Clinical, immunological, and molecular analysis in a large cohort of patients with X-linked agammaglobulinemia: an Italian multicenter study. Clin Immunol 2002;104(3):221–30.
26. Quinti I, Soresina A, Guerra A, et al. Effectiveness of immunoglobulin replacement therapy on clinical outcome In patients with primary antibody deficiencies: results from a multicenter prospective cohort study. J Clin Immunol 2011;31(3):315–22.
27. Chapel HM, Spicketl GP, Ericson D, et al. The comparison of the efficacy and safety of intravenous versus subcutaneous immunoglobulin replacement therapy. J Clin Immunol 2000;20(2):94–100.
28. Borte M, Bernatowska E, Ochs HD, et al. Efficacy and safety of home-based subcutaneous immunoglobulin replacement therapy in paediatric patients with primary immunodeficiencies. Clin Exp Immunol 2011;164(3):357–64.
29. Hoffmann F, Grimbacher B, Thiel J, et al. Home-based subcutaneous immuno-globulin G replacement therapy under real-life conditions in children and adults with antibody deficiency. Eur J Med Res 2010;15(6):238–45.
30. Berger M, Rojavin M, Kiessling P, et al. Pharmacokinetics of subcutaneous immu-noglobulin and their use in dosing of replacement therapy in patients with primary immunodeficiencies. Clin Immunol 2011;139(2):133–41.
31. Lucas M, Lee M, Lortan J, et al. Infection outcomes in patients with common vari-able immunodeficiency disorders: relationship to immunoglobulin therapy over 22 years. J Allergy Clin Immunol 2010;125(6):1354–60, e4.
32. Orange JS, Grossman WJ, Navickis RJ, et al. Impact of trough IgG on pneumonia incidence in primary immunodeficiency: a meta-analysis of clinical studies. Clin Immunol 2010;137(1):21–30.

33. Khan S, Grimbacher B, Boecking C, et al. Serum trough IgG level and annual intravenous immunoglobulin dose are not related to body size in patients on regular replacement therapy. Drug Metab Lett 2011;5(2):132–6.
34. Yong PL, Boyle J, Ballow M, et al. Use of intravenous immunoglobulin and adjunctive therapies in the treatment of primary immunodeficiencies: a working group report of and study by the Primary Immunodeficiency Committee of the American Academy of Allergy Asthma and Immunology. Clin Immunol 2010; 135(2):255–63.
35. Roifman CM, Berger M, Notarangelo LD. Management of primary antibody deficiency with replacement therapy: summary of guidelines. Immunol Allergy Clin North Am 2008;28(4):875–6, x.
36. Shehata N, Palda V, Bowen T, et al. The use of immunoglobulin therapy for patients with primary immune deficiency: an evidence-based practice guideline. Transfus Med Rev 2010;24(Suppl 1):S28–50.
37. Rachid R, Bonilla FA. The role of anti-IgA antibodies in causing adverse reactions to gamma globulin infusion in immunodeficient patients: a comprehensive review of the literature. J Allergy Clin Immunol 2012;129(3):628–34.
38. Feldmeyer L, Benden C, Haile SR, et al. Not all intravenous immunoglobulin preparations are equally well tolerated. Acta Derm Venereol 2010;90(5):494–7.
39. Chapel HM, Christie JM, Peach V, et al. Five-year follow-up of patients with primary antibody deficiencies following an outbreak of acute hepatitis C. Clin Immunol 2001;99(3):320–4.
40. Quinti I, Pierdominici M, Marziali M, et al. European surveillance of immunoglobulin safety-results of Initial survey of 1243 patients with primary Immunodeficiencies In 16 countries. Clin Immunol 2002;104(3):231–6.
41. Spickett GP, Askew T, Chapel HM. Management of primary antibody deficiency by consultant immunologists in the United Kingdom: a paradigm for other rare diseases. Qual Health Care 1995;4(4):263–8.
42. Blore J, Haeney MR. Primary antibody deficiency and diagnostic delay. BMJ 1989;298(6672):516–7.
43. Seymour B, Miles J, Haeney M. Primary antibody deficiency and diagnostic delay. J Clin Pathol 2005;58(5):546–7.
44. Chapel HM. Consensus on diagnosis and management of primary antibody deficiencies. Consensus panel for the diagnosis and management of primary antibody deficiencies. BMJ 1994;308(6928):581–5.
45. Kainulainen L, Nlkoskelainen J, Ruuskanen O. Diagnostic findings in 95 Finnish patients with common variable immunodeficiency. J Clin Immunol 2001;21(2): 145–9.
46. Wang J, Cunningham-Rundles C. Treatment and outcome of autoimmune hematologic disease in common variable Immunodeficiency (CVID). J Autoimmun 2005;25(1):57–62.
47. Sordet C, Cantagrel A, Schaeverbeke T, et al. Bone and joint disease associated with primary immune deficiencies. Joint Bone Spine 2005;72(6):503–14.
48. Wood P. Primary antibody deficiency syndromes. Ann Clin Biochem 2009;46(Pt 2): 99–108.
49. Wood P, Stanworth S, Burton J, et al. Recognition, clinical diagnosis and management of patients with primary antibody deficiencies: a systematic review. Clin Exp Immunol 2007;149(3):410–23.
50. Mellemkjaer L, Hammarstrom L, Andersen V, et al. Cancer risk among patients with IgA deficiency or common variable immunodeficiency and their relatives: a combined Danish and Swedish study. Clin Exp Immunol 2002;130(3):495–500.

51. Gardulf A, Bjorvell H, Gustafson R, et al. The life situations of patients with primary antibody deficiency untreated or treated with subcutaneous gammaglobulin infusions. Clin Exp Immunol 1993;92(2):200–4.
52. Bergner M, Bobbitt RA, Carter WB, et al. The Sickness Impact Profile: development and final revision of a health status measure. Med Care 1981;19(8):787–805.
53. Berger M, Murphy E, Riley P, et al. Improved quality of life, immunoglobulin G levels, and infection rates in patients with primary immunodeficiency diseases during self-treatment with subcutaneous immunoglobulin G. South Med J 2010;103(9):856–63.
54. Howard V, Greene JM, Pahwa S, et al. The health status and quality of life of adults with X-linked agammaglobulinemia. Clin Immunol 2006;118(2-3):201–8.
55. Lederman HM, Winkelstein JA. X-linked agammaglobulinemia: an analysis of 96 patients. Medicine (Baltimore) 1985;64(3):145–56.
56. Aghamohammadi A, Montazeri A, Abolhassani H, et al. Health-related quality of life in primary antibody deficiency. Iran J Allergy Asthma Immunol 2011;10(1):47–51.
57. Tcheurekdjian H, Palermo T, Hostoffer R. Quality of life in common variable immunodeficiency requiring intravenous immunoglobulin therapy. Ann Allergy Asthma Immunol 2004;93(2):160–5.
58. Galli E, Barbieri C, Cantani A, et al. Treatment with gammaglobulin preparation for intravenous use in children with humoral immunodeficiency: clinical and immunologic follow-up. Ann Allergy 1990;64(2 Pt 1):147–50.
59. Gardulf A, Andersen V, Bjorkander J, et al. Subcutaneous immunoglobulin replacement in patients with primary antibody deficiencies: safety and costs. Lancet 1995;345(8946):365–9.
60. Hogy B, Kelnecke HO, Borte M. Pharmacoeconomic evaluation of immunoglobulin treatment in patients with antibody deficiencies from the perspective of the German statutory health insurance. Eur J Health Econ 2005;6(1):24–9.
61. Lippert B, Berger K, Bemtorp E, et al. Cost effectiveness of haemophilia treatment: a cross-national assessment. Blood Coagul Fibrinolysis 2005;16(7):477–85.
62. Wakim M, Shah A, Arndt PA, et al. Successful anti-CD20 monoclonal antibody treatment of severe autoimmune hemolytic anemia due to warm reactive IgM autoantibody in a child with common variable immunodeficiency. Am J Hematol 2004;76(2):152–5.
63. Mahevas M, Le Page L, Salle V, et al. Efficiency of rituximab In the treatment of autoimmune thrombocytopenic purpura,; associated with common variable immunodeficiency. Am J Hematol 2006;81(8):645–8.
64. El-Shanawany TM, Williams PE, Jolles S. Response of refractory immune thrombocytopenic purpura in a patient with common variable immunodeficiency to treatment with rituximab. J Clin Pathol 2007;60(6):715–8.
65. Al-Ahmad M, Al-Rasheed M, Al-Muhani A. Successful use of rituximab in refractory idiopathic thrombocytopenic purpura in a patient with common variable immunodeficiency. J Investig Allergol Clin Immunol 2010;20(3):259–62.
66. Gobert D, Bussel JB, Cunningham-Rundles C. Efficacy and safety of rituximab in common variable immunodeficiency-associated immune cytopenias: a retrospective multicentre study on 33 patients. Br J Haematol 2011;155(4):498–508.
67. Hatab AZ, Ballas ZK. Caseating granulomatous disease in common variable immunodeficiency treated with Infliximab. J Allergy Clin Immunol 2005;116(5):1161–2.

68. Thatayatikom A, Thatayatikom S, White AJ. Infliximab treatment for severe granulomatous disease in common variable immunodeficiency: a case report and review of the literature. Ann Allergy Asthma Immunol 2005;95(3):293–300.
69. Malbran A, Juri MC, Fernandez Romero DS. Common variable immunodeficiency and granulomatosis treated with infliximab. Clin Immunol 2010;134(3):359–60.
70. Kaplan AP, Joseph K. The bradykinin-forming cascade and its role in hereditary angioedema. Ann Allergy Asthma Immunol 2010;104(3):193–204.
71. Pickering RJ, Good RA, Kelly JR, et al. Replacement therapy in hereditary angioedema. Successful treatment of two patients with fresh frozen plasma. Lancet 1969;1(7590):326–30.
72. Cohen G, Peterson A. Treatment of hereditary angioedema with frozen plasma. Ann Allergy 1972;30(12):690–2.
73. Kunschak M, Engl W, Maritsch F, et al. A randomized, controlled trial to study the efficacy and safety of C1 inhibitor concentrate in treating hereditary angioedema. Transfusion 1998;38(6):540–9.
74. Kaplan AP. Enzymatic pathways in the pathogenesis of hereditary angioedema: the role of C1 inhibitor therapy. J Allergy Clin Immunol 2010;126(5):918–25.
75. Bork K, Frank J, Grundt B, et al. Treatment of acute edema attacks in hereditary angioedema with a bradykinin receptor-2 antagonist (Icatibant). J Allergy Clin Immunol 2007;119(6):1497–503.
76. Krause K, Metz M, Zuberbier T, et al. Successful treatment of hereditary angioedema with bradykinin B2-receptor antagonist icatibant. J Dtsch Dermatol Ges 2010;8(4):272–4.
77. Cicardi M, Banerji A, Bracho F, et al. Icatibant, a new bradykinin-receptor antagonist, in hereditary angioedema. N Engl J Med 2010;363(6):532–41.
78. Lumry WR, Li HH, Levy RJ, et al. Randomized placebo-controlled trial of the bradykinin B receptor antagonist icatibant for the treatment of acute attacks of hereditary angioedema: the FAST-3 trial. Ann Allergy Asthma Immunol 2011;107(6):529–37.
79. Zuraw BL, Busse PJ, White M, et al. Nanofiltered C1 inhibitor concentrate for treatment of hereditary angioedema. N Engl J Med 2010;363(6):513–22.
80. Hofstra JJ, Budde IK, van Twuyver E, et al. Treatment of hereditary angioedema with nanofiltered C1-esterase inhibitor concentrate (Cetor(R)): Multi-center phase II and III studies to assess pharmacokinetics, clinical efficacy and safety. Clin Immunol 2012;142(3):280–90.
81. van Doom MB, Burggraaf J, van Dam T, et al. A phase I study of recombinant human C1 inhibitor in asymptomatic patients with hereditary angioedema. J Allergy Clin Immunol 2005;116(4):876–83.
82. Zuraw B, Cieardi M, Levy RJ, et al. Recombinant human C1-inhibitor for the treatment of acute angioedema attacks in patients with hereditary angioedema. J Allergy Clin Immunol 2010;126(4):821–7, e14.
83. Lehmann A. Ecallantide (DX-88), a plasma kallikrein inhibitor for the treatment of hereditary angioedema and the prevention of blood loss in on-pump cardiothoracic surgery. Expert Opin Biol Ther 2008;8(8):1187–99.
84. Cieardi M, Levy RJ, McNeil DL, et al. Ecallantide for the treatment of acute attacks in hereditary angioedema. N Engl J Med 2010;363(6):523–31.
85. Levy RJ, Lumry WR, McNeil DL, et al. EDEMA4: a phase 3, double-blind study of subcutaneous ecallantide treatment for acute attacks of hereditary angioedema. Ann Allergy Asthma Immunol 2010;104(6):523–9.
86. Levi M, Choi G, Picavet C, et al. Self-administration of C1-inhibltor concentrate in patients with hereditary or acquired angioedema caused by C1-inhibitor deficiency. J Allergy Clin Immunol 2006;117(4):904–8.

87. Bygum A, Andersen KE, Mikkelsen CS. Self-administration of intravenous C1-inhlbitor therapy for hereditary angioedema and associated quality of life benefits. Eur J Dermatol 2009;19(2):147–51.

88. Tallroth GA. Long-term prophylaxis of hereditary angioedema with a pasteurized C1 inhibitor concentrate. Int Arch Allergy Immunol 2011;154(4):356–9.

89. Lunn M, Santos C, Craig T. Cinryze as the first approved C1 inhibitor in the USA for the treatment of hereditary angioedema: approval, efficacy and safety. J Blood Med 2010;1:163–70.

90. Cicardi M, Bork K, Caballero T, et al. Evidence based recommendations for the therapeutic management of angioedema owing to hereditary C1 inhibitor deficiency: consensus report of an International Working Group. Allergy 2012; 67(2):147–57.

Immunotherapies in Infectious Diseases

Vivek Kak, MD[a],*, Vidya Sundareshan, MD[b], Jignesh Modi, MD[b],
Nancy Misri Khardori, MD, PhD, FIDSA[c]

KEYWORDS

• Immunoglobulins • Interferons • Colony stimulating factors

Key Points

- The use of immunotherapy in treating infections involves modulation of the immune response to control the infection and destroy the infecting organism.

- The most common immunotherapies in infections include use of antibodies against various organisms, use of growth factors and cytokines to augment the native immune response, and enhance effector cell response to control infections.

- The increasing prevalence of antimicrobial resistance among pathogens as well as increasing prevalence of immunocompromised patients will lead to an increased role for immunotherapies in treatment of infectious diseases.

INTRODUCTION

The development of an infectious process involves the interaction between an infecting pathogen and the immune system of the host. The entry of a pathogen into a host leads to the activation of the immune system and the release of mediators. The aim of this initial response is to limit the infection and activate the phagocytic effector cells of the immune system (neutrophils and macrophages) to enhance the killing of the infecting organism. This immune response if inadequate can lead to development of an overwhelming infection, while an overwhelming release of the mediators can cause a systemic inflammatory response called sepsis syndrome.[1]

The treatment of an infection generally consists of antimicrobial chemotherapy to kill the invading organism. Immunotherapy to modulate the immune response is used as an adjunct to antimicrobial therapy. The use of immunotherapy in infectious diseases

The author is a member of the speakers' bureaus for Cubist Pharmaceuticals and Forest Pharmaceuticals.
[a] Allegiance Health, 1100 East Michigan Avenue, #305, Jackson, MI 49201, USA
[b] Division of Infectious Diseases, Department of Internal Medicine, Southern Illinois University School of Medicine, 801 North Rutledge, Post Office Box 9636, Springfield, IL 62794, USA
[c] Division of Infectious Diseases, Department of Internal Medicine and Microbiology and Molecular Cell Biology, Eastern Virginia Medical School, 700 West Olney Road, Norfolk, VA 23507, USA
* Corresponding author.
E-mail address: vkak@yahoo.com

Med Clin N Am 96 (2012) 455–474
doi:10.1016/j.mcna.2012.04.002
medical.theclinics.com

includes (1) modulating the immune response to a microbe (for example by using cyto-kines and cytokine inhibitors), (2) modifying a specific antigen-based response (eg, using interferons), and (3) minimizing end-organ damage using nonspecific anti-inflammatory agents (such as steroids) (**Box 1**).[2]

The second half of the 20th century was the golden age of antimicrobial therapy and vaccines and led to the hope that infectious diseases would be eradicated or treated easily. The widespread use of antimicrobial agents, however, has led to the develop-ment of drug resistance in multiple organisms, including infections that are truly not treatable by the current armamentarium of antimicrobial agents, such as totally drug resistant *Mycobacterium tuberculosis*, pan-resistant *Acinetobacter baumanii*.[3] In the absence of development of novel antimicrobial agents that can treat these infections, modulation of a patient's immune system using immunotherapies has become more important than ever.

This article will focus on the role of antibody preparations in treatment and prophylaxis of infections and use of colony stimulating factors and other cytokines in certain infections.

Advances in microbiology and the understanding of the host–microbe interaction in the late 19th and early 20th centuries led to development of vaccines and immune therapy. Immune therapy in that era referred to the use of serum or immunoglobulin for treatment and prophylaxis of infectious diseases. The principle of serum therapy was established in 1890 when it was shown that immunity against diphtheria toxin and tetanus toxin resulted from the presence of antibodies in blood that could be transferred to nonimmune animals by the serum of animals that had been intentionally injected with nonlethal doses of the toxins.[4] This discovery led to the development of a commercial sheep serum against diphtheria, the first widely available immuno-therapy against a human infection. The use of this serum therapy in diphtheria led to a reduction in mortality from 50% to 80% to less than 15%.[5] This success led to investigations of serum therapy in other infections, notably those caused by *Strepto-coccus pneumoniae* and *Neisseria meningitides*. The use of hyperimmune horse serum for acute pneumococcal pneumonia was successful in reducing mortality in seroype-1 pneumococcal pneumonia. However, the efficacy of this therapy was demonstrated only in individuals with type 1 pneumococcal disease and only if the

---

Box 1
Immunotherapeutic approaches in infectious diseases

1. Modulation of immune response (weakened or augmented)

    Blockade of cytokines

    Inhibition of signaling cascades

    Blockage of costimulatory factors

2. Change of antigen-specific response

    Induction of B cell tolerance

    Immune switching from type 1 to type 2 immune helper cell responses

    Induction of regulatory cell response using antigen delivery

3. Avoidance of end-organ damage

    Inhibition of coagulation pathway

    Inhibition of proinflammatory mediators

    Antagonism of cytokines and complement

treatment was given within 3 days of illness.[6] These studies validated the efficacy of immunotherapy in reducing mortality from infections. They also confirmed the role of early intervention to treat these infections and the importance of an accurate and specific diagnosis of the infecting pathogen. The routine use of serum therapy was limited by a number of side effects including serum sickness, anaphylaxis, and the risk of blood borne pathogen transmission. Its use in treatment of acute bacterial infections was largely abandoned by early 1940s and replaced by antimicrobial chemotherapy.[7] However, the use of immunoglobulin therapy has remained a mainstay for treatment of hepatitis A, poliomyelitis, measles, mumps, and pertussis.

The advances in immunology and vaccine development led to appreciation of the myriad mediators other than antibodies that are part of the immune response. This has led to the development of therapies using mediators like interferons, interleukins, and colony stimulatory factors.

ANTIBODY PREPARATIONS
Polyclonal and Hyperimmune Globulins

The history of use of antibody preparations in treatment and prevention of infections is over 120 years old.[5] Antibody preparations these days can be human- or animal plasma-derived, and they can be administered intravenously, intramuscularly, or subcutaneously. They can be polyclonal (pooled preparations with a broad spectrum of activity) or hyperimmune (preparations that have been obtained from immune individuals with enhanced activity against a specific organism).[8] Immunoglobulin products are often used as replacement therapy in individuals with primary and secondary immunodeficiency with the goal of decreasing morbidity and mortality from infectious complications. However, the mechanisms of action of immunoglobulins in infection are often not related to the increased antibody levels seen with supplementation and involve the modulation of the immune response, including an increase in the opsonization of bacteria by the complement system and down-regulation of the proinflammatory cytokines and increase of anti-inflammatory mediators such as soluble decoy receptors for various cytokines (**Box 2**).[9] The role of immunoglobulins in various types of infections will be discussed further.

Bacterial Infections

Respiratory infections
The incidence of respiratory tract infections due to encapsulated bacteria in individuals with primary immunodeficiency is markedly reduced by the use of immunoglobulin preparations. The administration of immune globulins with antibody activity against

---

Box 2
Possible mechanisms of action of immunoglobulins in infections

1. Enhancement of antimicrobial activity

    Increase in the neutrophilic oxidative burst

    Augmentation of serum opsonin activity

2. Toxin inactivation

    Increased clearance of endotoxins

    Neutralization of endotoxins and exotoxins and superantigens

3. Modulation of the immune response

    Activation of leukocytes

bacterial polysaccharides to Native American infants led to a significant decrease in the occurrence of invasive pneumococcal and *Haemophilus influenzae* type b infections. It was also shown to decrease the incidence of pneumococcal otitis media in children.[10,11] High doses of intravenous immunoglobulin (IVIG) therapy decrease the frequency of otitis media and serious bacterial infections in children with human immunodeficiency virus infection.[12] IVIG has also been used to treat children with recurrent pneumococcal otitis media.[13]

Diphtheria

The morbidity and mortality associated with diphtheria are primarily related to the action of its toxin on the heart and respiratory and the central nervous systems. The development of an effective vaccine has led to a marked decrease in actual disease due to this organism. In an acute infection, the use of equine diphtheria antitoxin is indicated along with antimicrobial therapy. The dose is dependent on the severity, site, and duration of infection as shown in **Table 1**. Since the antitoxin is of equine origin, skin testing for hypersensitivity before use is indicated. The antitoxin is available from the Centers for Disease Control and Prevention (CDC).[8] Postexposure prophylaxis of diphtheria, however, involves use of vaccination and antimicrobial therapy rather than using antitoxin.

Tetanus

The use of immunoglobulin to prevent and treat tetanus dates back to 1890 when horse serum obtained from immunized horses was used in the treatment of severe tetanus.[14] This has been replaced largely by human tetanus immunoglobulin (TIG); however, in some areas of the world, only equine antibodies are available. TIG is used in unimmunized or incompletely immunized individuals who sustain high-risk wounds such as contaminated wounds, wounds with devitalized tissues, and deep puncture wounds. The recommended prophylactic dose is 250 IU intramuscularly along with active immunization with tetanus toxin. If TIG is not available, 3000 to 5000 units of equine antitoxin can be used.[15] Human polyclonal IVIG can also be used, but because of its variable level of antitetanus antitoxin, a minimal dose of 100 mg/kg is suggested for tetanus prophylaxis.[16]

The treatment of established tetanus involves antibiotic therapy to decrease organism burden and immunoglobulin therapy to neutralize unbound toxin. The dose of TIG in established tetanus is 3000 to 6000 IU and dose of equine antitoxin is 50,000 to 100,000 units. A portion of the dose can also be used to infiltrate the wound site.[17] TIG is also indicated in treatment of tetanus neonatorum. The intrathecal use of TIG in neonatal tetanus has been suggested, although its efficacy has not been proven in this setting.[18]

Botulism and Clostridium difficile disease

The ingestion or absorption of the neurotoxin produced by *Clostridium botulinum* leads to botulism. The disease can occur as foodborne botulism due to ingestion of

Table 1
Diphtheria antitoxin

Site of Disease	Duration of Disease	Dose (Intravenously)
Pharyngeal or laryngeal disease	48 h	20,000–40,000 IU
Nasopharygeal disease	48 h	40,000–60,000 IU
Neck edema	Any duration	80,000–120,000 IU
Extensive disease	>72 h	80,000–120,000 IU

contaminated food, wound botulism from a contaminated wound, and infant botulism from ingestion of C botulinum spores that subsequently multiply and produce toxin in the gut.[19] Foodborne and wound botulism in the United States are treated with an investigational heptavalent equine antitoxin available through the CDC.[20] Infant botulism can be treated by the human immunoglobulin preparation, BabyBIG (botulinum immune globulin), which is available through the California Infant Botulism Treatment and Prevention Program.[8] BabyBIG is an orphan drug that consists of human-derived botulism antitoxin antibodies and is approved by US Food and Drug Administration (FDA) for the treatment of infant botulism types A and B.

The incidence of clostridium difficile disease has increased in the United States over the last decade.[21] Data from human studies has shown that individuals with low serum antibody levels to C difficile toxin A are at a greater risk for developing C difficile diarrhea.[22,23] This has led to use of immunoglobulin therapy in severe or relapsing C difficile diarrhea. A review of the clinical experience reported that use of IVIG in a dose ranging from 150 to 400 mg/kg improved the severity of clinical disease.[24]

Toxic Shock Syndrome

The development of toxic shock syndrome either from Streptococcus pyogenes or Staphylococcus aureus infections is related to the production of toxins that act as superantigens and lead to the release of various cytokines and development of sepsis syndrome.[25] IVIG preparations contain antibodies to both staphylococcal and streptococcal superantigens and have been used in toxic shock syndrome.[25,26] Although there are no prospective data that have conclusively shown decreases in mortality with the use of IVIG in toxic shock syndrome, clinicians do use it in severe toxic shock syndrome, usually as a single dose of 400 mg/kg.[27] A randomized prospective trial evaluating use of IVIG in streptococcal toxic shock syndrome did show a decrease in sepsis-related organ failure with the use of IVIG, but the trial was terminated early due to slow patient recruitment.[28]

Sepsis syndrome

The global immunomodulating effects of immunoglobulins in infection and the mortality associated with the severe inflammatory response seen in sepsis have led to numerous studies of IVIG as an adjunct to modify the inflammatory response in severe sepsis.[9] Multiple small studies and trials that have supported the use of IVIG in sepsis. A recent meta-analysis and a Cochrane review of the available data suggested a significant mortality benefit with IVIG when compared with placebo. The relative risk ratio in these studies with the use of IVIG compared with placebo ranged from 0.66 to 0.81.[29–31] However, the weakness of the original studies and the derived meta-analyses lie in their small study size, and the underlying heterogeneity in the underlying causes that led to sepsis limits drawing firm conclusions about the routine use of IVIG in sepsis.

Viral Infections

Hepatitis A

Immunoglobulin use in the prevention of hepatitis A dates to the 1940,s when it was found that its use ended epidemics of hepatitis A is closed living circumstances.[32] Immunoglobulin can be used to prevent disease before possible exposure and for postexposure prophylaxis. When administered within 2 weeks of exposure to hepatitis A, immunoglobulin is 85% to 90% effective in preventing disease.[33] This protection involves immunoglobulin preventing early disease, while the subclinical viremia from the exposure provides long-lasting immunity. The dose of immunoglobulin for postexposure prophylaxis is 0.02 mg/kg.[34,35] Since 1995, hepatitis A vaccine has been used for postexposure prophylaxis; thus these days, immunoglobulin use for postexposure prophylaxis is generally recommended for those individuals who cannot be vaccinated because of age (<12 months), those with an allergy to the vaccine components or those who refuse vaccination.[36] The use of immunoglobulin is also recommended for infants who are born to mothers with acute hepatitis A to prevent transmission.

Hepatitis B

Hepatitis B immune globulin (HBIG) prepared from the serum of donors with high titers of antibody to hepatitis B surface antigen is a highly effective prophylactic agent against development of hepatitis B. In studies, HBIG given before or after exposure (via needle stick or sexual or mucus membrane) has been shown to be 80% to 90% effective in preventing disease.[37] The postexposure prophylaxis of hepatitis B should be started within 24 hours of exposure but can be given up to 96 hours after exposure, and the dose is 0.06 mg/kg. The postexposure HBIG should be supplemented with hepatitis B vaccination to provide long-lasting (>6 month) immunity.[38] The use of HBIG is also routinely recommended in the immediate postpartum period to infants born to mothers with hepatitis B infection. The dose is usually 0.5 mL and is combined with first dose of hepatitis B vaccine.[37]

HBIG has a role in limiting the occurrence of postliver transplant hepatitis B in patients with known chronic hepatitis B infection.[39] The likelihood of reactivation of hepatitis B in the transplanted organ exceeds 50% within 3 years after transplant. In a recent review, use of HBIG along with antiviral monotherapy was shown to reduce this reactivation to less than 10%.[40,41]

Respiratory syncytial virus

The high incidence of respiratory syncytial virus (RSV) and the absence of vaccination strategies have led to use of passive antibody therapies to prevent and modify the course of this disease in high-risk children. The use of prophylaxis with RSV immunoglobulin (RSV-IG), a hyperimmune immunoglobulin with high titers of RSV-neutralizing antibody in premature children, has shown a decrease in severe RSV infection and intensive care unit stay.[42,43] However, RSV-IG has not been shown to be effective in treatment of RSV infection in adults, with the exception of adult bone marrow transplant patients, in whom combined therapy with RSV-IG and ribavarin may be effective in RSV pneumonia.[44,45] The use of RSV-IG as a prophylactic agent in children has been largely supplanted by a monoclonal anti RSV antibody, palivizumab.[46]

Rabies

The postexposure prophylaxis of rabies involves use of both vaccine and rabies immunoglobulin in addition to cleansing of the wound.[47,48] The recommended dose of RIG is 20 IU/kg along with simultaneous initiation of active vaccination. This combination provides longer-term protection against rabies.[48] The full dose of the rabies immunoglobulin should be infiltrated around the wound, and the vaccine given in an anatomically distant site. If not given at the time of initial vaccination, rabies immunoglobulin can be administered up to day 7 after exposure.[49] If there are multiple wounds, the World Health Organization recommendations state that the rabies immunoglobulin can be diluted 2- to 3-fold using sterile saline to allow for thorough infiltration into all wounds.[50]

Measles

The use of immunoglobulin can prevent and modify measles if given within six days of exposure. Immunoglobulin at the dose of 0.25 mg/kg in healthy individuals provides postexposure prophylaxis against measles and is recommended for infants below 1 year of age, unimmunized pregnant women, and immunocompromised patients, since active vaccination is contradicted in these patients.[51] IVIG at a dose of 100 to 400 mg/kg can also be used for postexposure prophylaxis in immunocompromised patients and provides prophylaxis for 3 weeks after an exposure.[52] In other settings, postexposure prophylaxis can be obtained by the measles vaccine if given within 72 hours of exposure.

Cytomegalovirus

The acquisition of cytomegalovirus (CMV) leads to development of a latent infection that can be reactivated when the patient becomes immunodeficient. The control of CMV infection by the immune system involves neutralizing antibodies, and thus immunoglobulin use to control and treat reactivation CMV disease is attractive. This has led to the use of immunoglobulin in immunocompromised patients, especially those undergoing bone marrow or solid organ transplant to prevent as well as modify the course of end organ CMV disease, especially pneumonia.[53–55] The efficacy of immunoglobulin in this setting is difficult to assess, especially because of the widespread use of antiviral drugs such as ganciclovir and valganciclovir for both treatment and prophylaxis of CMV disease. The use of CMV immunoglobulin in the treatment of established CMV disease is unproven but based on the lower mortality seen with the combination use of immunoglobulin and antiviral drugs for CMV pneumonia in stem cell transplant recipients, certain authorities recommend the combined use of antiviral and immunoglobulin therapy for CMV pneumonia in bone marrow transplant patients.[56,57]

Varicella

Since 1969, the use of zoster immunoglobulin, a hyperimmune globulin prepared from individuals recovering from shingles, has been shown to be effective in preventing development of clinical varicella in exposed children when given within 72 hours after exposure.[58] After 1978, Varicella-zoster immune globulin (VZIG) given within 96 hours of exposure has been used to prevent varicella in susceptible individuals. The dose is variable with 125 U being used as a minimum dose, and 625 U as a maximum dose.[59] The use of immunoglobulin as a modality to prevent disease has, however, decreased since the availability of the varicella vaccine and availability of antiviral drugs for the herpes group of viruses.

Parvovirus B19/erythrovirus

Parvovirus B19 produces 5th disease in infants. It can infect red blood cell precursors and in immunocompromised individuals cause a chronic infection that most often manifests as a pure red blood cell aplasia. The immune response to parvovirus infection involves neutralizing antibody, and IVIG is an excellent source of parvovirus B19- IgG.[60] IVIG has thus been used in the treatment of parvovirus B19 infections including red blood cell aplasia in immunocompromised patients.[61] The usual dose is 400 mg/kg/d for 5 to 10 days.[62] In patients requiring chronic suppressive therapy, the dose is unclear, however a dose of 400 mg/kg once a month has been used.[63] IVIG has also been used in treating dilated cardiomyopathy caused by parvovirus B19 in a single case series.[64]

Enteroviral infections

Severe enteroviral diseases most often occur in immunodeficient individuals and neonates. Patients with agammaglobinemia may develop chronic enteroviral menin-goencephalitis (CEM) or vaccine-associated poliomyelitis.[65] The routine use of IVIG in patients with agammaglobinemia has reduced the occurrence of CEM. In a series of patients with CEM, use of IVIG both intraventricularly and intravenously led to improvement in 6 of 12 patients.[66] Based on these data and in the absence of controlled trials, infants with severe disseminated enteroviral infections may be candidates for IVIG as long as the IVIG preparation contains significant titers of antibodies against the infecting enteroviral serotype.[67]

Vaccinia

The use of vaccination is recommended for laboratory personnel working with vaccinia or related pox viruses.[68] The vaccine can lead to severe complications such as eczema vaccinatum and encephalitis in immunocompromised patients. Human vaccinia immunoglobulin (VIG) is used to treat these vaccine-related complications. VIG is available from the CDC and the dose is 0.6 mL/kg intramuscularly given as divided doses over 24 to 36 hours, and this can be repeated at intervals of 2 to 3 days.[68]

Monoclonal Antibodies

The use and success of polyclonal immunoglobulin preparations in preventing and modifying course of certain infections has led to the development of monoclonal antibodies against infectious agents. Since monoclonal antibodies by definition consist of a single type of immunoglobulin with activity against a specific target, they could be an attractive and effective addition to the antimicrobial armamentarium.[69] The development of monoclonal antibodies against various infectious agents has, however, lagged compared to their use in rheumatology and oncology mainly due to availability of antimicrobial agents, which are much cheaper than the monoclonal antibodies.

At the current time there is only 1 licensed monoclonal antibody for use in infectious disease. Palivizumab is a monoclonal antibody that binds to F protein of RSV, and it is used in the treatment and prevention of RSV pneumonia in high-risk infants.[46] It is also used in treatment of RSV pneumonia in adult stem cell transplant recipients. There are multiple other monoclonal antibodies against infectious diseases in the pipeline, including those against hepatitis C, human immunodeficiency virus (HIV), West Nile virus infections, and *C difficile* infections.[70]

INTERFERONS

Interferon-α (IFN-α) and interferon-β (IFN-β) are produced and released by cells infected with certain viruses, while interferon-γ (IFN-γ) is produced by natural killer cells in response to antigenic stimulation. IFN-α is produced by dendritic cells in response to viral infections and has a significant role in the inhibition of intracellular viral replication. It also activates cytotoxic T lymphocytes and natural killer cells against viral infected cells.[71] Based on their antiviral and immunomodulatory activity both IFN-α and INF-β have been used in treatment of viral infections, especially hepatitis B and hepatitis C. IFN-γ is an important immunomodulator, and it is involved in antigen presentation and cytokine production by antigen-presenting cells. It plays a vital role in control of intracellular pathogens such as mycobacteria, fungi, viruses, and intracellular bacteria.[72] The role of interferon in treatment of infections will be discussed.

Hepatitis B Virus

The development of chronic hepatitis B often involves failure of innate immune response to the virus and of development of adaptive immune response. Interferon therapy in hepatitis B can lead to the cellular clearance of viral proteins through disruption of the replication process.[73] In hepatitis Be antigen-positive patients, interferon stimulates an immune response, while in hepatitis Be antigen-negative patients, it acts a direct antiviral agent.[74] The success of this treatment can lead to loss of the viral DNA and successful antibody formation. IFN-α initially was available as standard INF-α dosed at 3 million units subcutaneously 3 times a week, but now it has largely been replaced by pegylated interferons. The addition of polyethylene glycol (PEG) to interferon created a drug with reduced immunogenicity and increased half-life compared with standard interferon.[75] Thus peglylated IFN-α2a is now used in treatment of chronic hepatitis B at a dose of 180 μg subcutaneously once a week for 24 weeks. The peglylated IFN-α2b can also be used at a weight-based dose of 1.5 μg/kg subcutaneously once a week for 24 weeks. Because of the possible decompensation of liver disease, interferon therapy is not recommended for patients with cirrhosis.[73] The response rate to interferon therapy in chronic hepatitis B is defined as loss of the hepatitis e antigen, and acquisition of the hepatitis e antibody is 32% to 33% with peginterferon alfa-2a.[76] The use of interferon therapy in chronic hepatitis B has often been overshadowed by the use of oral antiviral agents mainly because of the ease of their use and diminished occurrence of adverse effects compared with interferon.[77]

Hepatitis C Virus

The use of interferon in chronic hepatitis C leads to a rapid inhibition of hepatitis C RNA production followed by a second phase of clearance of infected cells.[78,79] The response of patients infected with hepatitis C genotype 1 to interferon-based regimens can be associated with the occurrence of single nucleotide polymorphism in the interleukin-28B (IL-28B) gene.[80] The IL-28B polymorphism encodes for IFN-γ3, which stimulates interferon gene induction and leads to inhibition of viral replication.[81]

The standard of care for treatment of chronic hepatitis C consists of peginterferon alfa-2a (dosed 180 μg subcutaneously weekly) or peginterferon alfa-2b (dosed at 1.5 μg/kg weekly) along with ribavarin in nongenotype 1 disease.[82] In the treatment of hepatitis C genotype 1 disease, the use of dual therapy (pegylated interferon and ribavarin) has been supplemented with the addition of the direct acting antivirals, either telaprevir or boceprevir.[83,84] The duration of treatment with interferons generally is between 24 and 48 weeks and depends on the kinetics of viral clearance during follow-up.

Human Papillomavirus

The human papillomaviruses (HPVs) are the cause of genital warts, cervical cancer, and anogenital cancers. They are also being implicated in the development of head and neck cancers. They have the ability to persist in the epithelium for decades by avoiding immune eradication. This is done by HPV reducing the expression of interferons.[85] Several trials of IFN-αn3 have shown a benefit of this modality over placebo. The usual dose consists of 250,000 IU (0.05 mL) given intralesionally per wart twice a week for up to 8 weeks.[86] The use of systemic interferon therapy may be considered in patients that have generalized extragenital HPV diseases such as recurrent respiratory papillomatosis.[87]

Another interferon-based topical treatment for HPV infections consists of imiquimod. Imiquimod is an interferon inducer and is indicated for topical treatment of external genital and perianal warts. It is used topically 3 times a week until the warts are cleared or until a maximum of 16 weeks.[88] The importance of interferon in the control of viral warts is also illustrated by published reports of their control by cimetidine, a drug that also induces the production of IFN-γ and IL-2.[89]

Fungal/Mycobacterial Infections and IFN-γ

IFN-γ is a potent activator of macrophage function and enhances the activity of macrophages against various intracellular pathogens including fungi and mycobacteria.[72] Its use has been shown to reduce the development of infections in patients with chronic granulomatous diseases.[90] It also is used as an adjunctive therapy for patients with refractory fungal and mycobacterial diseases including those patients with disseminated mycobacterial infections in the presence of genetic defects in the production of IFN-γ or its receptor expression.[91–93] There are no controlled studies looking at the use of IFN-γ in fungal infections, but there are case studies suggesting that IFN-γ can play a role as adjunctive treatment in patients with certain fungal infections.[94]

COLONY STIMULATING FACTORS

The uses of colony stimulating factors (CSFs) in infections constitute a form of augmentative therapy while treating or preventing infections. Their use is intended to enhance immune function against the pathogen as well as increase the amount of circulating peripheral blood cells. CSFs enhance bone marrow production and maturation of the cells operative in innate immunity (ie, neutrophils and macrophages). There are 3 types of recombinant human CSFs available, granulocyte CSF (G-CSF), granulocyte–macrophage CSF (GM-CSF), and macrophage CSF (M-CSF).[95]

G-CSF promotes the proliferation and differentiation of the neutrophil precursors and enhances neutrophil function. The deficiency of G-CSF is associated with reduced granulopoiesis as well as diminished immunologic function of neutrophils.[95] In patients with neutropenia, G-CSF is used to promote bone marrow recovery, as the susceptibility to serious fungal infections is proportional to the degree and duration of neutropenia.[96] It produces anti-inflammatory mediators compared with the other CSFs and is thought to protect against endotoxemia. It can downregulate the proinflammatory response in infections where neutrophils are the predominant effector cell.[97,98] GM-CSF has a broader spectrum of activity compared with G-CSF and promotes the proliferation and differentiation of mononuclear cells including lymphocytes, macrophages, and dendritic cells along with neutrophils.[97] G-CSF and GM-CSF have been widely used for primary as well as secondary prophylaxis in patients with various types of malignancies requiring myelosuppressive chemotherapy, as well as in congenital, cyclic, or idiopathic neutropenia. GM-CSF additionally has a role in prevention and treatment of neutropenia in patients undergoing autologous and allogeneic bone marrow transplantations. The M-CSF promotes the proliferation and differentiation of monocytes and macrophages. It has been used as an adjunct to antifungal therapy in patients with bone marrow transplants and established fungal infections.[99]

The use of CSFs is well established in patients with malignancy and neutropenia for prophylaxis of development of febrile neutropenia. There are multiple clinical trials showing benefit of CSFs in decreasing episodes of febrile neutropenia and infections with chemotherapy in malignant lymphomas, solid organ tumors, and hemopoietic stem cell transplantations, although a mortality benefit, or reduction in mortality related to infections has not been definitively documented.[100]

The concomitant use of G-CSF or GM-CSF along with antibiotics in treatment of febrile neutropenia in patients with malignancy has been shown to lead to a reduction in the duration of neutropenia as well as hospital length of stay, but has not been shown to decrease the overall mortality.[101] It is suggested that the use of CSFs in patients with established febrile neutropenia be reserved for patients with a high risk of infection-related complications or in those who are not improving with antimicrobial therapy.[102]

The use of G-CSF and GM-CSF is also common in patients with primary neutropenic disorders such as cyclic neutropenia and those with neutropenia due to marrow suppression because of infections such as HIV or hepatitis C or as an adverse effect of medications used to treat these infections. In patients with primary neutropenia, the routine use of G-CSF leads to decreases in infections, antibiotic use, and hospitalization.[103] In advanced HIV infections, direct suppression of neutrophil production by HIV can lead to neutropenia and increased risk of infections.[104,105] The use of G-CSFs in this setting increases neutrophil counts with a decrease in infections and improved mortality.[106] G-CSF has a role in treating drug-induced neutropenia such as that seen with interferon treatment of hepatitis C. In this setting, endogenous G-CSF production is suppressed by interferon, leading to neutropenia, and thus exogenous G-CSF to resolve neutropenia may be necessary in these patients.[107] The use of CSFs has also been studied in septic preterm neonates who are neutropenic and has been shown to reduce 14-day mortality compared with controls who did not receive a CSF.[108]

The use of CSFs in patients without neutropenia is based on the ability of G-CSF to enhance the function of the neutrophils as well as lead to a decrease of the proinflammatory cytokine release.[97] In patients with severe community-acquired pneumonia, a single dose of G-CSF was noted to lead to a reduction in apoptosis, increased cell surface marker expression, and anti-inflammatory cytokine release from neutrophils.[109] However, systematic reviews of addition of G-CSF to antimicrobial therapy in non-neutropenic patients have not shown any benefit in mortality compared with antimicrobial therapy alone.[110] It is postulated that G-CSF may have a role in patients with poor wound healing as well as diabetic foot ulcers, as its use leads to enhanced oxidative burst and phagocytosis comparable to healthy controls.[111]

The experience with the use of CSFs to treat established fungal infections is mainly limited to case series. However, in a randomized trial, the use of a combination of G-CSF and fluconazole compared with fluconazole alone in non-neutropenic patients with candidiasis showed a trend toward the benefit.[97] Several case reports also suggest that addition of G-CSF to antifungal therapy is useful in fungal infections such as aspergillosis, disseminated zygomycosis, mucormycosis, and fusariosis.[112–115]

Although the use of G-CSF is widespread in patients undergoing chemotherapy, a retrospective analysis of patients undergoing chemotherapy suggested a greater reduction of the risk of fungal infections in these patients with GM-CSF compared with G-CSF or no CSFs.[116] GM-CSF along with antifungal therapy has also been used to improve clinical response in patients with established fungal infection such as refractory *Aspergillus* infection.[117]

OTHER CYTOKINES
Interleukins

The interleukins are a group of cytokines that play an important role in the development of cell-mediated immunity, control of B cell differentiation, and development of the T helper cell type 1 pathway.[118] Among the interleukins, therapeutic studies for infections have looked at IL-2 and interleukin-12 (IL-12). IL-2 is mainly produced by T helper lymphocytes and enhances the production of T-helper and cytotoxic lymphocytes. It increases the production of interleukin-1 (IL-1) and enhances phagocytosis and intracellular killing of organisms.[119] IL-12 is required for early control of infection and for generation of acquired protective immunity. IL-12 also regulates the magnitude of the IFN-γ response to an infecting organism thus promoting resistance to the infection.[118]

Recombinant IL-2 was studied in patients infected with HIV receiving antiretroviral drugs. The use of IL-2 did lead to sustained increases in CD4+ cell counts but had no clinical or survival benefit.[120]

The use of IL-12 in patients with infections has been limited by the fact that IL-12 can produce an excessive inflammatory response in animals without neutropenia.[118] The use of IL-12 was associated with a beneficial effect in experimental candidiasis; however, the use of IL-12 immunotherapy in patients with bone marrow transplants showed an unexpected increase in severe fungal infections.[121] Thus, as of now there is no role for the use of interleukins in control prevention of infections.

Tumor necrosis factor-α (TNF-α) plays a pivotal role in the development of the inflammatory response during infections. It is produced primarily by monocytes and macrophages and plays a central role in the immune response to infections. It activates neutrophils, lymphocytes, and vascular endothelial cells and leads to the production of acute-phase proteins and development of fever.[1] The damage caused by an unchecked proinflammatory response in infections has led to interest in inhibition of this cytokine in certain infections. TNF-α production also plays a vital role in development of autoimmune disease and the FDA has approved various TNF-α antagonists for the treatment of inflammatory illnesses like rheumatoid arthritis and Crohn disease. The use of these drugs, however, is associated with an increased risk of infections such as those due to *Mycobacterium tuberculosis*, atypical mycobacteria, and others including *Aspergillus, Candida, Coccidioides immitis*, and *Histoplasma capsulatum*.[122] Thus the current TNF-α antagonists are not used during active infections. However, modulation of the levels of TNF-α, especially using drugs such as thalidomide, is used in the treatment of complications of source infections.

Thalidomide causes a partial inhibition of production of TNF-α. It also acts as a costimulatory signal for T cell activation and can lead to an increased production of IL-12 and interferon-γ.[123] The use of thalidomide can lead to a decrease in the acute proinflammatory symptoms seen in certain infections. This use was first described in Hansen disease patients with erythema nodosum leprosum (ENL), an acute inflammatory condition seen in patients with lepromatous leprosy with decrease in the clinical signs associated with this syndrome.[124] The use of thalidomide in patients with tuberculosis can lead to accelerated weight gain.[125] Other uses of thalidomide in infections include its use in treatment of oral apthous ulcers, wasting syndrome, and diarrhea in patients with HIV infection.[126] The adverse effects of thalidomide, especially teratogenic potential and development of peripheral neuropathy, limit its use in the clinical setting.

ACTIVATED PROTEIN C

The development of severe sepsis in infections is often accompanied with derangement of the coagulation cascade. Protein C is an important modulator of the coagulation pathway and is activated from soluble protein C after thrombin interacts with thrombomodulin. Activated protein C (APC) has anti-inflammatory activity through its interaction with the endothelial protein C receptor (EPCR), which is found on endothelial cells, neutrophils, monocytes, and eosinophils. During sepsis, patients tend to have decreased APC levels, and this has been associated with an increase in the risk of death.[127] This observation led to the studies of recombinant APC (rhAPC) therapy in patients with sepsis.[128] The initial studies suggested that use of drotrecogin alfa led to a statistically significant reduction in mortality in patients with sepsis.[128] These optimistic results led to approval of drotrecogin alfa by the FDA for patients with severe sepsis and high risk of death. However, further analysis and studies did not confirm the initial optimistic results, and the drug was withdrawn from the market in late 2011.[129,130]

CORTICOSTERIODS

The use of adjunctive steroid therapy is well established in infections where containment of tissue damage through control of inflammation is required. Thus the standard of care for acute bacterial meningitis includes the use of steroids before the first dose of antibacterial therapy. The use of steroid in this setting reduces both the mortality and neurologic complications from bacterial meningitis.[131] The use of steroids should be considered in extrapulmonary tuberculosis, especially tuberculous meningitis and pericarditis.[132] Adjunctive corticosteroid therapy may provide significant clinical and radiographic benefits in selected patients with advanced pulmonary tuberculosis.[133]

In a large trial and other small studies, administering hydrocortisone at a dose of 50 to 100 mg 3 to 4 times a day for 1 week has been shown to be beneficial in patients with sepsis and inadequate adrenal reserve.[134]

SUMMARY

The history of immunotherapy in infectious diseases predates the development of antimicrobial chemotherapy by over half a century, and until the 1940s, immunotherapy in the form of immunoglobulins was the only therapeutic option for the treatment of a variety of infections. The use of immunotherapy is undergoing a comeback due to the development of antimicrobial drug resistance in various organisms, increased number of immunocompromised hosts, and emergence of novel pathogenic microbes. The current spectrum of immunotherapy in infectious diseases mainly involves augmentative/immunomodulating agents such as immunoglobulins, interferons, and CSFs. Monoclonal antibody preparations targeting conserved epitopes of important pathogens along with therapeutic vaccines that modulate the immune response to pathogens are on the horizon.

REFERENCES

1. Kak V. Mediators of systemic inflammatory response syndrome and the role of activated protein C in sepsis syndrome. Infect Dis Clin North Am 2011;25(4): 835–50.
2. Masihi KN. Immunomodulators in infectious diseases; panoply of possibilities. Int J Immunopharmacol 2000;22:1083–91.
3. Berghman LR, Abi-Ghanem D, Waghela SD, et al. Antibodies: an alternative for antibiotics. Poultry Science 2005;84:660–6.
4. Winau F, Winau R. Emil von Behring and serum therapy. Microbes Infect 2002;4: 185–8.
5. Buchwald UK, Pirofski L. Immune therapy for infectious diseases at the dawn of the 21st century: the past, present, and future role of antibody therapy, therapeutic vaccination, and biologic response modifiers. Curr Pharm Des 2003;9: 945–68.
6. Finland M. The serum treatment of lobar pneumonia. N Engl J Med 1930;201: 1244.

7. Casadevall A. Antibody-based therapies for emerging infectious diseases. Emerg Infect Dis 1996;2:200–8.
8. Keller MA, Stiehm ER. Passive immunity in prevention and treatment of infectious diseases. Clin Microbiol Rev 2000;13(4):602–14.
9. Berlot G, Bacer B, Piva M, et al. Immunoglobulins in sepsis. Adv Sepsis 2007; 6(2):41–6.
10. Santoshan M, Reid R, Ambrosino DN, et al. Prevention of *Haemophilus influenza* type b infections in high risk infants treated with bacterial polysaccharide immune globulin. N Engl J Med 1987;317:923–9.
11. Shurin PA, Rehmus JM, Johnson CE, et al. Bacterial polysaccharide immune globulin for prophylaxis of acute otitis media in high-risk children. J Pediatr 1993;123:801–10.
12. National Institute of Child Health and Human Development (NICHHD) intravenous immunoglobulin study group. Intravenous immunoglobulin for the prevention of bacterial infections in children with symptomatic human immunodeficiency virus infection. N Engl J Med 1991;325:73–80.
13. Ishizaka A, Sakiyama Y, Otsu M, et al. Successful intravenous immunoglobulin for recurrent pneumococcal otitis media in young children. Eur J Pediatr 1994;153:174–8.
14. Grundbacher FJ. Behring's discovery of diphtheria and tetanus antitoxins. Immunol Today 1992;13:188–90.
15. Kretsinger K, Broder KR, Cortese MM, et al. Preventing tetanus, diphtheria, and pertussis among adults: use of tetanus toxoid, reduced diphtheria toxoid and acellular pertussis vaccine recommendations of the Advisory Committee on Immunization Practices (ACIP) and recommendation of ACIP, supported by the Healthcare Infection Control Practices Advisory Committee (HICPAC), for use of Tdap among health-care personnel. MMWR Recomm Rep 2006;55(RR-17):1–37.
16. Lee DC, Lederman HM. Antitetanus toxoid antibodies in intravenous immune gamma globulin: an alternative to tetanus immune globulin. J Infect Dis 1992; 166:642–5.
17. Afshar M, Raju M, Ansell D, et al. Narrative review: tetanus—a health threat after natural disasters in developing countries. Ann Intern Med 2011;154(5):329–35.
18. Begue RE, Lindo-Soriano I. Failure of intrathecal tetanus antitoxin in the treatment of tetanus neonatorum. J Infect Dis 1991;164:619–20.
19. Shapiro RL, Hatheway C, Swerdlow DL. Botulism in the United States: a clinical and epidemiological review. Ann Intern Med 1998;129:221–8.
20. Investigational heptavalent botulinum antitoxin (HBAT) to replace licensed botulinum antitoxin AB and investigational botulinum antitoxin E. MMWR Morb Mortal Wkly Rep 2010;59(10):299.
21. Archibald LK, Banerjee SN, Jarvis WR. Secular trends in hospital-acquired *Clostridium difficile* disease in the United States, 1987–2001. J Infect Dis 2004; 189(9):1585–9.
22. Kim PH, Iaconis JP, Rolfe RD. Immunization of adult hamsters against *Clostridium difficile*-associated ileocecitis and transfer of protection to infant hamsters. Infect Immun 1987;55(12):2984–92.
23. Gerding DN, Johnson S. Management of *Clostridium difficile* infection: thinking inside and outside the box. Clin Infect Dis 2010;51(11):1306–13.
24. Abougergi MS, Kwon JH. Intravenous immunoglobulin for the treatment of *Clostridium difficile* infection: a review. Dig Dis Sci 2011;56(1):19–26.
25. Parsonnet J. Nonmenstrual toxic shock syndrome: new insights into diagnosis, pathogenesis and treatment. Curr Clin Top Infect Dis 1996;16:1–20.

26. Barry W, Hudgins L, Donta ST, et al. Intravenous immunoglobulin therapy for toxic shock syndrome. JAMA 1992;267(24):3315–31.

27. Stevens DL. Rationale for the use of intravenous gamma globulin in the treatment of streptococcal toxic shock syndrome. Clin Infect Dis 1998;26(3):639–64.

28. Darenberg J, Ihendyane N, Sjolin J, et al. Intravenous immunoglobulin G therapy in streptococcal toxic shock syndrome: a European randomized, double-blind, placebo-controlled trial. Clin Infect Dis 2003;37(3):333–40.

29. Turgeon AF, Hutton B, Fergusson DA, et al. Meta-analysis: intravenous immunoglobulin in critically ill adult patients with sepsis. Ann Intern Med 2007;146(3): 193–203.

30. Laupland KB, Kirkpatrick AW, Delaney A. Polyclonal intravenous immunoglobulin for the treatment of severe sepsis and septic shock in critically ill adults: a systematic review and meta-analysis. Crit Care Med 2007;35(12):2686–92.

31. Alejandria MM, Lansang MA, Dans LF, et al. Intravenous immunoglobulin for treating sepsis and septic shock. Cochrane Database Syst Rev 2002;1: CD001090.

32. Havens WP, Paul JR. Prevention of infectious hepatitis with gamma globulin. JAMA 1945;129:270–1.

33. Liu JP, Nikolova D, Fei Y. Immunoglobulins for preventing hepatitis A. Cochrane Database Syst Rev 2009;2:CD004181.

34. Advisory Committee on Immunization Practices (ACIP) Centers for Disease Control and Prevention (CDC). Update: prevention of hepatitis A after exposure to hepatitis A virus and in international travelers. Updated recommendations of the Advisory Committee on Immunization Practices (ACIP). MMWR Morb Mortal Wkly Rep 2007;56(41):1080–4.

35. Fiore AE, Wasley A, Bell BP. Prevention of hepatitis A through active or passive immunization: recommendations of the Advisory Committee on Immunization Practices (ACIP). MMWR Recomm Rep 2006;55(RR-7):1–23.

36. Victor JC, Monto AS, Surdina TY, et al. Hepatitis A vaccine versus immune globulin for postexposure prophylaxis. N Engl J Med 2007;357(17):1685–94.

37. Mast EE, Weinbaum CM, Fiore AE, et al. A comprehensive immunization strategy to eliminate transmission of hepatitis B virus infection in the United States: recommendations of the Advisory Committee on Immunization Practices (ACIP) part II: immunization of adults. MMWR Recomm Rep 2006;55(RR-16): 1–33.

38. Mitsui T, Iwano K, Suzuki S, et al. Combined hepatitis B immune globulin and vaccine for postexposure prophylaxis of accidental hepatitis B virus infection in hemodialysis staff members: comparison with immune globulin without vaccine in historical controls. Hepatology 1989;10(3):324–7.

39. Terrault NA, Zhou S, Combs C, et al. Prophylaxis in liver transplant recipients using a fixed dosing schedule of hepatitis B immunoglobulin. Hepatology 1996;24:1327–33.

40. Katz LH, Tur-Kaspa R, Guy DG, et al. Lamivudine or adefovir dipivoxil alone or combined with immunoglobulin for preventing hepatitis B recurrence after liver transplantation. Cochrane Database Syst Rev 2010;7:CD006005.

41. Chen J, Yi L, Jia JD, et al. Hepatitis B immunoglobulins and/or lamivudine for preventing hepatitis B recurrence after liver transplantation: a systematic review. J Gastroenterol Hepatol 2010;25(5):872–9.

42. Groothuis JR, Simoes EA, Hemming VG, et al. Respiratory syncytial virus (RSV) infection in preterm infants and the protective effects of RSV immune globulin (RSVIG). Pediatrics 1995;95:463–7.

43. The Prevent Study Group. Reduction of respiratory syncytial virus hospitalization among premature infants and infants with bronchopulmonary dysplasia using respiratory syncytial virus immune globulin prophylaxis. Pediatrics 1997;99: 93–9.

44. Whimbey E, Champlin RE, Englund JA, et al. Combination therapy with aerosolized ribavirin and intravenous immunoglobulin for respiratory syncytial virus disease in adult bone marrow transplant recipients. Bone Marrow Transplant 1995;16(3):393–9.

45. Ghosh S, Champlin RE, Englund J, et al. Respiratory syncytial virus upper respiratory tract illnesses in adult blood and marrow transplant recipients: combination therapy with aerosolized ribavirin and intravenous immunoglobulin. Bone Marrow Transplant 2000;25(7):751–75.

46. The Impact-RSV study group. Palivizumab, a humanized respiratory syncytial virus monoclonal antibody, reduces hospitalization from respiratory syncytial virus infection in high-risk infants. Pediatrics 1998;102:531–7.

47. Lin FT, Chen SB, Wang YZ, et al. Use of serum and vaccine in combination for prophylaxis following exposure to rabies. Rev Infect Dis 1988;10(Suppl 4):S766–70.

48. Manning SE, Rupprecht CE, Fishbein D, et al. Human rabies prevention—United States, 2008: recommendations of the Advisory Committee on Immunization Practices. MMWR Recomm Rep 2008;57(RR-3):1–28.

49. Khawplod P, Wilde H, Chomchey P, et al. What is an acceptable delay in rabies immune globulin administration when vaccine alone had been given previously? Vaccine 1996;14(5):389–91.

50. World Health Organization. WHO recommendations on rabies post-exposure treatment and the correct technique. 1. Guide for rabies post-exposure treatment. Geneva (Switzerland): World Health Organization; 1997. p. 1–10.

51. American Academy of Pediatrics. Measles. Red book report of the committee on infectious diseases. Elk Grove Village (IL): American Academy of Pediatrics; 1997.

52. Gershon AA. Measles virus. In: Mandel GL, editor. Principles and practice of infectious diseases. New York: Churchill Livingstone Incorporated; 1997. p. 2035–6.

53. Snydman DR, Werner BG, Heinze-Lacey B, et al. Use of cytomegalovirus immune globulin to prevent cytomegalovirus disease in renal-transplant recipients. N Engl J Med 1987;317(17):1049–54.

54. Snydman DR, Werner BG, Dougherty NN, et al. Cytomegalovirus immune globulin prophylaxis in liver transplantation. A randomized, double-blind, placebo-controlled trial. Ann Intern Med 1993;119(10):984–91.

55. Winston DJ, Ho WG, Lin CH, et al. Intravenous immune globulin for prevention of cytomegalovirus infection and interstitial pneumonia after bone marrow transplantation. Ann Intern Med 1987;106(1):12–8.

56. Verdonck LF, de Gast GC, Dekker AW, et al. Treatment of cytomegalovirus pneumonia after bone marrow transplantation with cytomegalovirus immunoglobulin combined with ganciclovir. Bone Marrow Transplant 1989;4(2):187–9.

57. Emanuel D, Cunningham I, Jules-Elysee K, et al. Cytomegalovirus pneumonia after bone marrow transplantation successfully treated with the combination of ganciclovir and high-dose intravenous immune globulin. Ann Intern Med 1988;109(10):777–82.

58. Brunell PA, Ross A, Miller LH, et al. Prevention of varicella by zoster immune globulin. N Engl J Med 1969;280:1191–4.

59. Marin M, Guris D, Chaves SS, et al. Prevention of varicella: recommendations of the Advisory Committee on Immunization Practices (ACIP). MMWR Recomm Rep 2007;56(RR-4):1–40.

60. Schwarz TF, Roggendorf M, Hottentrager B, et al. Immunoglobulins in the prophylaxis of parvovirus B19 infection. J Infect Dis 1990;162:1214.
61. Mouthon L, Guillevin L, Tellier Z. Intravenous immunoglobulins in autoimmune- or parvovirus B19-mediated pure red-cell aplasia. Autoimmun Rev 2005;4(5):264–9.
62. Frickhofen N, Abkowitz JL, Safford M, et al. Persistent B19 parvovirus infection inpatients infected with human immunodeficiency virus type 1 (HIV-1): a treatable cause of anemia with AIDS. Ann Intern Med 1990;113:926–33.
63. Koduri PR, Kumapley R, Valladares J, et al. Chronic pure red cell aplasia caused by parvovirus B19 in AIDS: use of intravenous immunoglobulin- a report of eight patients. Am J Hematol 1987;61:16–20.
64. Dennert R, Velthuis S, Schalla S, et al. Intravenous immunoglobulin therapy for patients with idiopathic cardiomyopathy and endomyocardial biopsy-proven high PVB19 viral load. Antivir Ther 2010;15(2):193–201.
65. Ochs HD, Winkelstein J. Disorders of the B-cell system. In: Steihm ER, editor. Immunologic disorders in infants and children. 4th edition. Philadelphia: The W.B. Saunders Company; 1996. p. 296–338.
66. McKinney RE, Katz SL, Wilfert CM. Chronic enteroviral meningoencephalitis in agammaglobulinemic patients. Rev Infect Dis 1987;9(2):334–56.
67. Abzug MJ, Keyserling HL, Lee ML, et al. Neonatal enterovirus infection: virology, serology, and effects of intravenous immune globulin. Clin Infect Dis 1995;20:1201–6.
68. Center for Disease Control. Vaccinia (smallpox) vaccine recommendation of the immunization practices advisory Committee (ACIP). Morbid Mortal Weekly Rep 1991;40(RR-14):1–21.
69. Saylor C, Dadachova E, Casadevall A. Monoclonal Antibody-based therapies for microbial diseases. Vaccine 2009;27(6):G38–46.
70. ter Meulen J. Monoclonal antibodies in infectious diseases: clinical pipeline in 2011. Infect Dis Clin North Am 2011;25:789–802.
71. Holland SM. The interferons. In: Holland S, editor. Cytokine therapeutics in infectious diseases. 1st edition. Philadelphia: Lippincott Williams & Wilkins; 2001. p. 221–50.
72. Segal BH, Kwon-Chung J, Walsh TJ, et al. Immunotherapy for fungal infections. Clin Infect Dis 2006;42(4):507–15.
73. Keeffe EB, Dieterich DT, Han SH, et al. A treatment algorithm for the management of chronic hepatitis B virus infection in the United States: 2008 update. Clin Gastroenterol Hepatol 2008;6(12):1315–41.
74. Borden EC, Sen GC, Uze G, et al. Interferons at age 50: past, current and future impact on biomedicine. Nat Rev Drug Discov 2007;6(12):975–90.
75. Shiffman ML. Pegylated interferons: what role will they play in the treatment of chronic hepatitis C? Curr Gastroenterol Rep 2001;3(1):30–7.
76. Craxi A, Di Bona D, Camma C, et al. Interferon alpha for hBeAg positive hepatitis B: systemic review. J Hepatol 2003;39(S1):S99–105.
77. Lok AS, Mcmahon BJ. Chronic hepatitis B: update 2009. Hepatology 2009;50(3):661–2.
78. Stegmann KA, Bjorkstrom NK, Veber H, et al. Interferon-alpha-induced trail on natural killer cells is associated with control of hepatitis C virus infection. Gastroenterology 2010;138(5):1885–97.
79. Herrmann E, Lee JH, Marinos G, et al. Effect of ribavirin on hepatitis C viral kinetics in patients treated with pegylated interferon. Hepatology 2003;37(6):1351–8.

80. Ge D, Fellay J, Thompson AJ, et al. Genetic variation in IL28b predicts hepatitis C treatment-induced viral clearance. Nature 2009;461(7262):399–401.
81. Afdhal NH, McHutchison JG, Zeuzem S, et al. Hepatitis C pharmacogenetics: state of the art in 2010. Hepatology 2011;53(1):336–45.
82. Chander G, Sulkowski MS, Jenckes MW, et al. Treatment of chronic hepatitis C: a systemic review. Hepatology 2002;36(5):S135–44.
83. Bacon BR, Gordon SC, Lawitz E, et al. Boceprevir for previously treated chronic HCV genotype 1 infection. N Engl J Med 2011;364(13):1207–17.
84. McHutchison JG, Everson GT, Gordon SC, et al. Telaprevir with peginterferon and ribavirin for chronic HCV genotype 1 infection. N Engl J Med 2009; 360(18):1827–38.
85. Beglin M, Melar-New M, Laimins L. Human papillomaviruses and the interferon response. J Interferon Cytokine Res 2009;29(9):629–35.
86. Yang J, Pu YG, Zeng ZM, et al. Interferon for the treatment of genital warts: a systematic review. BMC Infect Dis 2009;9(1):156.
87. Gerein V, Rastorguev E, Gerein J, et al. Use of interferon-alpha in recurrent respiratory papillomatosis: 20-year follow-up. Ann Otol Rhinol Laryngol 2005; 114(6):463–71.
88. Stanley MA. Imiquimod and the imidazoquinolones: mechanism of action and therapeutic potential. Clin Exp Dermatol 2002;27:571–7.
89. Mitsuishi T, Iida K, Kawana S. Cimetidine treatment for viral warts enhances IL-2 and IFN-gamma expression but not IL-18 expression in lesional skin. Eur J Dermatol 2003;13(5):445–8.
90. Gallin JI, Malech HL, Weening RS, et al. A controlled trial of interferon gamma to prevent infection in chronic granulomatous disease. N Engl J Med 1991;14: 1023–6.
91. Sternfeld T, Nigg A, Belohradsky BH, et al. Treatment of relapsing. *Mycobacterium avium* infection with interferon-gamma and interleukin-2 in an HIV-negative patient with low CD4 syndrome. Int J Infect Dis 2010;14(S3):e198–201.
92. Seneviratne SL, Doffinger R, Macfarlane J, et al. Disseminated *Mycobacterium tuberculosis* infection due to interferon gamma deficiency. Response to replacement therapy. Thorax 2007;62(1):97–9.
93. Jouanguy E, Altare F, Lamhamedi S, et al. Interferon-γ-receptor deficiency in an infant with fatal bacilli Calmette-Guerin infection. N Engl J Med 1996;335: 1956–61.
94. Phillips P, Forbes JC, Speert DP. Disseminated infection with *Pseudollescheria boydii* in a patient with chronic granulomatous disease: response to gamma-interferon plus antifungal therapy. Pediatr Infect Dis J 1991;10:536–9.
95. Page AV, Liles WC. Colony-stimulating factors in the prevention and management of infectious diseases. Infect Dis Clin North Am 2011;25:803–17.
96. Nemunaitis J, Buckner CD, Dorsey KS, et al. Retrospective analysis of infectious disease in patients who received recombinant granulocyte-macrophage colony-stimulating factor versus patients not receiving a cytokine who underwent autologous bone marrow transplant for lymphoid cancer. Am J Clin Oncol 1998;21: 341–6.
97. Root RK, Dale DC. Granulocyte colony-stimulating factor and granulocyte-macrophage colony-stimulating factor: comparisons and potential for use in the treatment of infections in non-neutropenic patients. J Infect Dis 1999; 179(Suppl 2):S342–52.
98. Arpinati M, Green CL, Heimfeld S, et al. Granulocyte colony-stimulating factor mobilizes T helper 2 inducing dendritic cells. Blood 2000;95:2482–90.

99. Nemunaitis J, Shannon-Dorcy K, Appelbaum FR, et al. Long-term follow-up of patients with invasive fungal disease who received adjunctive therapy with recombinant human macrophage colony-stimulating factor. Blood 1993;82: 1422–7.

100. Bohlius J, Herbst C, Reiser M, et al. Granulopoiesis-stimulating factors to prevent adverse effects in the treatment of malignant lymphoma. Cochrane Database Syst Rev 2008;4:CD003189.

101. Clark OA, Lyman G, Castro AA, et al. Colony stimulating factors for chemotherapy induced febrile neutropenia. Cochrane Database Syst Rev 2000;4:CD003039.

102. Aapro MS, Bohlius J, Cameron DA, et al. 2010 update of EORTC guidelines for the use of granulocyte-colony stimulating factor to reduce the incidence of chemotherapy-induced febrile neutropenia in adult patients with lymphoproliferative disorders and solid tumors. Eur J Cancer 2011;47:8–32.

103. Dale DC, Bonilla MA, Davis MW, et al. A randomized controlled phase III trial of recombinant human granulocyte colony-stimulating factor (filgrastim) for treatment of severe chronic neutropenia. Blood 1993;81:2496–502.

104. Moore RD, Keruly JC, Chaisson RE. Neutropenia and bacterial infection in acquired immunodeficiency syndrome. Arch Intern Med 1995;155:1965–70.

105. Ortega M, Almela M, Soriano A, et al. Bloodstream infections among human immunodeficiency virus-infected adult patients: epidemiology and risk factors for mortality. Eur J Clin Microbiol Infect Dis 2008;27:969–76.

106. Keiser P, Rademacher S, Smith JW, et al. Granulocyte colony-stimulating factor use is associated with decreased bacteremia and increased survival in neutropenic HIV-infected patients. Am J Med 1998;104:48–55.

107. Koskinas J, Zacharakis G, Sidiropoulos J, et al. Granulocyte colony stimulating factor in HCV genotype-1 patients who develop Peg-IFN-alpha2b related severe neutropenia: a preliminary report on treatment, safety and efficacy. J Med Virol 2009;81:848–52.

108. Kuhn P, Messer J, Paupe A, et al. A multicentre, randomized, placebo-controlled trial of prophylactic recombinant granulocyte-colony stimulating factor in preterm neonates with neutropenia. J Pediatr 2009;155:324–30.

109. Droemann D, Hansen F, Aries SP, et al. Neutrophil apoptosis, activation and anti-inflammatory cytokine response in granulocyte colony-stimulating factor-treated patients with community-acquired pneumonia. Respiration 2006;73:340–6.

110. Cheng AC, Stephens DP, Currie BJ. Granulocyte-colony stimulating factor (G-CSF) as an adjunct to antibiotics in the treatment of pneumonia in adults. Cochrane Database Syst Rev 2007;2:CD004400.

111. Cruciani M, Lipsky BA, Mengoli C, et al. Granulocyte-colony stimulating factors as adjunctive therapy for diabetic foot infections. Cochrane Database Syst Rev 2009;3:CD006810.

112. Dornbusch HJ, Urban CE, Pinter H, et al. Treatment of invasive pulmonary aspergillosis in severely neutropenic children with malignant disorders using liposomal amphotericin B(AmBisome), granulocyte colony stimulating factor, and surgery: report of five cases. Pediatr Hematol Oncol 1995;171:577–86.

113. Gonzalez CE, Couriel DR, Walsh TJ. Disseminated zygomycosis in a neutropenic patient: successful treatment with amphotericin B lipid complex and granulocyte colony-stimulating factor. Clin Infect Dis 1997;24:192–6.

114. Sahin B, Paydas S, Cosar E, et al. Role of granulocyte colony-stimulating factor in the treatment of mucormycosis. Eur J Clin Microbiol Infect Dis 1996;15:866–9.

115. Lewis R, Hogan H, Howell A, et al. Progressive fusariosis: unpredictable posaconazole bioavailability, and feasibility of recombinant interferon-gamma plus

granulocyte macrophage-colony stimulating factor for refractory disseminated infection. Leuk Lymphoma 2008;49:163–5.

116. Peters BG, Adkins DR, Harrison BR, et al. Antifungal effects of yeast derived rhu-GM-CSF in patients receiving high-dose chemotherapy given with or without autologous stem cell transplantation: a retrospective analysis. Bone Marrow Transplant 1996;18:93–102.

117. Abu J, Haidar R, Bitar F, et al. *Aspergillus* vertebral osteomyelitis in a child with a primary monocytes killing defect: response to GM-CSF therapy. J Infect 2000; 41:97–100.

118. Romani L, Puccetti P, Bistoni F. Interleukin-12 in infectious diseases. Clin Microbiol Rev 1997;10:611–36.

119. Olejniczak K, Kasprzak A. Biological properties of interleukin 2 and its role in pathogenesis of selected diseases–a review. Med Sci Monit 2008;14(10): RA179–89.

120. INSIGHT-ESPRIT Study Group, SILCAAT Scientific Committee, Abrams D, et al. Interleukin-2 therapy in patients with HIV infection. N Engl J Med 2009;361(16): 1548–59.

121. Toren A, Or R, Ackerstein A, et al. Invasive fungal infections in lymphoma patients receiving immunotherapy following autologous bone marrow transplantation (ABMT). Bone Marrow Transplant 1997;20:67–9.

122. Medina Rodríguez F. Biologic therapy and infections. Reumatol Clin 2006;2(6): 302–12.

123. Corral LG, Kaplan G. Immunomodulation by thalidomide and thalidomide analogues. Ann Rheum Dis 1999;58:107–13.

124. Sampaio EP, Kaplan G, Miranda A, et al. The influence of thalidomide on the clinical and immunologic manifestation of erythema nodosum leprosum. J Infect Dis 1993;168:408–14.

125. Tramontana JM, Utaipat U, Molloy A, et al. Thalidomide treatment reduces tumor necrosis factor alpha production and enhances weight gain in patients with pulmonary tuberculosis. Mol Med 1995;1:384–97.

126. Calabrese L, Fleisher AB. Thalidomide: current and potential clinical application. Am J Med 2000;6:487–95.

127. Levi M, Ten Cate H. Disseminated intravascular coagulation. N Engl J Med 1999;341:586–92.

128. Bernard GR, Vincent JL, Laterre PF, et al. Efficacy and safety of recombinant human activated protein C for severe sepsis. N Engl J Med 2001;344:699–709.

129. Abraham E, Laterre PF, Garg R, et al. Drotrecogin alfa (activated) for adults with severe sepsis and a low risk of death. N Engl J Med 2005;353:1332–41.

130. Nadel S, Goldstein B, Williams MD, et al. Drotrecogin alfa (activated) in children with severe sepsis: a multicentre phase III randomized controlled trial. Lancet 2007;369(9564):836–43.

131. Van de Beek D, de Gans J, Mcintyre P, et al. Steroids in adults with acute bacterial meningitis: a systemic review. Lancet Infect Dis 2004;4:139–43.

132. Dooley DP, Carpenter JL, Rademacher S. Adjunctive corticosteroid therapy for tuberculosis: a critical reappraisal of the literature. Clin Infect Dis 1997;25(4): 872–87.

133. Smego RA, Ahmed N. A systematic review of the adjunctive use of systemic corticosteroids for pulmonary tuberculosis. Int J Tuberc Lung Dis 2003;7(3):208–13.

134. Oppert M, Schindler R, Husung C, et al. Low dose hydrocortisone improves shock reversal and reduces cytokine levels in early hyperdynamic septic shock. Crit Care Med 2005;33:2457–64.

Immunotherapies in Rheumatologic Disorders

Anne V. Miller, MD*, Sriya K.M. Ranatunga, MD, MPH

- Rheumatoid arthritis • Systemic lupus erythematosus
- Vasculitis • Disease-modifying antirheumatic drugs
- Biologic response modifiers • Biologics

Key Points

- Autoimmune diseases with rheumatologic manifestations are characterized by self-perpetuating dysregulations of the innate and adaptive arms of the immune system.
- Both nonbiologic and biologic therapies used in the rheumatic diseases target these immune dysregulations to reduce damage from ongoing inflammation.
- Although most of the available immunotherapies in rheumatology have been developed for rheumatoid arthritis, an increasing number are being tested for efficacy in other autoimmune disorders.

INTRODUCTION

Inflammation, with its overt and easily recognizable features of pain, swelling, redness, and warmth, has long been recognized as a feature common to the rheumatic diseases. The absence of the "usual culprits" of infection and trauma as a cause of such symptoms, coupled with a growing understanding of immunologic mechanisms, has led to the realization that such symptoms result from the misdirection of our own immunologic defenses against self tissues and organs.

Over the past several decades, rheumatology has directed its focus to understanding and countering the immune dysregulation underlying these autoimmune diseases. Older therapies, effective though poorly understood, are being scrutinized anew and are yielding the immune-modulating mechanisms behind their efficacy. New therapies, the "biologics," are drugs tailored to address specific immune defects and imbalances.

Med Clin N Am 96 (2012) 475–496
doi:10.1016/j.mcna.2012.04.003
0025-7125/12/$ – see front matter **medical.theclinics.com**

This article discusses the current immunotherapies of the rheumatic diseases, correlating our current understanding of their mechanisms with dysfunctions believed to be present in the various major autoimmune syndromes.

THE DISEASES AS THERAPEUTIC TARGETS

Although the pathogenesis of most major autoimmune diseases is often reduced to "genetic predisposition + trigger = autoimmune disease," this simplified equation belies the complexity of their defects and dysregulations, and the fact that these differ in the various diseases. As these defects in various diseases become better understood, therapeutic targets emerge.

Systemic lupus erythematosus (SLE), for example, has long been known to be characterized by the presence of (often multiple) autoantibodies that cause direct and indirect damage to tissues and organs. Harder to define has been the trigger leading to the production of these autoantibodies. A combination of clearance defects, defective receptor signaling (including Toll-like receptors [TLRs] 7 and 9), and lack of suppressive activity are thought to allow the prolonged exposure of self-antigens to break immune tolerance, causing continuing activation of both innate and adaptive immune responses.[1,2] Therapeutic targets in SLE therefore include autoantibody-producing B cells, malfunctioning TLRs, cytokines, activated T cells, and general lymphoproliferation or lymphoid function.

Rheumatoid arthritis (RA) is thought to begin with antigen-dependent T-cell activation likely by endogenous trigger(s), followed by fibroblast and macrophage activation with subsequent cytokine production and angiogenesis, followed by an influx of inflammatory cells.[3] Therapeutic targets in RA therefore include participants in T-cell activation (both B and T cells), cytokines and, again, general lymphoproliferation. Similar involvement and targeting of various innate and adaptive mechanisms are being sought in the other phenotypes of autoimmunity.

- Most, if not all, of the autoimmune rheumatic diseases involve dysfunction in both the innate and adaptive arms of the immune system.
- Therapeutic agents in the rheumatic diseases modulate the dysfunction of these components.
- Existing and emerging therapies designed or known to work for a given disease indication are often found to have unpredicted efficacy in other diseases, broadening our understanding of their pathogenesis.

THE THERAPIES AND THEIR EFFECTS

The immunomodulating therapies used in the rheumatic diseases have evolved from a modest handful of naturally derived and chemically synthesized agents to a much larger arsenal that now includes bioengineered recombinant and monoclonal antibody products, the biologic response modifiers or biologics. All modulate biologic processes, some at precise loci and others via multiple mechanisms. These therapies, their mechanisms, and their uses are described here (**Box 1**).

Nonbiologic (Chemical and Naturally Derived) Immunomodulators

Glucocorticoids
Since the first clinical trials in 1948 of Compound E, isolated from bovine adrenal glands and later renamed cortisone, the glucocorticoids (GCs) have been recognized for their profound anti-inflammatory and immunosuppressant effects, and as a group have become some of the most widely prescribed medicines in clinical practice.[4]

Box 1
Nonbiologic (chemical or naturally derived) and biologic immunomodulators in the rheumatic diseases

Chemical or naturally derived agents

    Glucocorticoids

    Methotrexate

    Sulfasalazine

    Hydroxychloroquine

    Leflunomide

    Cyclosporine

    Mycophenolate mofetil

    Azathioprine

    Cyclophosphamide

    Colchicine

    Minocycline

Biologic response modifiers

    Etanercept

    Infliximab

    Adalimumab

    Certilizumab

    Golimumab

    Abatacept

    Rituximab

    Tocilizumab

    Anakinra

    Belimumab

Unfortunately, at high doses and with prolonged dosing, their metabolic effects of insulin resistance, osteoporosis, and atherosclerosis have limited their usefulness.

Endogenous GCs in physiologic concentrations perform a myriad of functions, including immunosuppression, which serves to protect the host from damage caused by self-generated inflammatory reactions, and metabolic effects such as regulation of glucose uptake and gluconeogenesis. These effects are largely mediated through ubiquitous cytoplasmic GC receptors (GCR), which are readily bound by GC as it diffuses into a cell. The resulting complex can enter the nucleus and interact with the genome, activating DNA transcription (transactivation, via direct effects on regulatory regions of DNA) or blocking it (transrepression, via inactivation of transcription proteins such as nuclear factor [NF]-κB). Transactivation is thought to mediate the metabolic effects of GCs; transrepression is thought to mediate their anti-inflammatory effects, which include suppression of cytokine synthesis.[5] These genomic effects take place over a time frame of 15 minutes to several hours.[6]

A faster-acting route of GC action occurs through nongenomic pathways, which bypass DNA signaling altogether.[7] These effects include changes in the activity of intracellular kinases, the activation of T-cell receptors, the inhibition of release of the inflammatory prostaglandins,[8,9] as well as various metabolic effects. These nongenomic actions take place in a matter of minutes and may require larger doses of GCs (>30 mg/d of prednisone or its equivalent).

Because of the predictable and undesirable metabolic side effects caused by immunosuppressant doses of steroids, a goal of current research is to identify therapeutic agents that can more selectively trigger the pathways that lead to clinically desirable anti-inflammatory and immunosuppressive effects.

- GCs, including prednisone and methylprednisolone, are used in nearly all the inflammatory rheumatic diseases to suppress both the early phases of innate immune activation and later adaptive phases via a combination of fast-acting (nongenomic) and slower-acting (genomic) effects.
- Because of their predictable and undesirable metabolic side effects, GCs are most useful in the rheumatic diseases when immediate or life-threatening immune suppression is necessary, or as a bridge therapy until safer, sloweracting agents take effect.
- When long-term use of GCs is unavoidable, attention to their metabolic effects, including bone mass preservation, is warranted.

Methotrexate

In the 1940s, a designer drug aimed at inhibiting folate metabolism, methotrexate (MTX), a folic acid analogue, was introduced as a cancer chemotherapy. Although it was shown to have efficacy in RA in 1951,[10] its widespread use was delayed by the demonstration of the remarkable anti-inflammatory effects of the GCs. As the side effects of the GCs became evident, the search for steroid-sparing alternatives reignited interest in MTX and other agents. Since its introduction as a therapy for RA in the 1970s, MTX has become the cornerstone of treatment for moderate to severe RA, against which all subsequent therapies have been and continue to be compared.

The high doses of MTX used in cancer chemotherapy inhibit purine and pyrimidine metabolism and amino acid synthesis by blocking folate-dependent pathways. Used in lower doses in RA, its efficacy was at first attributed to the same mechanism. However, when folic acid, universally administered in RA to avert depression of bone marrow synthesis, failed to significantly attenuate its anti-inflammatory effects, additional/alternative mechanisms were sought.

Because of MTX's prolonged effect despite its short half-life in the serum, its metabolites, particularly the MTX polyglutamates, were examined. These compounds have been found to inhibit the enzyme AICAR (5-amino-1-β-D-ribofuranosyl-imidazole-4-carboxamide) transformylase. One effect of this inhibition is an increase in levels of adenosine, a potent anti-inflammatory mediator with multiple reported effects including inhibition of cytokine transcription, leukocyte adhesion, and clonal expansion of T and B cells.[11–13] Blockade of adenosine receptors by caffeine or theophylline has been shown to reduce MTX's effect in a rat model of RA.[14] Similar studies in humans with RA have had mixed results.[15,16]

MTX polyglutamation is a slow process, taking up to 4 months to reach a steady state.[17] This finding is consistent with the clinically observed timeline of the MTX effect.

MTX is effective in RA as monotherapy in a significant percentage of patients; in inadequate responders, improved response can occur when administered in combination with other agents, including sulfasalazine (SSA), hydroxychloroquine (HCQ), and/or biologics. Its use may prolong survival. It is used off-label in psoriatic arthritis,

SLE, polymyositis and dermatomyositis, polymyalgia rheumatica, sarcoidosis, and in various vasculitides.

MTX is generally taken orally or subcutaneously, with up to 10% to 15% improved absorption via the subcutaneous route at higher doses. Because it is largely excreted by the kidneys, its dosage should be decreased with significant renal disease. Administration of medications that interfere with folate metabolism or transport, such as trimethoprim or probenecid, can increase the risk of side effects with MTX.

Adverse effects include mucositis, cytopenia, and macrocytosis, all believed to be related to folate antagonism and reduced with daily folate or weekly folinic acid supplementation. Hepatotoxicity can occur and is more frequent with alcohol use. Untreated viral hepatitis precludes its use. Pulmonary toxicity, usually a hypersensitivity pneumonitis with symptoms of dry cough and fever, may occur in 2% to 8% of patients, usually within the first year. Rarely, a lymphoma responsive to the discontinuance of MTX can develop. A teratogen, MTX is contraindicated in pregnancy. Despite these potential side effects MTX has the highest continuation rate of the disease-modifying agents used in RA, due to its efficacy and general tolerability.[18]

- Methotrexate is the primary disease-modifying agent used in RA.
- Coadministration of daily folic acid reduces hematologic and mucosal side effects.
- Patients should be monitored for hematologic, liver, and pulmonary toxicity.
- Concomitant use of trimethoprim or probenecid may increase toxicity.
- Methotrexate is contraindicated in pregnancy.

Sulfasalazine

Aside from plant-derived salicylates, the use of which dates to antiquity, and gold compounds, which are no longer standard therapy for RA, one of the oldest immunomodulating antirheumatic drugs currently in use is SSA. Specifically designed for RA as a combination of the antibacterial sulfapyridine and the anti-inflammatory salicylic acid, this agent was first shown to have efficacy in RA in the 1940s. Like MTX, its debut was overshadowed by the dramatic effects of cortisol in 1949; it was essentially shelved as a treatment for RA until the 1980s, when well-constructed trials conclusively demonstrated its effectiveness.[19,20]

Both the parent compound and its sulfapyridine moiety have immunosuppressant activity. Uncleaved SSA has been shown to increase intracellular adenosine concentrations, which downregulate inflammation via adenosine receptors, a mechanism it shares with MTX.[21] It also inhibits the nuclear transcription factor NF-κB, which is integral to cytokine generation[22] and inhibits white blood cell adhesion and function.[23] The sulfapyridine moiety has also been shown to have efficacy in RA; though its mechanism is unknown, it is not believed to be related to its antimicrobial activity.

SSA is currently recognized as a relatively fast-acting, effective agent for mild to moderate RA and juvenile idiopathic arthritis, similar in efficacy to leflunomide and at least low-dose MTX.[24–26] It is used off-label in the spondyloarthropathies. Although it is generally well tolerated when begun with gradually increasing doses, it can cause hepatotoxicity and bone marrow suppression, for which monitoring is necessary. It has no significant drug interactions and is considered safe for use in pregnancy.

- SSA is a relatively fast-acting, effective agent for mild to moderate RA.
- Although generally well tolerated when begun with gradually increasing doses, SSA should be monitored for hematologic and liver toxicity.
- SSA can be used in pregnancy.

Hydroxychloroquine

Although use of the antimalarials in cutaneous lupus dates to the 1890s with J.S. Payne's description of the efficacy of quinine in inducing pallor in a patient with photosensitive malar rash,[27] it was not until the 1950s that their usefulness in cutaneous lupus erythematosus and, subsequently, SLE became widely recognized. For years chloroquine, followed by the less toxic HCQ, were limited to use in mild RA and for the joint and skin manifestations of SLE. With a broadening understanding of its mechanisms of action, HCQ has become a cornerstone of therapy in SLE, reducing its morbidity and mortality.

HCQ, like quinine and the other antimalarials, is a weak base capable of easily gaining entry into cells and gravitating to the acidic compartments of lysosomes and other cytoplasmic vesicles, raising their pH incrementally and altering protein processing. This long-recognized effect, by hindering antigen presentation, receptor recycling, and protein excretion, is thought to lead to a downstream reduction in autoantibody formation and T-cell activation.[28,29]

More recently, HCQ has been shown to disrupt even earlier events in the immune-activation cascade by inhibiting the function of TLRs 3, 7, and 9 stationed on the lysosomal membranes. By inhibiting the triggering of these TLRs by self DNA, RNA, and immune complexes, HCQ interrupts and deescalates the ongoing inflammatory processes of RA and SLE.[30–32]

HCQ is now considered a mainstay of therapy in lupus and should be considered in all patients with this diagnosis. Its clinical effects in SLE include improvement in rash and joints, reduction in flares, improved renal outcomes, a reduction in vascular events, and improved mortality.[33–36] It also has efficacy in mild to moderate RA and has been shown in multiple studies to have a protective effect against arterial and venous thrombosis in SLE patients.[37] HCQ has been shown to have a potential antithrombotic role in the antiphospholipid (APL) antibody syndrome, possibly by interfering with the binding of APL antibodies to the endogenous anticoagulant annexin A5.[38] It also has a favorable effect on lipid profiles and glucose metabolism, which may improve the cardiovascular profiles of our patients with these atherogenic diseases.

HCQ has an excellent safety profile and is one of the safest of the antirheumatic therapies. For this reason, it is generally continued during pregnancy to prevent disease flares.[39] Ocular toxicity is one caveat. Retinal toxicity has been shown to increase after 5 to 7 years of use or after an accumulated dose of 1000 g. A baseline retinal assessment assessing visual fields plus either a multifocal electroretinogram, spectral domain optical coherence tomography, or fundus autofluorescence is now recommended at the onset of therapy, with a follow-up at 5 years (sooner if other risk factors are present).[40]

- HCQ reduces inflammation and reduces mortality in SLE by multiple mechanisms, and is considered a mainstay of therapy.
- HCQ has efficacy in mild to moderate RA and can be used in combination with other agents.
- HCQ has an excellent safety profile and is generally continued in lupus patients during pregnancy to reduce disease flares.
- Ocular toxicity risk increases after 5 to 7 years of use and should be monitored.

Leflunomide

Approved in 1998 for the treatment of RA, leflunomide is believed to work primarily by inhibiting the proliferation of activated lymphocytes by blocking dihydroorotate dehydrogenase, an enzyme involved in pyrimidine, specifically uridine (RNA), synthesis.[41] It is equipotent to MTX in efficacy and inhibition of erosive disease,[42] but with a higher incidence of discontinuance attributable to its side effects. In addition to RA, for which it is approved by the Food and Drug Administration (FDA), leflunomide has been effective in off-label usage in psoriatic arthritis, systemic lupus, juvenile polyarthritis, and refractory dermatomyositis.

Its most frequent potential side effects, occurring in up to 15% of patients, include rash, alopecia, diarrhea (minimized by omitting loading doses), and transaminase elevations. It should be avoided with preexisting liver disease. It is unclear whether, like MTX, leflunomide is associated with an increased risk of interstitial pulmonary disease.[43] Prudence would suggest that it be avoided in patients with preexisting lung disease. Neuropathy and cytopenia have been reported. It is a teratogen and is contraindicated in pregnancy.

Because its active metabolite, teriflunomide, can persist in the serum for up to 2 years because of its extensive enterohepatic recirculation, the administration of cholestyramine is used when expedited elimination of the drug is necessary (eg, with adverse reactions or in anticipation of pregnancy).

- Leflunomide, an oral agent with FDA approval for the treatment of RA, has an efficacy and side-effect profile similar to that of MTX.
- Patients should be monitored for hepatotoxicity.
- Leflunomide is contraindicated in pregnancy and with preexisting liver disease.
- Cholestyramine is effective in eliminating the active metabolites of leflunomide from the serum when necessary.

Cyclosporine

Cyclosporine (CSP), a mainstay of antirejection therapy for organ transplants, also has an FDA indication for use in severe, active RA unresponsive or inadequately responsive to MTX. Several studies, but not all, suggest that MTX and CSP are more effective in combination than either drug alone.[44–47] In the form of an emulsion, CSP eye drops are used in the keratoconjunctivitis sicca of Sjögren syndrome.

CSP, by binding the intracellular enzyme calcineurin, inhibits the transcription and production of interleukin (IL)-2 and other inflammatory cytokines triggered by T-cell activation, reducing downstream inflammation. Its effectiveness in RA suggests a strong T-cell component in RA pathogenesis.

Side effects include acute (reversible) and chronic (irreversible) renal toxicity, hypertension, tremor, increased infections, and increased malignancy. It does not cause myelosuppression. Although it is not a teratogen, it can cause growth restriction and prematurity and should only be used in pregnancy when its benefits outweigh its risks. Multiple drug interactions exist that can increase or decrease cyclosporine levels, affecting effectiveness and toxicity.

Although enthusiasm for the use of CSP in RA has waned with the advent of the biologic therapies, it remains an option as monotherapy or in combination with MTX or leflunomide for patients who cannot tolerate or have contraindications to the use of biologics or standard disease-modifying antirheumatic drugs (DMARDs).

- CSP blocks inflammatory cytokine transcription in T cells by binding intracellular calcineurin.
- CSP, though effective, is a third-line agent in the treatment of RA because of its side effect profile and drug interactions.
- Patients on CSP should be monitored for renal dysfunction and hypertension.

Mycophenolate mofetil

Mycophenolate mofetil (MMF), another drug originally approved by the FDA for prevention of transplant rejection and often used in conjunction with cyclosporine in transplant patients, has found increasing application in the rheumatic diseases. MMF is an inhibitor of the synthesis of guanosine monophosphate (GMP), a purine required for DNA and RNA synthesis. Because lymphocytes lack alternative pathways for synthesis of GMP, MMF selectively inhibits the proliferation of T and B lymphocytes and the production of their associated cytokines.[48] MMF also inhibits the production of cytokines by macrophages and dendritic cells, including tumor necrosis factor (TNF)-α.[49]

MMF, in off-label use, has been shown to be as effective as cyclophosphamide in the induction phase of treatment of moderately severe proliferative lupus nephritis[50]; it is also useful in maintaining remission in severe lupus nephritis after induction of remission with cyclophosphamide. MMF appears to be significantly more effective than cyclophosphamide in black and Latino patients.[51] It is also used off-label in inflammatory myositis.

Side effects are relatively mild, perhaps related to the specificity of its cellular effects, and include cytopenia and gastrointestinal symptoms. MMF is classified as Pregnancy Risk Category D because of increased first trimester losses and associated congenital malformations.

- MMF is as effective as cyclophosphamide in the treatment of moderately severe lupus nephritis.
- Patients on MMF should be monitored for cytopenia.

Cytotoxic agents

Azathioprine (AZA) is a prodrug whose active metabolite 6-mercaptopurine (6-MP) is a purine mimic that blocks purine synthesis and DNA repair. It inhibits cellular proliferation, particularly of rapidly dividing cells such as lymphocytes and hematopoietic cells. Although it gained FDA approval for active RA, its efficacy was found to be inferior to that of MTX.[52] Since the advent of biologic agents (below), its use in RA has become third line. It is also used off-label in SLE, inflammatory myositis, psoriatic arthritis, and Behçet disease, and to maintain remission in systemic vasculitis.

Bone marrow suppression, hepatotoxicity, nausea, and vomiting are its most common side effects. Bone marrow toxicity occurs more frequently in individuals deficient in the enzyme thiopurine methyltransferase (TMPT), which metabolizes 6-MP to less marrow-toxic metabolites. Renal insufficiency as well as the use of xanthine oxidase inhibitors such as allopurinol or febuxostat can also lead to elevated levels and increased toxicity. Determination of the patient's TMPT genotype before administration, cautious use with renal insufficiency, avoidance of xanthine oxidase inhibitors, and, most importantly, incremental dosing with close monitoring for toxicity can reduce the risk of side effects. It is Pregnancy Risk Category D.

Cyclophosphamide (CYC), an alkylating agent, is a potent and relatively fast-acting antiproliferative agent whose bone marrow and bladder toxicity and potential for late malignancy have restricted its use to refractory and organ-threatening or life-threatening rheumatic conditions such as lupus cerebritis, lupus nephritis, systemic vasculitis, or early interstitial pulmonary inflammation (eg, systemic sclerosis). It is administered either orally (daily) or intravenously (every 3–4 weeks). Dosing is determined by weight and renal function.

Toxicities include bone marrow suppression, with nadirs occurring at 7 to 14 days, loss of fertility in both males and females, bladder toxicity and cancer, and infections. Patients receiving intravenous CYC should receive mercaptoethane sulfonate before and after administration to prevent bladder toxicity; oral regimens should be taken in the morning with liberal fluids to assure elimination from the bladder before bedtime. Patients on CYC should receive Pneumocystis prophylaxis. It is Pregnancy Risk Category D.

- AZA is used (on label) as a third-line agent in RA, and (off label) in SLE, the inflammatory myopathies, psoriatic arthritis, and Behçet, and to maintain remission in systemic vasculitis.
- Because of its toxicities, CYC is reserved for use in severe and organ-threatening or life-threatening conditions such as lupus cerebritis and nephritis, systemic vasculitis, or early interstitial pulmonary inflammation.
- Both should be screened carefully for toxicity: AZA for bone marrow toxicity and hepatotoxicity; CYC for bone marrow toxicity and bladder toxicity, and long-term cancer risks.

Colchicine

Although the benefits of colchicum (more recently renamed colchicine), an alkaloid derived from the autumn crocus *Colchicum autumnale*, have been recognized for more than 2000 years, our understanding of its immunomodulating effects continues to grow. While its binding to cellular microtubules has long been understood to impair neutrophil migration, these same microtubules are also involved in cell division, signal transduction, regulation of gene expression, and in secretion. Colchicine's many effects include inhibition of leukocyte adhesion, phagocytosis, and cytokine secretion; inhibition of phospholipase-2 activation; modulation of pyrin, which affects inflammasome activation; and downregulation of cytokine receptors.[53] Its therapeutic effect correlates with its level in leukocytes, where it is preferentially sequestered, rather than plasma levels.[54,55]

Colchicine is indicated for the treatment of acute gouty flares and familial Mediterranean fever. Off-label uses include prophylaxis against gouty flares while instituting urate-lowering therapy, pseudogout flares and prophylaxis, the mucocutaneous manifestations of Behçet disease, and recurrent pericarditis.

Colchicine is excreted through several pathways: hepatobiliary excretion, small intestinal excretion (via the P-glycoprotein transporter), hepatic deactivation (via CYP3A4, 5%–20%), and renal excretion (10%–20%). Hepatic or renal dysfunction or the use of drugs or foods that compete with these pathways can lead to subacute toxicity. The list of these drugs and foods is long and includes many in common use (**Box 2**).

Colchicine has a narrow therapeutic window. Side effects of acute overadministration include nausea, vomiting, and diarrhea. For this reason, acute gout is no longer

Box 2
Common drugs that can increase colchicine levels and risk of toxicity
Clarithromycin
Erythromycin
Cyclosporine
Verapamil
Diltiazem
Ketoconazole
Itraconazole
Amprenavir
Fosamprenavir
Grapefruit juice

treated with intravenous or hourly oral colchicine. Subacutely, often related to worsening renal function or the administration of drugs that compete for its elimination pathways, a colchicine-related neuromyopathy can occur.

- Colchicine is indicated for use in acute gout and familial Mediterranean fever; it is used off label for prevention of gout and pseudogout flares, recurrent pericarditis, and Behçet.
- Colchicine has a narrow therapeutic window. To minimize acute gastrointestinal side effects, usage in gout flares is limited to three 0.6-mg tablets daily on day 1, and twice a day thereafter.
- Subacutely, neuromyopathy can result from renal insufficiency and/or drug interactions.

Minocycline

Minocycline, which inhibits metalloproteinase-9 production and T-cell proliferation and cytokine production,[56] has shown efficacy in mild to moderate RA in off-label use, with results in one trial favoring minocycline over hydroxychlorquine[57,58] It is generally well tolerated; potential side effects include nausea, vomiting, diarrhea and, less commonly, skin hyperpigmentation or photosensitivity. Induction of autoimmunity, including a lupus-like syndrome or antineutrophil cytoplasmic antibody–positive vasculitis has been reported.[59,60] A summary of the nonbiologic immunomodulators used in the rheumatic diseases is provided in **Table 1**.

Biologic Response Modifiers or Biologics

Biologic response modifiers, or biologics, are purified, modified, and/or reconstructed proteins derived from the genetic sequences of living cells, which are used to modify a patient's immune response. In the case of the rheumatic diseases, they are used to suppress overly active (and destructive) inflammatory responses by very specifically targeting key mediators, such as cytokines (eg, TNF-α, interleukins), cells, or cellular interactions.

The first biologic available for use in the rheumatic diseases was the TNF inhibitor etanercept (Enbrel), which was approved in 1998 for severe RA. Since then, several additional anticytokines, an anti–B-cell therapy, and a T-cell/B-cell coactivation signal inhibitor have been added (see **Box 1**). These agents, especially when combined with standard agents such as MTX or leflunomide, have significantly increased treatment success in RA and other inflammatory arthropathies, as measured by disease activity scores, functional assessments, and radiographic progression.

Tumor necrosis factor inhibitors

Five TNF inhibitors have been approved by the FDA for treatment in the rheumatic diseases: etanercept (Enbrel), infliximab (Remicade), adalimumab (Humira), certolizumab (Cimzia), and golimumab (Simponi). Their FDA indications include RA (all), psoriatic arthritis (all but certolizumab), ankylosing spondylitis (all but certolizumab), and juvenile idiopathic arthritis (etanercept, adalimumab). Off-label trials suggest efficacy in refractory sarcoidosis,[61–63] Kawasaki disease,[64] Behçet disease, and others.[65] All are given parenterally.

Although all the TNF inhibitors reduce inflammation by counteracting TNF activity, they differ in other ways. Etanercept is a human immunoglobulin G (IgG)-TNF receptor fusion protein that is administered subcutaneously, binding to circulating TNF and inactivating it. The remaining 4 are anti-TNF monoclonal antibodies (wholly or in part) that neutralize both circulating and membrane-bound TNF. These agents contain varying proportions of mouse protein. Infliximab is chimeric, containing approximately

Table 1
Summary of nonbiologic (chemical or naturally-derived) immunomodulators used in the rheumatic diseases

Agent	Description	Mechanism	Route	Usage
Glucocorticoid	Steroid hormone	Genomic and nongenomic effects	PO, IM, IV	Life- or organ-threatening inflammation; bridge, until safer agents "kick in"
Methotrexate	Folate analogue	Increases adenosine, inhibits folate metabolism	PO, SQ, IM	FDA: RA, JIA OL: PM/DM, SLE, PsA, PMR, certain vasculitides, sarcoidosis
Sulfasalazine	Sulfonamide + salicylate	Increases adenosine, inhibits NF-κB, other	PO	FDA: RA, JIA OL: Spondyloarthropathy
Hydroxychloroquine	Antimalarial (4-aminoquinoline derivative)	Lowers compartmental pH; modulates Toll-like receptor activity, other	PO	FDA: SLE, RA OL: JIA, SjS, APLS, palindromic rheumatism
Leflunomide	Isoxazole derivative	Inhibits pyrimidine synthesis, other	PO	FDA: RA OL: PsA, JIA, SLE, DM
Cyclosporine	Fungal metabolite	Inhibits T-cell activation by blocking calcineurin activation	PO, drops	FDA: RA OL: SLE FDA: KCS-SjS
Mycophenolate mofetil	Antibiotic from *Penicillium* sp	Inhibits DNA and RNA synthesis in lymphocytes	PO	OL: lupus nephritis, DM
Azathioprine	Purine analogue	Inhibits DNA repair, inhibits DNA and RNA synthesis	PO	FDA: RA OL: DM, PM, lupus, PsA nephritis, Behçet, vasculitis maintenance
Cyclophosphamide	Synthetic agent	Alkylating agent	PO, IV	OL: SLE nephritis, cerebritis; vasculitis; early ILD (SSc)
Colchicine	Naturally occurring, plant source	Interferes with microtubular function	PO	FDA: gout, fMf OL: pseudogout, Behçet, pericarditis
Minocycline	Tetracycline group antibiotic	Metalloproteinase-9 inhibitor	PO	FDA: RA

Abbreviations: APLS, antiphospholipid syndrome; DM, dermatomyositis; FDA, Federal Drug Administration approved usage; fMf, familial Mediterranean fever; IM, intramuscular; IV, intravenous; JIA, juvenile idiopathic arthritis; KCS-SjS, keratoconjunctivitis sicca/Sjögren syndrome; OL, off label; PO, oral; PM, polymyositis; PMR, polymyalgia rheumatica; PsA, psoriatic arthritis; RA, rheumatoid arthritis; SLE, systemic lupus erythematosus; SSc, systemic sclerosis; SQ, subcutaneous.

25% mouse protein; certolizumab is humanized (~5% mouse protein); golimumab and adalimumab are fully human.

As with naturally occurring foreign proteins, TNF inhibitors can themselves be immunogenic. Human antichimeric antibodies (HACA) develop in a significant number of infliximab patients, particularly when given at the lower dose ranges, and correlate with the risk of infusion reactions. Concomitant methotrexate (MTX) significantly reduces HACA. For this reason, infliximab is not recommended as monotherapy. Human antihuman antibodies have been found in patients treated with adalimumab, correlate with diminished effectiveness, and appear to be reduced with concomitant MTX use.[66,67] Certolizumab, which lacks an Fc antibody component, may theoretically be less antigenic.

The TNF inhibitors share boxed warnings for the potential of serious as well as opportunistic infections, activation of latent tuberculosis and, in adolescents, lymphoma and other malignancies. Other potential side effects include injection site or infusion reactions, neutropenia, demyelinating disease, cutaneous reactions such as psoriasis, induction of autoimmunity, and the development of heart failure. Infliximab is contraindicated at doses greater than 5 mg/kg in patients with New York Heart Association class III/IV heart failure. The incidence of nonmelanoma skin cancer appears to be increased with TNF-inhibitor use; the data on the incidence of solid tumors is mixed, with large Swedish registry studies failing to find an increase.[68] The TNF inhibitors are Pregnancy Risk Category B (**Table 2**).

- All of the 5 listed TNF inhibitors are indicated for use in RA; several have additional antirheumatic applications.
- Infliximab, a chimeric monoclonal antibody containing significant mouse protein, should be used in conjunction with MTX to minimize the production of human antichimeric antibodies.
- Before the institution of a TNF inhibitor, patients should be screened for latent tuberculosis.
- Patients on a TNF inhibitor should be monitored for infection and heart failure. Infrequent side effects include neutropenia, demyelinating disease, skin cancer, and induction of autoimmunity.

Table 2
FDA-approved tumor necrosis factor (TNF)-α inhibitors in rheumatology

TNF-α Inhibitor	Description	Mechanism	Route	Usage
Etanercept (Enbrel)	TNF receptor-human fusion protein	Decoy receptor for soluble TNF	SQ	FDA: RA, JIA, AS, PsA OL: Behcet
Infliximab (Remicade)	Chimeric (mouse/human) anti-TNF monoclonal antibody	Antibody to TNF	IV	FDA (with methotrexate): RA, AS, PsA OL: Behçet, sarcoid
Adalimumab (Humira)	Human monoclonal antibody	Antibody to TNF	SQ	FDA: RA, JIA, AS, PsA OL: Behcet
Certolizumab (Cimzia)	Pegylated, humanized, Fab' fragment	Antibody to TNF	SQ	FDA: RA
Golimumab (Simponi)	Human monoclonal antibody	Antibody to TNF	SQ	FDA: RA, AS, PsA

Abbreviations: AS, ankylosing spondylitis; FDA, Federal Drug Administration approved usage; IV, intravenous; JIA, juvenile idiopathic arthritis; OL, off-label usage; PsA, psoriatic arthritis; RA, rheumatoid arthritis; SQ, subcutaneous.

Abatacept (Orencia)

Abatacept, or CTLA4-Ig, is a fusion protein that blocks the second signal of T-cell activation by antigen-presenting B cells. Abatacept is comprised of a human IgG1 Fc fragment fused to a T-cell surface receptor, CTLA4. Following intravenous or subcutaneous administration, circulating abatacept (CTLA4-Ig) binds the B-cell component of the second activation signal, B7, preventing it from binding either of its 2 T-cell membrane-bound ligands, CTLA4 and CD28. As a result, T-cell–mediated cytokine release and promotion of B-cell activities are suppressed.

Abatacept is approved by the FDA for use in moderate to severe RA that has been inadequately responsive to one or more standard (nonbiologic) DMARDs. It may be given as monotherapy, although its efficacy is enhanced when given concomitantly with standard disease-modifying agents such as MTX; it should not be given with other biologic agents because of an increased incidence of infection. It can take 6 months to achieve full effect.

The major side effect of Abatacept is the risk of serious infections, particularly bronchial and pulmonary. It is Pregnancy Risk Factor C.

- Abatacept (Orencia) blocks the second signal of T-cell activation by B cells, suppressing T-cell–mediated cytokine release and promotion of B-cell activities.
- It is indicated for RA that has been unresponsive to standard DMARDs.
- Abatacept may be used as monotherapy or in combination with standard (nonbiologic) DMARDs.
- Patients on abatacept should be monitored for infections.

Rituximab (Rituxan)

Rituximab is a chimeric monoclonal antibody, which targets the CD20 surface protein that transiently appears on maturing B cells. The resulting depletion of B cells results in a reduction of autoantibodies (as well as functional antibodies) and T-cell/B-cell interactions, potentially suppressing both humoral and cellular autoimmunity. It is approved by the FDA for use in conjunction with MTX in refractory RA unresponsive to TNF therapy and in granulomatosis with polyangiitis (GPA, formerly known as Wegener's granulomatosis).

Following intravenous infusion, B-lymphocyte depletion occurs within 2 to 4 weeks and persists for 6 to 12 months. In RA, reduction in joint activity appears to correlate with the degree of B-cell depletion[69]; patients seropositive for the antibodies RF (rheumatoid factor) and CCP (cyclic citrullinated peptide) appear more responsive.[70] Responders and partial responders can be retreated as frequently as every 24 weeks, usually with good response.[71,72]

Infusion reactions are the most common side effect of rituximab; most are thought to be related to an interaction of the drug with B cells, with resultant cytokine release, and can be managed with pretreatment with antihistamines, steroids, and a gradually increasing rate of infusion. However, anaphylaxis and death can occur. Severe infections are infrequent but have been reported, including several cases of progressive multifocal leukoencephalopathy (JC virus).[73] Tuberculosis reactivation can occur. Because hypogammaglobulinemia can develop, especially with retreatment(s), vaccinations should precede therapy and measurement of IgG should be considered before retreatment.[71,74] Rituximab is Pregnancy Risk Factor C.

- Rituximab, a chimeric monoclonal antibody that depletes B cells, is indicated for use with MTX in RA that has not adequately responded to TNF inhibition and in GPA.

- Responders and partial responders can be retreated as frequently as every 24 weeks.
- Rituximab carries boxed warnings for potentially fatal infusion reactions, severe infections, and possible reactivation of tuberculosis.
- Patients should be monitored for hypogammaglobulinemia.
- Vaccinations in patients receiving rituximab should be given at least 4 weeks before administration or following B-cell repletion.
- Patients should be screened for latent tuberculosis before institution of rituximab.

Interleukin-1β inhibitors

IL-1β is a "first-wave" response cytokine, initially thought to play a major role in RA, that has been found to be a key mediator of inflammation in gout and many autoinflammatory diseases, including periodic fevers such as familial Mediterranean fever. IL-1β inhibition has shown dramatic efficacy in the treatment of these syndromes. To date, FDA indications are limited to RA (anakinra) and a group of autoinflammatory diseases, the cryopyrin-associated periodic syndromes (rilonacept, canakinumab). Trials are under way to define their usefulness in gout.

Anakinra (Kineret) is an IL-1 receptor antagonist whose efficacy in RA proved to be inferior to that of the anti-TNF agents. In addition, site reactions to daily subcutaneous injections were not infrequent. Interest in anakinra was rekindled, however, with the identification of IL-1 as the key mediator of inflammation in gout and autoinflammatory diseases. Encouraging results in mice led to a trial of anakinra in 10 human gout patients who had not responded to or could not take nonsteroidal anti-inflammatory agents. Within 48 hours, all patients experienced a 50% to 100% decrease in symptoms and signs of inflammation, with no adverse effects.[75]

Rilonacept (Arcalyst), synthesized from the fusion of human IgG1 Fc fragment with human IL-1 receptor, functions as an "IL-1 trap" to bind and inactivate IL-1. It has been shown to decrease gouty flares during urate-lowering therapy,[76] while canakinumab (Ilaris), a humanized monoclonal antibody to IL-1, is effective in relieving acute gouty flares and in reducing flares during initiation of urate-lowering therapy.[77,78]

To date, none of the IL-1 inhibitors are approved for use in gout.

- Anakinra (Kineret), a once-daily injectable IL-1 inhibitor, is indicated for use in RA unresponsive to standard (nonbiologic) DMARDs. It may be used alone or in combination with standard DMARDs.
- Injection site reactions and, less frequently, infections are potential side effects.
- As a group, the IL-1 inhibitors have potential in gout management but are not indicated for this diagnosis at present.

Tocilizumab

IL-6 is a proinflammatory cytokine produced by T and B lymphocytes, monocytes, and fibroblasts whose effects include the induction of synovial neovascularization, osteoclast activation, and the upregulation of metalloproteinases. At the hepatocyte, it upregulates the production of C-reactive protein (CRP) and hepcidin; the latter, through its effects on iron absorption and mobilization, is believed to play a key role in the anemia of chronic disease.[79–81] IL-6 also promotes the differentiation of pro-inflammatory Th17 cells.

Tocilizumab (TCZ) is a humanized monoclonal antibody that targets soluble and membrane-bound IL-6. Its current FDA indication is for use in RA that has been unresponsive to at least one TNF inhibitor and systemic juvenile idiopathic arthritis. It is administered intravenously and may be used as monotherapy or in combination with standard (nonbiologic) DMARDs.

In addition to its significant efficacy in reducing the synovitis and radiographic progression of RA, TCZ improves systemic features of inflammation including anemia, anorexia, fever, and fatigue. Not surprisingly in view of the hepatic effects of IL-6, TCZ rapidly lowers CRP.

Side effects of tocilizumab include infection, reversible elevations of transaminases (particularly when given with MTX), neutropenia, tuberculosis reactivation, and increases in total cholesterol and triglyceride levels. In addition, gastrointestinal perforations at a rate of 0.26 per 100 patients have been reported.[82] TCZ is Pregnancy Risk Factor C.

- Tocilizumab (TCZ) is an intravenously administered humanized monoclonal antibody that targets IL-6: it is indicated for use in patients with RA that has been unresponsive to at least one TNF inhibitor or systemic juvenile idiopathic arthritis (JIA). It may be given with (nonbiologic) DMARDs or as monotherapy.
- TCZ improves systemic inflammatory features of fatigue, anemia of chronic disease, and elevated CRP.
- Side effects include infection, elevated transaminases, neutropenia, elevations in cholesterol and triglycerides, and, rarely, gastrointestinal perforation.
- Patients should be screened for tuberculosis before administration of tocilizumab.

Belimumab

Belimumab is an intravenously administered human monoclonal antibody directed against B-lymphocyte stimulator (BLys), resulting in a reduction in the number of B cells and short-lived plasma cells. Its indication is as an additive therapy in inadequately controlled, autoantibody-positive SLE patients.

Its use in 2 large clinical trials showed modest but significant efficacy in patients who had moderate levels of disease activity. Because patients with severe renal or central

Table 3
Other FDA-approved biologic response modifiers

Other Biologic	Description	Mechanism	Route	FDA-Approved Usage
Anakinra (Kineret)	Human IL-1 receptor antagonist protein	IL-1 receptor antagonist	SQ	RA
Abatacept (Orencia)	Human IgG1 heavy chain fused with soluble (human) CTLA4	Blocks second T-cell signal (T-cell activation) by B cells	SQ, IV	RA, JIA
Rituximab (Rituxan)	Chimeric (mouse/human) monoclonal antibody	Antibody to CD-20 (anti–B cell)	IV	With MTX: RA; With glucocorticoids: GPA, MPA
Tocilizumab (Actemra)	Humanized monoclonal antibody	Antibody to IL-6 receptor	IV	RA, sJIA
Belimumab (Benlysta)	Human monoclonal antibody	Antibody to B-lymphocyte stimulator (BLys)	IV	With standard therapy: antibody-positive SLE

Abbreviations: CTLA4, cytotoxic T lymphocyte–associated antigen 4; FDA, Federal Drug Administration approved usage; GPA, granulomatosis with polyangiitis (Wegener granulomatosis); IL, interleukin; IV, intravenous; JIA, juvenile idiopathic arthritis; MPA, microscopic polyangiitis; MTX, methotrexate; RA, rheumatoid arthritis; sJIA, systemic juvenile rheumatoid arthritis; SLE, systemic lupus erythematosus; SQ, subcutaneous.

Table 4
Antirheumatic immunotherapy usage by disease

	RA	(s)JIA	SLE	PsA	AS	PMR	SSc	SjS	PM/DM	Vasc	Gout	Sar	Beh
Standard Agents													
Glucocorticoids	X	X	X	X	X	(ol)	(ol)	(ol)	X	(ol)	(ol)	(ol)	(ol)
Methotrexate	X	X	(ol)	(ol)		(ol)	(ol)	(ol)	(ol)	(ol)		(ol)	(ol)
Sulfasalazine	X	X		(ol)	(ol)								
Hydroxychloroquine	X	(ol)	X	(ol)				(ol)	(ol)				
Leflunomide	X	(ol)	(ol)	(ol)					(ol)			(ol)	
Cyclosporine	X		(ol)	(ol)				X	(ol)	(ol)			
Mycophenolate			(ol)					(ol)	(ol)	(ol)			
Azathioprine	X		(ol)	(ol)				(ol)	(ol)	(ol)		(ol)	(ol)
Cyclophosphamide			(ol)				(ol)	(ol)	(ol)	(ol)		(ol)	(ol)
Colchicine											X		(ol)
Minocycline	(ol)												
TNF Inhibitors													
Etanercept (Enbrel)	X	X		X	X							(ol)	(ol)
Infliximab (Remicade)	X			X	X					(ol)		(ol)	(ol)
Adalimumab (Humira)	X	X		X	X								(ol)
Certolizumab (Cimzia)	X												
Golimumab (Simponi)	X			X	X								
Other Biologics													
Anakinra (Kineret)	X												
Abatacept (Orencia)	X	X		(ol)									
Rituximab (Rituxan)	X							(ol)		X			
Tocilizumab (Actemra)	X	X											
Belimumab (Benlysta)			X										

Abbreviations: AS, ankylosing spondylitis; Beh, Behçet disease; JIA, juvenile idiopathic arthritis; PM/DM, poly- and dermatomyositis; PMR, polymyalgia rheumatica; PsA, psoriatic arthritis; RA, rheumatoid arthritis; Sar, sarcoidosis; SLE, systemic lupus erythematosus; SjS, Sjögren syndrome; SSc, systemic sclerosis; Vasc, vasculitis types; X, FDA-approved use; (ol), off-label use.

nervous system (CNS) disease were excluded from the studies, its use in these subgroups is unproven. In addition, subgroups of black and Hispanic patients did not appear to respond, though numbers were too small to be conclusive.[83,84] Patients thought most likely to benefit are those with higher disease activity (excluding severe renal or CNS disease), anti-dsDNA positivity, low complements, or corticosteroid treatment at baseline.[85]

Side effects include nausea, vomiting, fever, and upper respiratory infection. Serious infections in clinical trials were similar to placebo. Infusion reactions occurred in fewer than 1% of patients. The FDA reported more deaths in patients who received belimumab treatment than in those treated with placebo during clinical trials.[86]

- Belimumab is a human monoclonal antibody directed against BLys that is indicated for use in moderately active, antibody-positive SLE patients inadequately controlled on standard therapy including steroids, HCQ, and immunosuppressives such as azathioprine or MMF.
- It has not been studied for efficacy in severe lupus nephritis or cerebritis.
- Postmarketing surveillance is ongoing (**Table 3**).

FUTURE TARGETS FOR IMMUNOTHERAPIES IN RHEUMATIC DISEASES

Potential targets for immunologic intervention continue to emerge as our colleagues in the basic sciences work to refine our understanding of the components of immune function and regulation. Cell types and subtypes, cytokines, intermediary pathway proteins, and membrane and cytosolic enzymes and receptors are the focus of ongoing translational research, and include:

- Glucocorticoid receptors specific for anti-inflammatory effects
- Cytokine-directed therapies, including additional anticytokines (IL-6, -12, -23, -15, -17, -18), inhibitory cytokines, and cytokine function blockers
- Cell-specific surface markers or receptors such as second-generation anti–B-cell therapies (eg, atacicept, ofatumumab, ocrelizumab)
- Small-molecule inhibitors of specific intracellular kinases, which activate signaling cascades. Such molecules are more easily manufactured and can be administered orally, offering the potential of more affordable therapies. Those under investigation for the treatment of RA include inhibitors of Janus kinases (JAKs), spleen tyrosine kinase (SyK), and p38 mitogen-activated protein kinases (MAPKs).
- Vaccines against cytokines, costimulatory molecules, and collagen.[87–90]

SUMMARY

For a summary of FDA and common off-label usages of the immunotherapies used in the rheumatic diseases, see **Table 4**. Although most of the available immunotherapies in rheumatology have been developed for RA, an increasing number are being tested for efficacy in the less common autoimmune disorders.

ACKNOWLEDGMENTS

The authors gratefully acknowledge the expert technical assistance provided by Rita Tramell, PhD in the preparation of this article.

REFERENCES

1. Mountz JD, Wu J, Cheng J, et al. Autoimmune disease. A problem of defective apoptosis. Arthritis Rheum 1994;37:1415–20.
2. Pisitkun P, Deane JA, Difilippantonio MJ, et al. Autoreactive B cell responses to RNA-related antigens due to TLR7 gene duplication. Science 2006;312:1669–72.
3. Weyand CM, Goronzy JJ. Pathogenesis of rheumatoid arthritis. Med Clin North Am 1997;81:29–55.
4. Hench PS, Kendall EC. The effect of a hormone of the adrenal cortex (17-hydroxy-11-dehydrocorticosterone; compound E) and of pituitary adrenocorticotropic hormone on rheumatoid arthritis. Proc Staff Meet Mayo Clin 1949;24:181–97.
5. Krane SM. Some molecular mechanisms of glucocorticoid action. Br J Rheumatol 1993;32(Suppl 2):3–5.
6. Haller J, Mikics E, Makara GB. The effects of non-genomic glucocorticoid mechanisms on bodily functions and the central neural system. A critical evaluation of findings. Front Neuroendocrinol 2008;29:273–91.
7. Boldizsar F, Talaber G, Szabo M, et al. Emerging pathways of non-genomic glucocorticoid (GC) signalling in T cells. Immunobiology 2010;215:521–6.
8. Croxtall JD, van Hal PT, Choudhury Q, et al. Different glucocorticoids vary in their genomic and non-genomic mechanism of action in A549 cells. Br J Pharmacol 2002;135:511–9.
9. Lowenberg M, Tuynman J, Bilderbeek J, et al. Rapid immunosuppressive effects of glucocorticoids mediated through Lck and Fyn. Blood 2005;106:1703–10.
10. Gubner R, August S, Ginsberg V. Therapeutic suppression of tissue reactivity. II. Effect of aminopterin in rheumatoid arthritis and psoriasis. Am J Med Sci 1951; 221:176–82.
11. Sajjadi FG, Takabayashi K, Foster AC, et al. Inhibition of TNF-alpha expression by adenosine: role of A3 adenosine receptors. J Immunol 1996;156:3435–42.
12. Rhodes JM, Bartholomew TC, Jewell DP. Inhibition of leucocyte motility by drugs used in ulcerative colitis. Gut 1981;22:642–7.
13. MacDermott RP, Schloemann SR, Bertovich MJ, et al. Inhibition of antibody secretion by 5-aminosalicylic acid. Gastroenterology 1989;96:442–8.
14. Montesinos MC, Yap JS, Desai A, et al. Reversal of the antiinflammatory effects of methotrexate by the nonselective adenosine receptor antagonists theophylline and caffeine: evidence that the antiinflammatory effects of methotrexate are mediated via multiple adenosine receptors in rat adjuvant arthritis. Arthritis Rheum 2000;43:656–63.
15. Nesher G, Mates M, Zevin S. Effect of caffeine consumption on efficacy of methotrexate in rheumatoid arthritis. Arthritis Rheum 2003;48:571–2.
16. Benito-Garcia E, Heller JE, Chibnik LB, et al. Dietary caffeine intake does not affect methotrexate efficacy in patients with rheumatoid arthritis. J Rheumatol 2006;33:1275–81.
17. Dalrymple JM, Stamp LK, O'Donnell JL, et al. Pharmacokinetics of oral methotrexate in patients with rheumatoid arthritis. Arthritis Rheum 2008;58: 3299–308.
18. Maradit-Kremers H, Nicola PJ, Crowson CS, et al. Patient, disease, and therapy-related factors that influence discontinuation of disease-modifying antirheumatic drugs: a population-based incidence cohort of patients with rheumatoid arthritis. J Rheumatol 2006;33:248–55.
19. McConkey B, Amos RS, Durham S, et al. Sulphasalazine in rheumatoid arthritis. Br Med J 1980;280:442–4.

20. Pullar T, Hunter JA, Capell HA. Sulphasalazine in rheumatoid arthritis: a double blind comparison of sulphasalazine with placebo and sodium aurothiomalate. Br Med J (Clin Res Ed) 1983;287:1102–4.
21. Morabito L, Montesinos MC, Schreibman DM, et al. Methotrexate and sulfasalazine promote adenosine release by a mechanism that requires ecto-5'-nucleotidase-mediated conversion of adenine nucleotides. J Clin Invest 1998;101:295–300.
22. Wahl C, Liptay S, Adler G, et al. Sulfasalazine: a potent and specific inhibitor of nuclear factor kappa B. J Clin Invest 1998;101:1163–74.
23. Neal TM, Winterbourn CC, Vissers MC. Inhibition of neutrophil degranulation and superoxide production by sulfasalazine. Comparison with 5-aminosalicylic acid, sulfapyridine and olsalazine. Biochem Pharmacol 1987;36:2765–8.
24. Haagsma CJ, van Riel PL, de Jong AJ, et al. Combination of sulphasalazine and methotrexate versus the single components in early rheumatoid arthritis: a randomized, controlled, double-blind, 52 week clinical trial. Br J Rheumatol 1997;36:1082–8.
25. Roman Aleksandrovich Tkachev (on his 80th birthday). Zh Nevropatol Psikhiatr Im S S Korsakova 1978;78:1880–1 [in Russian].
26. Smolen JS, Kalden JR, Scott DL, et al. Efficacy and safety of leflunomide compared with placebo and sulphasalazine in active rheumatoid arthritis: a double-blind, randomised, multicentre trial. European Leflunomide Study Group. Lancet 1999;353:259–66.
27. Wallace DJ. The history of antimalarials. Lupus 1996;5(Suppl 1):S2–3.
28. Kaufmann AM, Krise JP. Lysosomal sequestration of amine-containing drugs: analysis and therapeutic implications. J Pharm Sci 2007;96:729–46.
29. Fox RI. Mechanism of action of hydroxychloroquine as an antirheumatic drug. Semin Arthritis Rheum 1993;23:82–91.
30. Manzel L, Strekowski L, Ismail FM, et al. Antagonism of immunostimulatory CpG-oligodeoxynucleotides by 4-aminoquinolines and other weak bases: mechanistic studies. J Pharmacol Exp Ther 1999;291:1337–47.
31. Kyburz D, Brentano F, Gay S. Mode of action of hydroxychloroquine in RA-evidence of an inhibitory effect on toll-like receptor signaling. Nat Clin Pract Rheumatol 2006;2:458–9.
32. Lafyatis R, York M, Marshak-Rothstein A. Antimalarial agents: closing the gate on Toll-like receptors? Arthritis Rheum 2006;54:3068–70.
33. Ruiz-Irastorza G, Egurbide MV, Pijoan JI, et al. Effect of antimalarials on thrombosis and survival in patients with systemic lupus erythematosus. Lupus 2006;15:577–83.
34. Siso A, Ramos-Casals M, Bove A, et al. Previous antimalarial therapy in patients diagnosed with lupus nephritis: influence on outcomes and survival. Lupus 2008;17:281–8.
35. Pons-Estel GJ, Alarcon GS, McGwin G Jr, et al. Protective effect of hydroxychloroquine on renal damage in patients with lupus nephritis: LXV, data from a multiethnic US cohort. Arthritis Rheum 2009;61:830–9.
36. Becker-Merok A, Nossent J. Prevalence, predictors and outcome of vascular damage in systemic lupus erythematosus. Lupus 2009;18:508–15.
37. Petri M. Use of hydroxychloroquine to prevent thrombosis in systemic lupus erythematosus and in antiphospholipid antibody-positive patients. Curr Rheumatol Rep 2011;13:77–80.
38. Rand JH, Wu XX, Quinn AS, et al. Hydroxychloroquine protects the annexin A5 anticoagulant shield from disruption by antiphospholipid antibodies: evidence for a novel effect for an old antimalarial drug. Blood 2010;115:2292–9.

39. Ruiz-Irastorza G, Ramos-Casals M, Brito-Zeron P, et al. Clinical efficacy and side effects of antimalarials in systemic lupus erythematosus: a systematic review. Ann Rheum Dis 2010;69:20–8.
40. Marmor MF, Kellner U, Lai TY, et al. Revised recommendations on screening for chloroquine and hydroxychloroquine retinopathy. Ophthalmology 2011;118: 415–22.
41. Fox RI. Mechanism of action of leflunomide in rheumatoid arthritis. J Rheumatol Suppl 1998;53:20–6.
42. Emery P, Breedveld FC, Lemmel EM, et al. A comparison of the efficacy and safety of leflunomide and methotrexate for the treatment of rheumatoid arthritis. Rheumatology (Oxford) 2000;39:655–65.
43. Suissa S, Hudson M, Ernst P. Leflunomide use and the risk of interstitial lung disease in rheumatoid arthritis. Arthritis Rheum 2006;54:1435–9.
44. Stein CM, Pincus T, Yocum D, et al. Combination treatment of severe rheumatoid arthritis with cyclosporine and methotrexate for forty-eight weeks: an open-label extension study. The Methotrexate-Cyclosporine Combination Study Group. Arthritis Rheum 1997;40:1843–51.
45. Gerards AH, Landewe RB, Prins AP, et al. Cyclosporin A monotherapy versus cyclosporin A and methotrexate combination therapy in patients with early rheumatoid arthritis: a double blind randomised placebo controlled trial. Ann Rheum Dis 2003;62:291–6.
46. Marchesoni A, Battafarano N, Arreghini M, et al. Radiographic progression in early rheumatoid arthritis: a 12-month randomized controlled study comparing the combination of cyclosporin and methotrexate with methotrexate alone. Rheumatology (Oxford) 2003;42:1545–9.
47. Hetland ML, Stengaard-Pedersen K, Junker P, et al. Combination treatment with methotrexate, cyclosporine, and intraarticular betamethasone compared with methotrexate and intraarticular betamethasone in early active rheumatoid arthritis: an investigator-initiated, multicenter, randomized, double-blind, parallel-group, placebo-controlled study. Arthritis Rheum 2006;54:1401–9.
48. Eugui EM, Mirkovich A, Allison AC. Lymphocyte-selective antiproliferative and immunosuppressive activity of mycophenolic acid and its morpholinoethyl ester (RS-61443) in rodents. Transplant Proc 1991;23:15–8.
49. Colic M, Stojic-Vukanic Z, Pavlovic B, et al. Mycophenolate mofetil inhibits differentiation, maturation and allostimulatory function of human monocyte-derived dendritic cells. Clin Exp Immunol 2003;134:63–9.
50. Kamanamool N, McEvoy M, Attia J, et al. Efficacy and adverse events of mycophenolate mofetil versus cyclophosphamide for induction therapy of lupus nephritis: systematic review and meta-analysis. Medicine (Baltimore) 2010;89: 227–35.
51. Isenberg D, Appel GB, Contreras G, et al. Influence of race/ethnicity on response to lupus nephritis treatment: the ALMS study. Rheumatology (Oxford) 2010;49: 128–40.
52. Jeurissen ME, Boerbooms AM, van de Putte LB, et al. Influence of methotrexate and azathioprine on radiologic progression in rheumatoid arthritis. A randomized, double-blind study. Ann Intern Med 1991;114:999–1004.
53. Terkeltaub RA. Colchicine update: 2008. Semin Arthritis Rheum 2009;38:411–9.
54. Niel E, Scherrmann JM. Colchicine today. Joint Bone Spine 2006;73:672–8.
55. Chappey ON, Niel E, Wautier JL, et al. Colchicine disposition in human leukocytes after single and multiple oral administration. Clin Pharmacol Ther 1993; 54:360–7.

56. Kloppenburg M, Breedveld FC, Miltenburg AM, et al. Antibiotics as disease modifiers in arthritis. Clin Exp Rheumatol 1993;11(Suppl 8):S113–5.
57. Tilley BC, Alarcon GS, Heyse SP, et al. Minocycline in rheumatoid arthritis. A 48-week, double-blind, placebo-controlled trial. MIRA Trial Group. Ann Intern Med 1995;122:81–9.
58. O'Dell JR, Blakely KW, Mallek JA, et al. Treatment of early seropositive rheumatoid arthritis: a two-year, double-blind comparison of minocycline and hydroxychloroquine. Arthritis Rheum 2001;44:2235–41.
59. Sethi S, Sahani M, Oei LS. ANCA-positive crescentic glomerulonephritis associated with minocycline therapy. Am J Kidney Dis 2003;42:E27–31.
60. Elkayam O, Yaron M, Caspi D. Minocycline-induced autoimmune syndromes: an overview. Semin Arthritis Rheum 1999;28:392–7.
61. Carter JD, Valeriano J, Vasey FB, et al. Refractory neurosarcoidosis: a dramatic response to infliximab. Am J Med 2004;117:277–9.
62. Pettersen JA, Zochodne DW, Bell RB, et al. Refractory neurosarcoidosis responding to infliximab. Neurology 2002;59:1660–1.
63. Pritchard C, Nadarajah K. Tumour necrosis factor alpha inhibitor treatment for sarcoidosis refractory to conventional treatments: a report of five patients. Ann Rheum Dis 2004;63:318–20.
64. Burns JC, Best BM, Mejias A, et al. Infliximab treatment of intravenous immunoglobulin-resistant Kawasaki disease. J Pediatr 2008;153:833–8.
65. Arida A, Fragiadaki K, Giavri E, et al. Anti-TNF agents for Behcet's disease: analysis of published data on 369 patients. Semin Arthritis Rheum 2011;41:61–70.
66. Bartelds GM, Wijbrandts CA, Nurmohamed MT, et al. Clinical response to adalimumab: relationship to anti-adalimumab antibodies and serum adalimumab concentrations in rheumatoid arthritis. Ann Rheum Dis 2007;66:921–6.
67. Bartelds GM, Krieckaert CL, Nurmohamed MT, et al. Development of antidrug antibodies against adalimumab and association with disease activity and treatment failure during long-term follow-up. JAMA 2011;305:1460–8.
68. Askling J, van Vollenhoven RF, Granath F, et al. Cancer risk in patients with rheumatoid arthritis treated with anti-tumor necrosis factor alpha therapies: does the risk change with the time since start of treatment? Arthritis Rheum 2009;60:3180–9.
69. Dass S, Rawstron AC, Vital EM, et al. Highly sensitive B cell analysis predicts response to rituximab therapy in rheumatoid arthritis. Arthritis Rheum 2008;58:2993–9.
70. Chatzidionysiou K, Lie E, Nasonov E, et al. Highest clinical effectiveness of rituximab in autoantibody-positive patients with rheumatoid arthritis and in those for whom no more than one previous TNF antagonist has failed: pooled data from 10 European registries. Ann Rheum Dis 2011;70:1575–80.
71. Keystone E, Fleischmann R, Emery P, et al. Safety and efficacy of additional courses of rituximab in patients with active rheumatoid arthritis: an open-label extension analysis. Arthritis Rheum 2007;56:3896–908.
72. Thurlings RM, Vos K, Gerlag DM, et al. Disease activity-guided rituximab therapy in rheumatoid arthritis: the effects of re-treatment in initial nonresponders versus initial responders. Arthritis Rheum 2008;58:3657–64.
73. Tan CS, Koralnik IJ. Progressive multifocal leukoencephalopathy and other disorders caused by JC virus: clinical features and pathogenesis. Lancet Neurol 2010;9:425–37.
74. Popa C, Leandro MJ, Cambridge G, et al. Repeated B lymphocyte depletion with rituximab in rheumatoid arthritis over 7 yrs. Rheumatology (Oxford) 2007;46:626–30.

75. So A, De ST, Revaz S, et al. A pilot study of IL-1 inhibition by anakinra in acute gout. Arthritis Res Ther 2007;9:R28.
76. Schumacher HR Jr, Sundy JS, Terkeltaub R, et al. Rilonacept (IL-1 Trap) in the prevention of acute gout flares during initiation of urate-lowering therapy: results of a Phase 2 clinical trial. Arthritis Rheum 2012;64(3):876–84.
77. Schlesinger N, Mysler E, Lin HY, et al. Canakinumab reduces the risk of acute gouty arthritis flares during initiation of allopurinol treatment: results of a double-blind, randomised study. Ann Rheum Dis 2011;70:1264–71.
78. So A, De MM, Pikhlak A, et al. Canakinumab for the treatment of acute flares in difficult-to-treat gouty arthritis: results of a multicenter, phase II, dose-ranging study. Arthritis Rheum 2010;62:3064–76.
79. Palmqvist P, Persson E, Conaway HH, et al. IL-6, leukemia inhibitory factor, and oncostatin M stimulate bone resorption and regulate the expression of receptor activator of NF-kappa B ligand, osteoprotegerin, and receptor activator of NF-kappa B in mouse calvariae. J Immunol 2002;169:3353–62.
80. Suzuki M, Hashizume M, Yoshida H, et al. IL-6 and IL-1 synergistically enhanced the production of MMPs from synovial cells by up-regulating IL-6 production and IL-1 receptor I expression. Cytokine 2010;51:178–83.
81. Hashizume M, Uchiyama Y, Horai N, et al. Tocilizumab, a humanized anti-interleukin-6 receptor antibody, improved anemia in monkey arthritis by suppressing IL-6-induced hepcidin production. Rheumatol Int 2010;30:917–23.
82. Genentech I. Highlights of prescribing information: Actemra® (tocilizumab). http://www.gene.com/gene/products/information/actemra/pdf/pi.pdf. Accessed February 26, 2012.
83. Navarra SV, Guzman RM, Gallacher AE, et al. Efficacy and safety of belimumab in patients with active systemic lupus erythematosus: a randomised, placebo-controlled, phase 3 trial. Lancet 2011;377:721–31.
84. Furie R, Petri M, Zamani O, et al. A phase III, randomized, placebo-controlled study of belimumab, a monoclonal antibody that inhibits B lymphocyte stimulator, in patients with systemic lupus erythematosus. Arthritis Rheum 2011;63:3918–30.
85. van Vollenhoven RF, Petri MA, Cervera R, et al. Belimumab in the treatment of systemic lupus erythematosus: high disease activity predictors of response. Ann Rheum Dis Published Online First: 15 February 2012. DOI: 10.1136/annrheumdis-2011-200937.
86. U.S. Food and Drug Administration. FDA approves Benlysta to treat lupus. Available at: http://www.fda.gov/NewsEvents/Newsroom/PressAnnouncements/ucm246489.htm. Accessed February 27, 2012.
87. Semerano L, Assier E, Delavallee L, et al. Kinoid of human tumor necrosis factor-alpha for rheumatoid arthritis. Expert Opin Biol Ther 2011;11:545–50.
88. Delavallee L, Duvallet E, Semerano L, et al. Anti-cytokine vaccination in autoimmune diseases. Swiss Med Wkly 2010;140:w13108.
89. Xue H, Liang F, Liu N, et al. Potent antirheumatic activity of a new DNA vaccine targeted to B7-2/CD28 costimulatory signaling pathway in autoimmune arthritis. Hum Gene Ther 2011;22:65–76.
90. Zimmerman DH, Taylor P, Bendele A, et al. CEL-2000: a therapeutic vaccine for rheumatoid arthritis arrests disease development and alters serum cytokine/chemokine patterns in the bovine collagen type II induced arthritis in the DBA mouse model. Int Immunopharmacol 2010;10:412–21.

Immunotherapies in Neurologic Disorders

Donna Graves, MD, Steven Vernino, MD, PhD*

KEYWORDS

- Multiple sclerosis • Neuromyelitis optica • Myasthenia gravis
- Paraneoplastic neurologic disorders
- Intravenous immunoglobulin • Autoimmune encephalopathy

Key Points

- Immunotherapy is a major part of the current practice of neurology.

- Over the past 2 decades, major advances in immunotherapy for multiple sclerosis and neuromyelitis optica have greatly altered the course of these diseases.

- Several autoimmune neuromuscular disorders are caused by antibodies against membrane proteins. These disorders can now be definitively diagnosed and treated.

- Immunotherapy for inflammatory disorders of muscle and nerve are effective in stabilizing or reversing the clinical course.

- In recent years, a group of immunotherapy-responsive brain disorders have been identified; these autoimmune encephalopathies represent a potentially treatable cause of subacute dementia and seizures.

INTRODUCTION

Many neurologic diseases are treatable. Autoimmune inflammatory conditions account for many neurologic disorders, especially those that have a subacute or relapsing/remitting clinical course. Normally, components of the nervous system are immunologically privileged; for example, the central nervous system (CNS) is protected by the blood-brain barrier. When the immune system loses tolerance, the nervous system may become a target for autoimmunity. Neurologic autoimmunity can affect any part of the nervous system (brain, spinal cord, nerves, or muscle) and may have several different immune pathophysiologies. Some disorders result from frank inflammation in the target tissue (eg, myelitis or myositis). Other disorders are caused by pathogenic autoantibodies that have a functional effect on neuronal

---

Department of Neurology and Neurotherapeutics, UT Southwestern Medical Center, 5323 Harry Hines Boulevard, Dallas, TX 75390-9036, USA
* Corresponding author.
E-mail address: Steven.Vernino@utsouthwestern.edu

Med Clin N Am 96 (2012) 497–523
doi:10.1016/j.mcna.2012.05.001
medical.theclinics.com

function (eg, myasthenia gravis [MG] or autoimmune autonomic ganglionopathy [AAG]). Cell-mediated autoimmunity is the culprit in other disorders (eg, paraneoplastic cerebellar degeneration). Many common immune-mediated neurologic disorders (such as multiple sclerosis [MS]) have more complex pathophysiology, which is still not fully elucidated. A complete review of all the known primary neuroimmunologic disorders is beyond the scope of this review. Furthermore, the nervous system may be secondarily involved by systemic autoimmune inflammatory conditions, such as vasculitis, lupus, and sarcoidosis. Immunotherapy for those conditions generally follows the guidelines for the systemic illness, discussed elsewhere.

Increasingly, neurologists need to be able to diagnose and identify immune-mediated disorders. To treat these disorders, neurologists also must be comfortable using corticosteroids, immunosuppression, and other immunomodulatory therapies. This facet of neurology practice has evolved rapidly over the past 10 years. Options for immunotherapy of demyelinating disorders in particular have increased tremendously to include traditional immunosuppressants as well as novel biologicals developed to specifically target the immune pathophysiology of MS. Part of the increased use of immunotherapies in neurology is related to improved recognition of a broader spectrum of immune-mediated neurologic disorders as well as the development and application of novel therapeutics. Because autoimmune neurologic disorders are so diverse, specific evidence from randomized controlled trials is limited for most of the immunotherapies. The neuroimmunologic disorders can be broadly divided into 4 groups: demyelinating disorders (MS and neuromyelitis optica), antibody-mediated neuromuscular disorders (such as MG), inflammatory neuromuscular disorders (such as Guillain-Barré syndrome and dermatomyositis), and autoimmune encephalopathies. This review provides an overview of the immunotherapies currently used for neurologic disorders.

MS

MS is a leading cause of neurologic disability in young adults, affecting approximately 300,000 Americans and more than 1 million individuals worldwide. Although not typically a fatal disease, MS can lead to significant disability and have a devastating social impact through loss of employment, dependency on caregivers, and social isolation.[1] MS is an autoimmune disease affecting the CNS, characterized by focal areas of demyelination and inflammation as well as neurodegeneration.[2] The disease most commonly affects young women in their 20s and 30s but may begin earlier in childhood or later in life. The typical clinical course is one characterized by acute attacks of new neurologic symptoms followed by period of disease inactivity, namely relapsing-remitting MS (RRMS), which accounts for 85% of cases of MS. Management of MS must encompass both acute treatment of relapses as well as long-term preventative therapy.

Relapses are typically defined as new or worsening symptoms lasting at least 24 hours and not caused by another medical problem, such as infection, fever, or heat sensitivity. Relapses pose a significant risk of development of sustained disability and therefore appropriate management is imperative. Lublin and colleagues[3] showed that 42% of patients had a residual neurologic deficit and 28% had residual increase in disability persisting 2 months after an exacerbation.

IMMUNOTHERAPY FOR MS RELAPSES

Corticosteroids remain the first-line treatment of acute exacerbations. There is no consensus regarding optimal dosing; however, a regimen of 1000 mg intravenous

(IV) methylprednisolone daily for 3 to 5 days is considered standard. It is typically believed that oral corticosteroids are equal in efficacy, but the key is that one must use high-dose steroids. Many studies have evaluated the optimal dosing and route of administration without clear consensus.[4]

Plasma exchange (PE) may offer additional benefit for patients who do not respond adequately to steroids alone. A double-blind, sham-controlled, cross-over study from Mayo Clinic evaluated the use of PE in patients with acute relapses of CNS inflammatory demyelinating diseases who had failed to have significant improvement with corticosteroids. Forty-two percent of patients showed moderate or greater improvements in their neurologic disability after PE.[5]

IV immunoglobulin (IVIG) is commonly used in neurologic practice, but its usefulness in MS is speculative. Several studies have been performed evaluating the use of IVIG in the treatment of acute relapses; however, these have shown mixed results.[6,7] During pregnancy, the rate of acute MS exacerbations decreases, especially in the second and third trimester. However, in the months after pregnancy, relapse rates increase significantly.[8] IVIG is frequently used post partum to prevent acute relapses.[9]

DISEASE-MODIFYING IMMUNOTHERAPY FOR MS

The past 2 decades brought forth the approval of 7 preventative therapies for MS. The first disease-modifying therapy (DMT), interferon (IFN) β-1b (Betaseron), was approved in 1993. Since that time, we have seen the approval of 3 additional injectable therapies: glatiramer acetate (Copaxone), intramuscular (IM) IFN-β-1a (Avonex), and subcutaneous (SC) IFN-β-1b (Rebif). Mitoxantrone (Novantrone) is a chemotherapeutic agent that was approved for use in MS in 2002. More recently added to our armamentarium is natalizumab (Tysabri) and fingolimod (Gilenya). The mechanism of action, dosing, potential adverse reactions, and recommendations for monitoring for each of these agents are summarized in **Table 1**.

Although the disease course of MS is characterized by multiple attacks affecting different regions of the brain and spinal cord, many experts prefer to diagnose MS and implement treatment as early as possible. The term clinically isolated syndrome (CIS) has emerged to define the first demyelinating attack that is suggestive of MS, typically optic neuritis, transverse myelitis, or a brainstem syndrome. For some patients, this is an isolated event, but many others go on to have subsequent attacks and develop RRMS. Studies have shown that for patients with an initial demyelinating event that have even 1 lesion characteristic of MS on brain magnetic resonance imaging (MRI), the risk of having a second attack and thereby meeting diagnostic criteria for MS is 88%.[10] Several studies have been completed to evaluate the use of the DMTs in CIS (**Table 2**).[11–14] To date, only the first-line injectable therapies have been studied.

RRMS

RRMS is characterized by acute attacks of new or worsening symptoms followed by periods of recovery and disease. Because it is the most common form of MS, most evidence exists for the use of preventative therapies in RRMS.

First-generation injectable DMTs, including IFN-β-1b, IFN-β-1a, and glatiramer acetate, have more similarities than differences. All these agents have been shown to reduce the number of exacerbations by approximately 30%. In addition, these medications reduce the risk of new MRI activity. IFN-β-1a IM/SC was also shown to reduce the risk of sustained disability progression. Details from the pivotal trials leading to the approval of each of these therapies are shown in **Table 3**,[15–22] and

Table 1
DMTs for MS

DMT	Dose/Route	Mode of Action	Side Effects	Monitoring Laboratory Tests	Pregnancy Category
IFN-β-1a (Avonex)	30 μg IM weekly	Promotes T_H1 to T_H2 shift	Flulike symptoms, depression, thyroid dysfunction, liver enzyme abnormalities	CBC, LFTs, TSH	C
IFN-β-1a (Rebif)	22 μg or 44 μg SC 3 times a week	Promotes T_H1 to T_H2 shift	Skin site reactions, flulike symptoms, depression, thyroid dysfunction, liver enzyme abnormalities	CBC, LFTs, TSH	C
IFN-β-1b (Betaseron/ Extavia)	250 μg SC every other day	Decreases T_H1 and T_H17 production, increases IL-10 production, decreases MHC II expression	Skin site reactions, flulike symptoms, depression, thyroid dysfunction, liver enzyme abnormalities	CBC, LFTs, TSH	C
Glatiramer acetate (Copaxone)	20 mg SC once a day	Promotes T_H2 suppressor cells, possibly promotes brain-derived neurotrophic factor	Skin site reactions, immediate postinjection reaction, lipoatrophy	None	B
Mitoxantrone (Novantrone)	12 mg/m^2 IV every 3 mo with a lifetime cumulative dose of no more than 140 mg/m^2; frequency may vary	Topoisomerase-2 inhibitor, which leads to intercalation of DNA and decreased lymphocyte production	Hair loss, cardiotoxicity, leukemia, infertility, increased risk of infections, leukopenia, anemia, nausea, vomiting, thrombocytopenia	CBC, LFTs, U/A, LVEF	X
Natalizumab (Tysabri)	300 mg IV every 28 d	Blocks VLA-4 interaction with VCAM1, thereby preventing leukocyte extravasation across the BBB	Transient headache fatigue, recurrent UTIs, PML, hypersensitivity reaction	CBC, LFTs	C
Fingolimod (Gilenya)	0.5 mg orally once a day	S1P receptor modulator, which leads to the sequestration of lymphocytes within the lymph nodes	First-degree AV block with first dose, bradycardia, macular edema, hypertension, shingles, pelvic floor dysfunction in selected patients, skin cancer, back pain	CBC, LFTs, OCT, PFTs	C

Abbreviations: AV, atrioventricular; BBB, blood-brain barrier; CBC, complete blood count; IL, interleukin; LFT, liver function test; LVEF, left ventricular ejection fraction; MHC, major histocompatibility complex; OCT, optical coherence tomography; PFT, pulmonary function test; PML, progressive multifocal leukoencephalopathy; S1P, sphingosine-1 phosphate; TSH, thyroid-stimulating hormone; U/A, urine analysis; UTI, urinary tract infection; VCAM1, vascular cell adhesion molecule 1;

Table 2 The use of DMTs in CIS		
Trial	**Drug**	**Result**
ETOMS[11]	IFN-β-1b	Conversion risk at 2 y was 34% with IFN-β-Ia SC vs 45% with placebo
CHAMPS[12]	IFN-β-Ia IM	Conversion risk at 2 y was 21% with IFN-β-Ia IM vs 39% with placebo
BENEFIT[13]	IFN-β-1b	Conversion risk at 2 y 28% with IFN-β-1b vs 45% with placebo
PreCISe[14]	Glatiramer acetate	Conversion risk at 2 y was 25% with glatiramer acetate vs 43% with placebo

studies comparing the various DMTs are shown in **Table 4**.[23–27] In general, the injectable DMTs are safe and well tolerated. Because of the risk of hematologic abnormalities and hepatotoxicity, a blood count and liver function tests should be monitored with the IFN therapies.

Another issue to consider with the IFNs is the production of neutralizing antibodies (NAbs), which may negate the effect of these medications. The issue of NAbs and their practicality is controversial; however, experts suggest that both the NAb titer and clinical status of the patient should be considered in the decision regarding the impact of the presence of NAbs on changing DMTs. They also suggested reevaluation of the NAbs status before making a change in therapy unless patients were clearly performing poorly clinically.[28]

Natalizumab (Tysabri) is a monoclonal antibody that binds to very late antigen 4 and blocks its binding with vascular cell adhesion molecule 1, thereby inhibiting the autoreactive T cells from crossing over the blood-brain barrier to enter the CNS. In the AFFIRM pivotal trial using natalizumab as monotherapy, there was a 67% relative relapse reduction over the 2 years of the study compared with placebo. Furthermore, an 83% reduction in new and enlarging T2 lesions and 92% reduction in new enhancing lesions was seen compared with the placebo-treated group.[19] The SENTINEL study evaluated the use of natalizumab in combination with IM IFN-β-1a compared with an active comparator arm using IM IFN-β-1a as monotherapy. This study found a 54% reduction in annualized relapse rate (ARR) as well as an 83% reduction in the number of new/enlarging T2 lesions and 89% reduction in the number of gadolinium enhancing lesions.[20] Two cases of progressive multifocal leukoencephalopathy (PML) were noted during this trial, which led to the voluntary withdrawal of natalizumab from the market in 2005. Since its reintroduction in 2006, 193 cases of PML have been reported from the more than 92,000 patients who have now been treated with this medication (update as of September 30, 2011).

Fingolimod (Gilenya) is the first oral DMT approved for RRMS. It works as a sphingosine-1 phosphate (S1P) receptor modulator, which leads to the sequestration of lymphocytes within the lymph nodes. In the 24-month phase III FTY720 Research Evaluating Effects of Daily Oral Therapy in Multiple Sclerosis (FREEDOMS) trial comparing placebo with oral fingolimod at doses of 1.25 mg and the 0.5 mg daily dose now approved by the US Food and Drug Administration (FDA), there was a significant reduction in ARR with both doses of fingolimod (0.16 at 1.25 mg and 0.18 at 0.5 mg) compared with placebo (0.40), which represented a relative reduction of 60% and 54%, respectively. Furthermore, fingolimod also reduced the risk of disability progression with a probability of disability progression (confirmed after 3 months) of 17.7% at

Table 3
Pivotal studies for DMTs

DMT	Pivotal Study	Number of Patients	Treatment Arms		Results
IFN-β-1b (Betaseron/Extavia)	The IFNB Multiple Sclerosis Study Group[15]	372	IFN-β-1b 250 mg IFN-β-1b 50 mg Placebo	ARR 0.84 1.17 1.27	Time to first relapse 296 d 180 d 153 d
Glatiramer acetate (Copaxone)	Johnson et al[17]	251	Glatiramer acetate 2.0 mg daily Placebo	ARR 0.59 0.84	Time to first relapse 198 d 287 d
IFN-β-la IM (Avonex)	Jacobs et al[16]	301	IFN-β-la IM 30 μg weekly Placebo	ARR 0.61 0.9	% with EDSS progression 21.90% 34.90%
IFN-β-la SC (Rebif)	PRISMS[18]	560	IFN-β-la 44 mcg SC 3 x w IFN-β-la 22 mcg SC 3 x w Placebo	ARR 0.87 0.91 1.28	Time of first relapse 9.6 mo 7.6 mo 4.5 mo
Natalizumab (Tysabri)	AFFIRM[19]	942	NTZ 300 mg 4 wks Placebo	ARR 0.26 0.81	% with EDSS progression 17% 29%
	SENTINEL[20]	1171	NTZ 300 mg every 4 wks + IFN β-1a IM 30 mcg weekly IFN-β-la IM 30 mcg weekly	0.38 0.82	23% 29%
Fingolimod (Gilenya)	FREEDOMS[21]	1033	FTY 1.25 mg daily FTY 0.25 mg daily Placebo	ARR 0.16 0.18 0.4	% with EDSS progression 16.60% 17.70% 24.10%
	TRANSFORMS[22]	1153	FTY 1.25 mg daily FTY 0.5 mg daily IFN-β-la IM 30 μg weekly	ARR 0.2 0.16 0.33	

Abbreviations: ARR, annualized relapse rate; EDSS, expanded disability scale score.

Table 4
Trials comparing DMTs

Trial	DMTs Compared	Number of Patients	Duration	Result	References
EVIDENCE	IFN-β-1a IM vs IFN-β-1a SC	677	24-wk randomized treatment phase; 48-wk follow-up	IFN-β-1a SC 75% relapse free 48% no new/enlarging T2 lesions IFN-β-1a IM 63% relapse free 33% no new/enlarging T2 lesions	Panitch et al[23]
INCOMIN	IFN-β-1b SC vs IFN-β-1a IM	188	24 mo	IFN-β-1b SC 51% relapse free 55% no new/enlarging T2 lesions IFN-β-1a IM 36% relapse free 26% no new/enlarging T2 lesions	Durelli et al[24]
REGARD	IFN-β-1a SC vs glatiramer acetate	764	96 wk	No difference in time to first relapse *Secondary outcomes* No difference in number of T2 active lesions Number of glutamic acid decarboxylase-enhancing lesions was significantly less in the IFN-β-1a SC group	Mikol et al[25]
BEYOND	IFN-β-1b SC vs glatiramer acetate	2244	2 y	No difference between relapse risk: ARR = 0.36, IFN-β-1b SC 250 μg ARR = 0.33, IFN-β-1b SC 500 μg ARR = 0.34, GA SC 20 mg	O'Connor et al[26]
BECOME	IFN-β-1b SC vs glatiramer acetate	75	2 y	No difference in total number of enhancing and new nonenhancing T2 lesions.	Cadavid et al[27]

the 0.5-mg dose and 16.6% at the 1.25-mg dose compared with 24.1% with placebo. Almost 90% of patients receiving fingolimod, at either dose, were free of enhancing lesions over the course of 2 years and approximately 50% were free of new or enlarging T2 lesions.[21] The Trial Assessing Injectable Interferon Versus FTY720 Oral in RRMS (TRANSFORMS) trial comparing fingolimod with IM IFN-β-1a showed a 52% relative reduction in ARR in the patients treated with 0.5 mg fingolimod versus IFN. This study showed a similar beneficial effect on MRI markers compared with IFN-β-1a; however, there was no statistically significant difference in the disability progression between the fingolimod and IFN-β-1a groups.[22]

Mitoxantrone (Novantrone) inhibits topoisomerase-2, causing intercalation of DNA and thereby preventing lymphocyte proliferation. In 2002, the FDA approved mitoxantrone for use in rapidly worsening relapsing MS and secondary progressive MS (SPMS). Several studies have shown clear benefit of this medication in reducing relapse rates and disability; however, concerns regarding secondary lymphoid cancers and cardiotoxicity have led to decreased use of this medication.[29]

SPMS

After presenting with a pattern of RRMS early in the disease course, many patients go on to develop fewer acute relapses and over time develop a more insidious progression of neurologic decline. This stage is referred to as SPMS, and approximately 60% of patients progress to this stage within 2 decades from onset of disease.[30]

In a randomized study of 194 patients with worsening RRMS and SPMS treated with mitoxantrone or placebo, patients treated with mitoxantrone (12 mg/m^2) showed a benefit in disability, ambulation, and relapses at the 24-month end point.[31] The use of IFN-β-1b or IFN-β-1a for patients with SPMS has shown mixed results.

PRIMARY PROGRESSIVE MS

Approximately 10% of patients with MS have a disease course that is progressive from onset without relapses or remissions, termed primary progressive MS (PPMS). Typically, these patients present with insidious onset of asymmetric leg weakness or gait imbalance. Diagnosis requires 1 year of disease progression as well as supportive findings from imaging or cerebrospinal fluid (CSF) studies.[28] There are no FDA-approved therapies for PPMS and to date no study has shown clear benefit of DMTs for this group of patients. Post-hoc analysis from the PROMiSe study evaluating the use of glatiramer acetate in PPMS showed slowed clinical progression in a subset of male patients who displayed more rapid deterioration before study entry; however, the study failed to reach its primary end point of delay in sustained disability overall.[32] Rituximab (a monoclonal antibody directed against CD20+ B cells) was studied in a randomized placebo-controlled study in PPMS. Over the 96-week trial, no significant difference was found in the primary end point of time to disability progression.[33]

PEDIATRIC MS

Although MS is typically thought of as a disease of young adults, it is increasingly recognized in childhood, with up to 10% of cases occurring before the age of 18 years. There are no FDA-approved medications for the treatment of MS in pediatrics; however, each of the DMTs has been studied in pediatric cohorts as well. MS can have a significant impact on physical functioning, cognition, and overall quality of life even at this early stage, and it is imperative that preventative therapies be used even in young patients.[34]

NEUROMYELITIS OPTICA OR DEVIC DISEASE

Eugène Devic and his student Fernand Gault first described *neuromyélite optique* (neuromyelitis optica [NMO]) in the nineteenth century, a disease characterized by severe acute transverse myelitis and optic neuritis. For years, the definition of NMO was restricted to fulminant cases of transverse myelitis and optic neuritis occurring simultaneously or close to one another, and many believed the disease to be a variant of MS. It is now recognized that NMO is a relapsing disease that is distinct from MS. NMO carries a unique pathophysiology and different clinical, imaging, and CSF characteristics from those seen in MS. It is critical to distinguish NMO from MS because NMO requires different treatment approaches.[35] The discovery of NMO IgG, an autoantibody that binds to the water channel aquaporin 4, has helped to distinguish NMO from other autoimmune disorders of the CNS. It is now recognized that there is a spectrum of disorders that share similarities with NMO, referred to as NMO spectrum disorders (NMOSD, **Box 1**). A progressive course as seen in later stages of MS is rare in NMO. Instead, disability is driven by clinical relapses. Therefore, relapse prevention is key to NMO management because most patients who remain relapse-free remain neurologically stable.[35]

NMO relapses are characteristically severe, marked by complete vision loss or profound motor and sensory dysfunction resulting from extensive spinal cord lesions. Without treatment, more than 50% of patients are functionally blind or require assistance for ambulation because of recurrent attacks.[36] Therefore, exacerbations require prompt recognition and treatment of these acute events.

Corticosteroids, despite the lack of evidence-based studies, are typically considered as a first-line therapy for acute relapses of NMO. Solumedrol is typically administered as 1 g IV for 3 to 5 days with or without an oral taper. Studies have shown that 80% of patients with NMO respond to short courses of high-dose steroids.[37]

PE, as discussed earlier, can have a dramatic impact on severe acute CNS demyelinating attacks that have been refractory to corticosteroids. Studies support the use of PE in NMO as well. Given the humoral mechanisms involved in NMO, one would expect PE to be most effective in this disease. Watanabe and colleagues[38] reported moderate improvements in 3 of 6 patients with NMO treated with PE after having no

---

Box 1
NMO Spectrum Disorder

NMO

Incomplete/partial forms of NMO

    Single or recurrent longitudinally extensive transverse myelitis (LETM)

    Recurrent optic neuritis with negative brain MRI

Asian optic-spinal MS

Optic neuritis or LETM associated with coexisting systemic autoimmune disease

Optic neuritis or LETM associated with distinct neuroimaging patterns such as hypothalamic lesions or periependymal brain stem lesions

Adapted from Wingerchuk DM, Lennon VA, Lucchinetti CF, et al. The spectrum of neuromyelitis optica. Lancet Neurol 2007;6(9):805–15.

response to high-dose IV methylprednisolone after an acute exacerbation. Furthermore, these patients began to experience recovery after only 1 or 2 exchanges, showing the pathogenetic role of the humoral immune system in NMO and the need for early intervention. In another study of 4 patients with NMO in the midst of an acute exacerbation and refractory to high-dose steroids, PE resulted in improvement in all patients by 6-month follow-up.[39] The use of PE early in an acute exacerbation of NMO, often in conjunction with the use of steroids, is now considered first-line therapy.

There are no FDA-approved preventative therapies for NMO, and the rarity of this disease makes this task difficult. However, several medications seem to be effective in the treatment of this disease (**Table 5**). The European Federation of Neurologic Societies recently released guidelines regarding the diagnosis and management of NMO (**Table 6**).[40] Many patients with NMO are initially mistakenly diagnosed with MS. It is critical to recognize NMO as a distinct entity, because the DMTs used in the treatment of MS are not effective in the treatment of NMO and many of the DMTs can be harmful. Several case reports have shown that IFN-β can result in more frequent and severe exacerbations in patients with NMO.[41–44] In a case report of a woman initially diagnosed with MS, IFN-β-1a was shown to dramatically increase aquaporin 4 antibody titers, which correlated with relapses of her disease. Her diagnosis was revised, and antibody titers decreased after initiation of methotrexate and prednisolone therapy. In another study of 26 patients with NMO receiving either immunosuppressive (cyclophosphamide, mitoxantrone, or azathioprine [AZA]) or DMT (IFN), patients treated with DMT experienced shorter relapse-free periods than those treated with immunosuppressants (mean 9.0 vs 40.2 months; $P = .0001$).[45]

Azathioprine (Imuran) is a purine antagonist that inhibits DNA and RNA synthesis that has been used in the treatment of a variety of autoimmune diseases. In a retrospective chart review performed at the Mayo Clinic, 99 patients with either NMO (n = 86) or NMOSD (n = 13) who were treated with AZA were identified. Seventy patients were included in the study and found to have a decrease in ARR from 2.18 before AZA to 0.64 after initiation of AZA. A dosing regimen of at least 2.0 mg/kg/d was associated with the lowest ARR, and an increase in mean corpuscular volume of more than 5 fL was needed to reduce the ARR.[41] A prospective study of 7 newly diagnosed patients with NMO treated with AZA and prednisone showed significant improvements in disability (average Expanded Disability Status Scale [EDSS] score 8.2 at baseline and 4.0 at 18-month follow-up). Furthermore, no patient had an acute relapse or new symptoms during the 18-month follow-up.[46,47]

Bichuetti and colleagues evaluated 36 patients with NMO and compared treatment with AZA (n = 29) versus other treatments including IFN-β (n = 2), methotrexate 7.5 mg weekly (n = 1), cyclophosphamide (n = 2), prednisone (n = 1), and IVIG (n = 1). Patients receiving AZA had the lowest ARR at 0.6, compared with 1.5 in the other treatment group and 2.1 in the pretreatment groups. The mean disability remained unchanged (EDSS score 4.2) in the AZA group but increased in the other group (4.2 before treatment to 6.5 after treatment).[48]

Mycophenolate mofetil (MMF) (Cellcept) is a selective noncompetitive inhibitor of inosine 5-monophosphate dehydrogenase and thereby inhibits de novo synthesis of guanine ribonucleotide and results in T-cell and B-cell depletion. Although MMF is widely used as a preventative therapy for NMO and many experts consider it first-line treatment, evidence-based studies regarding its use are limited.[49] A recent study, evaluating the use of MMF in the treatment of 24 patients with NMO or NMOSD, found a positive effect on relapse rate and disability independent of treatment duration or addition of corticosteroid therapy.[50]

Rituximab (Rituxan) is a humanized monoclonal antibody that binds to CD20 antigen on the surface of pre-B and mature B lymphocytes and results in apoptosis of B cells. This therapy is approved for treatment of B-cell lymphoma, but is increasingly used as an immunotherapeutic agent to treat disorders associated with humoral autoimmunity. Cree and colleagues[51] performed an open-label, prospective study of 8 patients with NMO who had been refractory to other therapies. Patients were treated with rituximab at a dose of 375 mg/m^2 weekly for 4 weeks. Six of 8 patients remained relapse free over a 12-month follow-up period. The median EDSS score decreased from 7.5 (before treatment) to 5.5 (after treatment). In a larger, retrospective study of 25 patients with NMO, rituximab was found to lower the median ARR from 1.7 before treatment to 0 after initiation of therapy. Varying treatment regimens were used, but most commonly a regimen of either 375 mg/m^2 weekly for 4 weeks or 2 doses of 1000 mg given at 2-week intervals was used.[52] The number of circulating CD19+ B cells should be monitored, and redosing is recommended when levels recover to more than 1%.

Mitoxantrone (Novantrone) has been evaluated in a small prospective study of patients with NMO and was associated with both clinical and radiographic improvements.[53] Another study by Kim and colleagues[54] showed disability scores improved in 18 of 20 (90%) patients with NMO, with an improvement of 1 or more points on the EDSS in 12 of 18 (60%). Both studies suggest a need for induction of treatment with 6 monthly infusions, as relapses were typically seen when an induction of only 3 months was used.

Cyclophosphamide (Cytoxan) is an alkylating chemotherapeutic agent that leads to cross-linking of DNA and apoptosis of rapidly dividing cells, such as leukocytes. Studies involving the use of cyclophosphamide in NMO are largely limited to case reports showing its use in patients with NMO associated with other autoimmune diseases such as systemic lupus erythematosus and Sjögren syndrome.[55,56] Mok and colleagues[57] describe a single case of a patient with lupus-related NMO treated successfully with cyclophosphamide that had otherwise been refractory to IVIG, MMF, tacrolimus, and rituximab.

MG AND OTHER ANTIBODY-MEDIATED NEUROMUSCULAR DISORDERS

Acquired MG is an autoimmune disorder of the neuromuscular junction. The pathophysiology of MG has been firmly established: autoantibodies specific for the nicotinic acetylcholine receptor (AChR) interfere with synaptic transmission between the motor nerve and muscle. This situation leads to the characteristic clinical features of fatigable weakness. Based on this understanding of MG, several other neuromuscular disorders have been identified as antibody-mediated disorders (**Table 7**). Clinical features coupled with neurophysiologic and serologic testing allow the clinician to make the diagnosis of MG, Lambert-Eaton syndrome (LES), autoimmune neuromyotonia (NMT), or autoimmune autonomic ganglionopathy (AAG). Because these disorders are associated with reversible changes in synaptic function, the prognosis for improvement is generally good.

Occasionally, symptomatic management is sufficient. However, most patients with these disorders require immunotherapy aimed at reducing the levels of pathogenic antibodies. The approach to treatment of the various antibody-mediated disorders is similar and largely based on studies in patients with MG. In the acute setting, treatments that remove pathogenic antibodies or modulate the antibody response are effective in producing clinical improvement lasting several weeks. PE and IVIG seem to be equally effective in improving muscle strength in patients with MG.[58–60]

Table 5
Summary of studies regarding immunosuppressive therapies in NMO

Medication	Patients (n)	Type of Study	Follow-Up (mo)	Dosing Regimen	Results	Other Notable Features
AZA						
Costanzi et al,[46] 2011	99	Retrospective, chart review	22 (median)	No standard dosing regimen	Median ARR decreased from 2.18 (pre-AZA) to 0.64 (post-AZA); EDSS did not change	52 patients treated with prednisone during the study
Mandler et al,[47] 1998	7	Prospective	18 (mean)	2 mg/kg/d + prednisone 1 mg/kg/d	EDSS improved from 8.2 at baseline to 4.0 at 18 mo	Baseline EDSS was taken within months of an acute exacerbation
Bichuetti et al,[48] 2010	36	Retrospective, chart review	47.2 (mean)	No standard regimen; mean AZA dosing 2 mg/kg/d	ARR decreased from 2.1 to 0.6 (AZA) or 1.5 (other treatments)	Undisclosed number were also treated with prednisone Other treatment group was diverse
Mycophenolate mofetil						
Jacob et al,[50] 2009	24	Retrospective, chart review	28 (median)	No standard dosing; median dose 2000 mg/d	Median ARR improved from 1.3 to 0.09 91% of patients had EDSS stabilize or improve	9 patients received concomitant prednisone
Rituximab						
Jacob et al,[52] 2008	25	Retrospective, multicenter review	19 (median)	375 mg/m² weekly for 4 wk (n = 18) or 1000 mg at 2-wk interval for 2 doses (n = 4)	Median ARR improved from 1.7 (range 0.5–5) to 0 (range 0–3.2) Disability stabilized or improved in 20/25 patients (80%)	5 patients had concomitant treatment with prednisone or AZA 20% of patients reported infections

Cree et al,[51] 2005	8	Open-label prospective	12 (mean)	375 mg/m² weekly for 4 wk or 1000 mg × 2 doses at a 2-wk interval	6 of 8 patients remained relapse free over an average follow-up of 12 mo. Median EDSS 7.5 (before treatment) and 5.5 (after treatment)	Previous treatment with immunomodulatory therapies (n = 6), AZA (n = 3), mitoxantrone (n = 1)
Mitoxantrone						
Weinstock-Guttman et al,[53] 2006	5	Prospective	24	12 mg/m² monthly for 3 mo or 6 mo	Mean ARR decreased from 2.4 to 0.4 Trend toward improvement in EDSS from 4.40 to 2.25 at 2-y follow-up	2 of 5 patients experienced relapses after a 3-mo treatment so the protocol was later changed to 6 mo
Kim et al,[54] 2011	20	Retrospective, multicenter review	17 (median)	12 mg/m² monthly for 3 mo or 6 mo	Median ARR decreased from 2.8 to 0.7 50% of patients were relapse free EDSS improved from 5.6 to 4.4	2 patients had persistent neutropenia

Abbreviations: AZA, azathioprine; EDSS, Expanded Disability Status Scale score.

Table 6
European Federation of Neurological Societies panel recommendations for preventative management of NMO

	Drug Name	Regimen
First-line therapy		
	Azathioprine	Oral 2.5–3 mg/kg/d
Plus	Prednisolone	Oral 1 mg/kg/d, tapered when azathoprine becomes effective (after 2–3 mo)
OR		
	Rituximab	Option 1: IV 375 mg/m² weekly for 4 wk (lymphoma protocol) Option 2: 1000 mg infused twice, with a 2-wk interval between the infusions (rheumatoid arthritis protocol) Options 1 and 2 reinfusion after 6–12 mo; however, optimal treatment duration unknown
Second-line therapy	Alphabetical order	
	Cyclophosphamide	IV 7–25 mg/kg/ every month over a period of 6 mo, especially considered in case of association with systemic lupus erythematosus/Sjögren syndrome
OR		
	Mitoxantrone	IV 12 mg/m² monthly for 6 mo, followed by 12 mg/m² every 3 mo for 9 mo
OR		
	Mycophenolate mofetil	By mouth 1–3 g per day
Other therapies Escalation therapy	IVIG, methotrexate	
AND	Intermittent PE	

Data from Sellner J, Boggild M, Clanet M, et al. EFNS guidelines on diagnosis and management of neuromyelitis optica. Eur J Neurol 2010;17(8):1019–32.

Table 7
Antibody-mediated neuromuscular disorders

	Clinical Symptoms	Associated Antibody
MG	Fatigable weakness, ptosis, diplopia	Muscle AChR MUSK
LES	Proximal weakness, dry mouth	VGCC
NMT	Muscle twitching and stiffness	VGKC complex
AAG	Orthostatic hypotension, constipation, gastroparesis, heat intolerance	Ganglionic AChR

Abbreviations: MUSK, muscle-specific kinase; VGCC, voltage-gated calcium channel; VGKC, voltage-gated potassium channel.

Data from Vernino S. Autoimmune and paraneoplastic channelopathies. Neurotherapeutics 2007;4(2):305–14.

In case series, these acute treatments are also effective for the other antibody-mediated neuromuscular disorders.[61–63] Typically, a course of PE consists of 3 to 6 exchanges administered either on consecutive or alternate days. The optimal treatment using IVIG has not been established for MG. Common dosing protocols include 0.4 g/kg/dose administered on 5 consecutive days or 2 g/kg divided over 2 to 4 days. PE and IVIG are effective, but costly, short-term treatments.

For chronic management of these antibody-mediated disorders, a variety of immunotherapeutic agents are used. Immunotherapy for MG is reviewed in detail here. Treatments for the other antibody-mediated disorders are similar and reviewed elsewhere.[61,64–66]

Corticosteroids, given as daily or alternate-day oral therapy, are an effective treatment, but therapy may be limited by the frequent development of side effects over time. High initial doses of corticosteroids can transiently worsen MG. Therefore, IV pulse steroids are not commonly used, and the dose of oral steroids (prednisone) usually starts low and increases gradually until symptoms are controlled.[67] Occasionally, MG symptoms may be controlled with low doses of oral prednisone with minimal side effects (especially patients with mild disease and disease onset after age 40 years).[68] However, in most patients, additional immunosuppressive treatment is required to achieve long-term remission.

AZA is a well-established drug used in patients with immune-mediated neurologic disorders. Its use is typically aimed at reducing the dose of steroids or the frequency of IVIG and PE.[69] One randomized, double-blind study compared prednisone versus AZA plus prednisone versus placebo.[70] In this study, the prednisone dose required to maintain disease remission did not differ between the 2 groups at 1 year. However, by 3 years of treatment, many of the patients in the AZA group were able to discontinue prednisone. Further, patients in the prednisone with placebo group had a higher rate of clinical relapses. Based on this study, AZA (2.0–2.5 mg/kg/d) is commonly used to treat MG with the understanding that the clinical benefits may be delayed by more than a year. Common side effects of AZA include hepatotoxicity, nausea, vomiting, rash, pancreatitis, and leukopenia. Some patients are unable to tolerate AZA because of an acute allergic-type reaction with fever, malaise, and nausea. Long-term treatment with AZA raises the risk of malignancy as a potential complication.[71]

MMF is frequently used as an immunosuppressive agent for treatment of MG and other antibody-mediated disorders because of its favorable side effect profile and mechanism of action to inhibit T- lymphocyte and B-lymphocyte proliferation. MMF also decreases production of the inducible form of nitric oxide (reducing tissue damage by nitrites) and inhibits glycosylation and expression of certain adhesion molecules on lymphocytes. This situation leads to decreased lymphocytic and monocytic recruitment and penetration into sites of inflammation.[72,73] MMF was initially approved for the prophylaxis of organ rejection in adult renal, cardiac, and hepatic allograft recipients. Side effects are modest, including gastrointestinal problems (diarrhea, abdominal pain, and nausea), drug-induced fever, and leucopenia.[71,74] As with other chronic immunosuppression, there is an increased risk of malignancy, especially lymphoma.[75]

Two prospective, double-blind, placebo-controlled studies of MMF failed to show a significant benefit compared with prednisone over 3 months of treatment.[76,77] The lack of efficacy in these trials may have been caused by the short duration of follow-up, because agents like MMF and AZA may require more than 6 months to produce a meaningful immunosuppression. Retrospective studies indicate that MMF has a benefit for AChR antibody-positive MG starting after 6 months of treatment.[78,79]

Cyclosporine is a calcineurin inhibitor that produces immunosuppression by inhibiting T-cell function. The use of this drug in MG is supported by a randomized, placebo-controlled study of 39 patients in whom cyclosporine (5 mg/kg/d) was superior to placebo in improving strength and reducing steroid dose after 6 months of treatment.[80,81] Cyclosporine has a steroid-sparing effect, but major side effects often limit the long-term use of this drug. In the continuation phase of the controlled studies, 35% of patients had to discontinue the medication because of cumulative side effects (commonly nephrotoxicity). In 1 retrospective study, 96% of patients with MG showed a clinical response and reduced the dose of steroids, with a maximum clinical response 7 months after starting therapy; however, major side effects included increased creatinine levels in 28% and new malignancy in 11%.[82]

Tacrolimus (FK506), another calcineurin inhibitor, seems to be better tolerated than cyclosporine. In addition to its action as a T-cell immunomodulator, it is proposed that there is an additional beneficial action of the drug to improve calcium mobilization and efficiency of contraction in muscle. This drug has been used extensively for the treatment of MG in Japan. A large retrospective study of 212 patients with MG indicated a benefit of tacrolimus (0.1 mg/kg/d) to improve muscle strength beginning within 1 month of treatment.[83] However, 5% of patients had to discontinue the drug because of side effects. Retrospective case series in MG using lower-dose tacrolimus (2–3 mg/d) also showed a benefit in reducing daily prednisone dose and improving functional scores.[84,85] However, in a recent double-blind, placebo-controlled study of 80 patients, tacrolimus failed to show primary efficacy in reducing the required dose of prednisone in patients with MG. Some of the secondary analyses suggested a benefit, so tacrolimus (like MMF) is considered a valid immunotherapeutic agent for treatment of MG despite lack of class I evidence.[86]

Cyclophosphamide (Cytoxan) is an effective immunosuppressive agent and can be used as maintenance therapy in cases of refractory MG. The drug can be given as daily oral medication or by monthly pulse IV infusions; however, the high incidence of side effects generally limits its use to those with severe disease.[87] In particularly refractory cases of MG, an immunoablative treatment with cyclophosphamide has been proposed as a way of producing a long-lasting reduction in autoimmunity. Because hematopoietic stem cells are relatively resistant to cyclophosphamide, a high dose (50 mg/kg/d for 4 days) protocol followed by granulocyte colony-stimulating factor has been used in a few patients with MG to produce a durable disease remission without the need for bone marrow transplant.[88] At this time, this approach is limited to a small group of patients treated at specialized centers, because other effective treatment options are generally available for patients with MG or the other antibody-mediated disorders.

Rituximab has also been applied as an immunomodulatory agent for the antibody-mediated disorders. Its use is supported by several retrospective case series showing a benefit in patients with MG.[89–91] There are also case reports of rituximab for LES[89] and in AAG.[92] Common side effects of rituximab are fever, chills, nausea, vomiting, flushing, and bronchospasm. Other more significant side effects include neutropenia and increased risk of infections. Severe adverse events are rare, but those relevant to the treatment of neurologic disease include the possible development of PML and severe mucocutaneous reactions.[71]

OTHER AUTOIMMUNE NEUROMUSCULAR DISORDERS

Disorders characterized by inflammation of muscle include polymyositis, dermatomyositis, inclusion body myositis (IBM), necrotizing myopathy, and myositis associated with vasculitis or sarcoidosis. The inflammatory myopathies most commonly present as weakness of proximal muscles (sometimes with muscle pain) and increase of serum creatine kinase levels. Treatment of inflammatory myopathies is largely empiric and typically relies on the use of corticosteroids supplemented by other immunosuppressant therapy (**Table 8**). Because of the known clinical efficacy, corticosteroids are the first line of treatment but have never been subjected to controlled clinical trials. IBM is often resistant to steroid treatment. Second-line treatments include methotrexate and AZA. The response to therapy is best shown by objective improvement in muscle strength. The serum creatine kinase level is also a reliable measure of disease activity.

High-dose IVIG has been shown to be effective in patients with resistant dermatomyositis and polymyositis in several controlled studies.[93,94] Various studies have evaluated the effects of IVIG for the treatment of IBM[95] and have shown either no benefit or only mild response. At this point, IVIG therapy is not recommended for the routine treatment of IBM.[96]

Autoimmune inflammation can also affect the peripheral nerves. The classic presentations are acute inflammatory demyelinating polyradiculopathy (Guillain-Barré syndrome, [GBS]) and chronic inflammatory demyelinating polyradiculoneuropathy (CIDP). Several variants of these inflammatory neuropathies exist, including acute axonal motor or sensory neuropathies and multifocal motor neuropathy with conduction block. GBS is classically a monophasic illness presenting first with pain, numbness, and ascending weakness. In about 25% of cases, the bulbar or respiratory muscles are affected, and patients require intensive care. Most patients spontaneously stabilize and improve without immunotherapy. However, early immunotherapy can reduce the maximum severity of the illness and hasten recovery. Despite the immunologic nature of GBS, several trials have failed to show a clinical benefit of corticosteroids. In contrast, both PE and IVIG have been convincingly shown to be beneficial.[97]

Unlike GBS, the motor and sensory deficits in CIDP develop insidiously over months or years (arbitrarily, symptoms must progress for more than 8 weeks to establish the diagnosis of CIDP). Oral corticosteroids are considered effective treatment of CIDP, but high doses are often required, and long-term side effects make steroids less desirable. Additional immunosuppressive agents (such as AZA, cyclosporine) may be

Table 8
Immunotherapy for inflammatory myopathies

Therapeutic Agent	Indication	Route	Dose
Prednisone	First-line	Oral	Initially ~1 mg/kg; gradual taper > 4–6 wk and conversion to alternate day regimen
Methylprednisolone	Severe PM or DM	IV	1000 mg/d for 3 d
Methotrexate	Second-line	Oral	7.5–15 mg/once weekly
AZA	Second-line	Oral	2–3 mg/kg/d in divided doses
Cyclophosphamide	Third-line	Oral IV	2–2.5 mg/kg/d 500-mg to 1000-mg pulse dose every 2–4 wk
Cyclosporine	Third-line	Oral	2–3 mg/kg/d in divided doses
Immunoglobulin	Third-line[a]	IV	0.4 g/kg/d for 5 d in initial course followed by monthly 3-d courses for 3–6 mo

[a] Second-line in patients with immunodeficiency.

added to reduce long-term exposure to steroids. Several randomized controlled trials have shown the benefit of IVIG and PE, with about 75% to 80% of patients showing improvement.[98–100] In current practice, most treatment protocols for CIDP use IVIG. A typical initial treatment is 2 g/kg given in divided doses over 2 to 5 days. Most patients require maintenance therapy with IVIG (0.4–1.0 g/kg given every 3–6 weeks). The optimal dose and frequency need to be determined for each patient.

Several other inflammatory neuropathies may be treated with immunotherapy. These neuropathies include multifocal motor neuropathy with conduction block, inflammatory lumbosacral plexus neuropathy, and idiopathic inflammatory brachial plexopathy (Parsonage-Turner syndrome).

IMMUNOTHERAPY FOR AUTOIMMUNE ENCEPHALOPATHIES

The autoimmune encephalopathies are a diverse group of immune-mediated disorders of the CNS (**Table 9**). Unlike demyelinating CNS disorders, these disorders typically affect cortical function, leading to seizures, impaired memory, behavioral changes, or impaired consciousness. Autoimmune ataxia and stiff person syndrome are also included in this group for the purpose of this discussion. The autoimmune encephalopathies can be generally divided into paraneoplastic conditions (those that occur in the context of cancer) and idiopathic autoimmune disorders.

Encephalopathies such as Morvan syndrome, paraneoplastic limbic encephalitis, and nonparaneoplastic autoimmune limbic encephalitis have characteristic clinical features. Serologic testing often facilitates diagnosis (see **Table 9**). Limbic encephalitis is characterized by the triad of short-term memory impairment, complex partial temporal lobe seizures, and psychiatric symptoms. Signal abnormalities in the mesial temporal lobes without contrast enhancement are the typical MRI findings. Morvan

Table 9 Autoimmune encephalopathies		
Syndrome	**Clinical Symptoms**	**Associated Antibody**
Limbic encephalitis	Seizures, memory loss, personality changes	Anti-Hu VGKC complex Anti-Ma2
Brainstem encephalitis	Sleep disturbance, ophthalmoplegia	GQ1b Anti-Ma2
Rasmussen encephalitis	Intractable seizures, hemiparesis	
Cerebellar degeneration	Speech and gait ataxia	Anti-Yo VGCC Glutamic acid decarboxylase
Paraneoplastic chorea	Involuntary movements	Anti-CRMP5
N-methyl-D-aspartate receptor encephalitis	Confusion, psychosis, dyskinesias, hypoventilation	N-methyl-D-aspartate receptor
Morvan syndrome	Fluctuating confusion, muscle twitching, severe insomnia, dysautonomia	VGKC complex
Hashimoto encephalopathy	Fluctuating confusion, tremor, transient aphasia	Thyroperoxidase
Stiff person syndrome	Muscle stiffness and spasms	Glutamic acid decarboxylase amphiphysin

syndrome presents with behavioral changes, hallucinations, severe insomnia, autonomic hyperactivity, and NMT (spontaneous muscle activity).

The term steroid-responsive encephalopathy (SRE) refers to autoimmune encephalopathy that may be associated with evidence of thyroid autoimmunity (this association is sometimes called Hashimoto encephalopathy). This entity has a broad range of clinical presentations but cognitive impairment with tremor, strokelike events (including transient aphasia), and normal thyroid hormone levels are common scenarios. In the absence of other diagnostic findings, a clinical response to steroids may be the only evidence of an autoimmune cause for encephalopathy. Patients typically improve with corticosteroid therapy but may relapse.[101,102] It is still unclear whether steroid responsiveness should be a necessary criterion to make this diagnosis.

There have been no controlled treatment trials for SRE. Treatment with IVIG, AZA, or other immunosuppressants may work for refractory cases or in patients who require intolerable maintenance doses of steroids. Different approaches to treatment of SRE have been recommended. A short course of high-dose IV corticosteroids (5 consecutive days of methylprednisolone, 1 g per day) or, less preferably, oral prednisone (1.0 mg/kg/d for 10–30 days) is a typical initial therapy. Most patients show a response to treatment within weeks, and some show a dramatic improvement after the first few doses. Many patients (up to 40%) are able to discontinue corticosteroids after initial treatment without relapses.[103] Patients who relapse usually require long-term corticosteroid treatment and the addition of a corticosteroid-sparing agent (such as AZA or MMF). Successful treatment with IVIG or PE has been reported in a few refractory cases.[103,104] Discontinuation of treatment can be considered in patients who remain stable for a year or more to assess for disease remission.

IMMUNOTHERAPY FOR PARANEOPLASTIC NEUROLOGIC DISORDERS

Paraneoplastic neurologic disorders (PND) represent remote immunologic effects of malignancy. Our current understanding of the pathophysiology of PND involves activation of humoral and cellular immunity by a malignancy (more than 50% of PND cases present before the diagnosis of cancer).[105] Some tumors express onconeural antigens (proteins that are usually restricted to the nervous system but become aberrantly expressed by the tumor). As a result, an autoimmune response against normal components of the nervous system develops.[105] The clinical presentations of PND are diverse because any part of the nervous system can be affected. In many cases of PND, autoantibodies against defined onconeural antigens can be found in the serum of CSF. These antibodies, when present, help confirm the diagnosis, direct the search for malignancy, and suggest appropriate immunotherapy.[105]

Current therapeutic modalities for PND are, for the most part, based on anecdotal case reports and uncontrolled small case series. Prospective studies of treatment efficacy in PNDs have been hampered by the heterogeneity of the clinical presentation as well as the rarity of these syndromes. The best approach in treatment of any paraneoplastic disorder is to identify and treat the underlying tumor and at the same time provide appropriate supportive care and symptomatic therapies. Immunomodulatory treatments for PND are gaining acceptance, even although few prospective studies have been performed. Therapies for the antibody-mediated neuromuscular disorders (eg, MG) were described earlier. For other PNDs, there are no proven or accepted treatment protocols.[106] For the most part, treatment results have been disappointing.[107,108] Some patients stabilize after cancer treatment. This situation seems to be the case with PNDs associated with anti-Hu, anti-CRMP5/CV2, anti-Ma2 antibodies, but the neurologic outcome for patients with cerebellar degeneration and anti-Yo antibodies is often poor despite optimal cancer treatment. It seems that paraneoplastic disorders in which antibodies are directed against cell surface antigens are more amenable to immunomodulatory treatment. In these syndromes, antibodies may produce a functional neuronal deficit rather than a cytotoxic immune response, which would irreversibly damage neurons. This category includes paraneoplastic encephalitis associated with ovarian teratoma and anti-N-methyl-D-aspartate receptor antibodies.[109,110] In other PND, the antibodies are directed against intracellular neuronal antigens. In these cases, the antibodies seem to be a marker of a cell-mediated immune response against the cancer cells. These disorders are often characterized by selective neuronal loss and less potential for neurologic recovery.

Immunomodulatory therapy can be considered in cases in which a malignancy has not been identified, in cases in which oncologic treatment has been completed, or in conjunction with cancer treatment. The immunosuppressive effects of chemotherapeutic agents may help dampen the immune response. However, concurrent use of chemotherapeutic agents and immunosuppressive agents can lead to increased toxicity.[111] Steroids, IVIG, PE, rituximab, and cyclophosphamide are therapies that have been reported. Data on treatment response are largely based on small retrospective studies and case reports.

There have been no placebo-controlled clinical trials, but a few systematic prospective series have been reported. Two studies were conducted using IVIG alone or IVIG in combination with pulse IV cyclophosphamide and methylprednisolone.[112,113] However, treatment was given for a variable duration and in combination with chemotherapy in many cases. Among patients with progressive neurologic disease, 35% to 40% of patients stabilized neurologically, and only 1 patient improved. The investigators concluded that this immunomodulatory treatment was not useful for patients with severe disability but may provide a useful stabilization of disability in patients who are still ambulatory.[112]

In a single-center, prospective, open-label study to evaluate the efficacy of initial PE in combination with either chemotherapy or oral cyclophosphamide,[114] a positive response was seen in 45% of the patients (measured as improvement in Rankin disability score and in activities of daily living) after 6 months. Most of the stabilization and recovery occurred gradually, so the beneficial effects of PE were uncertain. Hematologic side effects of cyclophosphamide were a problem in many cases. The conclusion was that immunosuppressive therapy should be considered early in the course of PNDs, even when there is no evidence of active malignancy. Similar to the IVIG studies mentioned earlier, patients with less severe disability and those with peripheral, as opposed to central, neurologic syndromes tended to have a better outcome.[111,112,114]

Based on the presumed pathophysiology, treatment with MMF or tacrolimus has also been applied to PND even although there are no prospective trials to establish efficacy. Albert and colleagues used tacrolimus at a dose of 0.15 mg/kg/d for 14 days, followed by 0.3 mg/kg/d for 7 days to treat paraneoplastic cerebellar degeneration.[115] Although this regimen decreased the number of activated T cells in the CSF, no clinical improvement was observed. MMF, a selective inhibitor of lymphocyte proliferation, is associated with less myelosuppression than cyclophosphamide and anecdotally seems to be safe in patients with PND who are undergoing chemotherapy. However, no data on efficacy are available.

Uncontrolled studies and case reports using rituximab for PND suggest usefulness of this drug.[116–118] In 1 study, a maximum of 4 monthly infusions of rituximab were used at 375 mg/m^2 in 9 patients with PND.[118] Three showed clinical improvement. Several other monoclonal antibody therapies have been developed recently as immunomodulatory treatments for MS and other systemic autoimmune diseases. Some of these biologicals may prove useful in PNDs.

STIFF PERSON SYNDROME

Stiff person syndrome (SPS, formerly known as stiff man syndrome) is an unusual disorder presenting with muscle stiffness and spasms. It seems that the disease results from impairment of central inhibition of motor control; antibodies against glutamic acid decarboxylase (GAD) are found in about 65% of patients. Most patients respond symptomatically to γ aminobutyric acid-ergic agonist medications (benzodiazepines), but immunotherapy is required in more severe cases. In a randomized controlled cross-over trial, IVIG produced a reduction in stiffness and an improvement in activity.[119] The duration of benefit varied but was generally short-lived, indicating a need for additional maintenance immunotherapy. Some patients can be managed with intermittent IVIG infusions. A few cases of successful treatment with rituximab have been reported.[120] Maintenance immunosuppression with mycophenolate or AZA can be considered. Corticosteroids are generally not used in SPS because most patients have or will develop diabetes.

SUMMARY

The current practice of neurology requires expertise in the use of immunotherapies. A wide variety of neuroimmunologic disorders can be diagnosed and treated. Treatment of the most common disorder of these disorders, MS, has advanced dramatically in the past decade. Diagnosis and treatment of immune-mediated neuromuscular disorders has also become more effective. For most other autoimmune and paraneoplastic disorders, immunotherapy is used without clear guidance from controlled clinical trials. This area of neurotherapeutics continues to develop rapidly.

REFERENCES

1. Pugliatti M, Sotgiu S, Rosati G. The worldwide prevalence of multiple sclerosis. Clin Neurol Neurosurg 2002;104(3):182–91.
2. Hauser SL, Oksenberg JR. The neurobiology of multiple sclerosis: genes, inflammation, and neurodegeneration. Neuron 2006;52(1):61–76.
3. Lublin FD, Baier M, Cutter G. Effect of relapses on development of residual deficit in multiple sclerosis. Neurology 2003;61(11):1528–32.
4. Fox R, Kinkel R. High-dose methylprednisolone in the treatment of multiple sclerosis. In: Cohen J, Rudick R, editors. Multiple sclerosis therapeutics. 3rd edition. London: Informa Healthcare; 2007. p. 515–33.
5. Weinshenker BG, O'Brien PC, Petterson TM, et al. A randomized trial of plasma exchange in acute central nervous system inflammatory demyelinating disease. Ann Neurol 1999;46(6):878–86.
6. Visser LH, Beekman R, Tijssen CC, et al. A randomized, double-blind, placebo-controlled pilot study of i.v. immune globulins in combination with i.v. methylprednisolone in the treatment of relapses in patients with MS. Mult Scler 2004; 10(1):89–91.
7. Sorensen PS, Haas J, Sellebjerg F, et al. IV immunoglobulins as add-on treatment to methylprednisolone for acute relapses in MS. Neurology 2004;63(11):2028–33.
8. Confavreux C, Hutchinson M, Hours MM, et al. Rate of pregnancy-related relapse in multiple sclerosis. Pregnancy in Multiple Sclerosis Group. N Engl J Med 1998;339(5):285–91.

9. Achiron A, Kishner I, Dolev M, et al. Effect of intravenous immunoglobulin treatment on pregnancy and postpartum-related relapses in multiple sclerosis. J Neurol 2004;251(9):1133–7.

10. Brex PA, Ciccarelli O, O'Riordan JI, et al. A longitudinal study of abnormalities on MRI and disability from multiple sclerosis. N Engl J Med 2002;346(3):158–64.

11. Comi G, Filippi M, Barkhof F, et al. Effect of early interferon treatment on conversion to definite multiple sclerosis: a randomised study. Lancet 2001;357(9268):1576–82.

12. Jacobs LD, Beck RW, Simon JH, et al. Intramuscular interferon beta-1a therapy initiated during a first demyelinating event in multiple sclerosis. CHAMPS Study Group. N Engl J Med 2000;343(13):898–904.

13. Kappos L, Polman CH, Freedman MS, et al. Treatment with interferon beta-1b delays conversion to clinically definite and McDonald MS in patients with clinically isolated syndromes. Neurology 2006;67(7):1242–9.

14. Comi G, Martinelli V, Rodegher M, et al. Effect of glatiramer acetate on conversion to clinically definite multiple sclerosis in patients with clinically isolated syndrome (PreCISe study): a randomised, double-blind, placebo-controlled trial. Lancet 2009;374(9700):1503–11.

15. The IFNB Multiple Sclerosis Study Group. Interferon beta-1b is effective in relapsing-remitting multiple sclerosis. I. Clinical results of a multicenter, randomized, double-blind, placebo-controlled trial. Neurology 1993;43(4):655–61.

16. Jacobs LD, Cookfair DL, Rudick RA, et al. Intramuscular interferon beta-1a for disease progression in relapsing multiple sclerosis. The Multiple Sclerosis Collaborative Research Group (MSCRG). Ann Neurol 1996;39(3):285–94.

17. Johnson KP, Brooks BR, Cohen JA, et al. Copolymer 1 reduces relapse rate and improves disability in relapsing-remitting multiple sclerosis: results of a phase III multicenter, double-blind placebo-controlled trial. The Copolymer 1 Multiple Sclerosis Study Group. Neurology 1995;45(7):1268–76.

18. PRISMS Study Group. Randomised double-blind placebo-controlled study of interferon beta-1a in relapsing/remitting multiple sclerosis. PRISMS (Prevention of Relapses and Disability by Interferon beta-1a Subcutaneously in Multiple Sclerosis) Study Group. Lancet 1998;352(9139):1498–504.

19. Polman CH, O'Connor PW, Havrdova E, et al. A randomized, placebo-controlled trial of natalizumab for relapsing multiple sclerosis. N Engl J Med 2006;354(9):899–910.

20. Rudick RA, Stuart WH, Calabresi PA, et al. Natalizumab plus interferon beta-1a for relapsing multiple sclerosis. N Engl J Med 2006;354(9):911–23.

21. Kappos L, Radue EW, O'Connor P, et al. A placebo-controlled trial of oral fingolimod in relapsing multiple sclerosis. N Engl J Med 2010;362(5):387–401.

22. Cohen JA, Barkhof F, Comi G, et al. Oral fingolimod or intramuscular interferon for relapsing multiple sclerosis. N Engl J Med 2010;362(5):402–15.

23. Panitch H, Goodin DS, Francis G, et al. Randomized, comparative study of interferon β-1a treatment regimens in MS THE EVIDENCE Trial. Neurology 2002;59: 1496–506.

24. Durelli L, Verdun E, Barbero P, et al. Every-other-day interferon beta-1b versus once-weekly interferon beta-1a for multiple sclerosis: results of a 2-year prospective randomized multicentre study (INCOMIN). The Lancet Neurology 2002;359:1453–60.

25. Mikol DD, Barkhof F, Chang P, et al. Comparison of subcutaneous interferon beta-1a with glatiramer acetate in patients with relapsing multiple sclerosis (the REbif vs Glatiramer Acetate in Relapsing MS Disease [REGARD] study): a multicentre, randomised, parallel, open-label trial. The Lancet Neurology 2008;7:903–14.

26. O'Connor P, Filippi M, Arnason B, et al. 250 mcg or 500 mcg interferon beta-1b versus 20 mg glatiramer acetate in relapsing-remitting multiple sclerosis: a prospective randomized, multicentre study. The Lancet Neurology 2009;8: 889–97.
27. Cadavid D, Wolansky LJ, Skurnick J, et al. Efficacy of treatment of MS with IFN β-1b or glatiramer acetate by monthly brain MRI in the BECOME study. Neurology 2009;72(23):1976–83.
28. Polman CH, Reingold SC, Banwell B, et al. Diagnostic criteria for multiple sclerosis: 2010 revisions to the McDonald criteria. Ann Neurol 2011;69(2):292–302.
29. Fox EJ. Management of worsening multiple sclerosis with mitoxantrone: a review. Clin Ther 2006;28(4):461–74.
30. Tremlett H, Yinshan Z, Devonshire V. Natural history of secondary-progressive multiple sclerosis. Mult Scler 2008;14(3):314–24.
31. Hartung HP, Gonsette R, Konig N, et al. Mitoxantrone in progressive multiple sclerosis: a placebo-controlled, double-blind, randomised, multicentre trial. Lancet 2002;360(9350):2018–25.
32. Wolinsky JS, Narayana PA, O'Connor P, et al. Glatiramer acetate in primary progressive multiple sclerosis: results of a multinational, multicenter, double-blind, placebo-controlled trial. Ann Neurol 2007;61(1):14–24.
33. Hawker K, O'Connor P, Freedman MS, et al. Rituximab in patients with primary progressive multiple sclerosis: results of a randomized double-blind placebo-controlled multicenter trial. Ann Neurol 2009;66(4):460–71.
34. Banwell B, Bar-Or A, Giovannoni G, et al. Therapies for multiple sclerosis: considerations in the pediatric patient. Nat Rev Neurol 2011;7(2):109–22.
35. Wingerchuk DM, Weinshenker BG. Neuromyelitis optica. Curr Treat Options Neurol 2008;10(1):55–66.
36. Wingerchuk DM, Weinshenker BG. Neuromyelitis optica: clinical predictors of a relapsing course and survival. Neurology 2003;60(5):848–53.
37. Wingerchuk DM, Hogancamp WF, O'Brien PC, et al. The clinical course of neuromyelitis optica (Devic's syndrome). Neurology 1999;53(5):1107–14.
38. Watanabe S, Nakashima I, Misu T, et al. Therapeutic efficacy of plasma exchange in NMO-IgG-positive patients with neuromyelitis optica. Mult Scler 2007;13(1):128–32.
39. Llufriu S, Castillo J, Blanco Y, et al. Plasma exchange for acute attacks of CNS demyelination: predictors of improvement at 6 months. Neurology 2009;73(12): 949–53.
40. Sellner J, Boggild M, Clanet M, et al. EFNS guidelines on diagnosis and management of neuromyelitis optica. Eur J Neurol 2010;17(8):1019–32.
41. Palace J, Leite MI, Nairne A, et al. Interferon beta treatment in neuromyelitis optica: increase in relapses and aquaporin 4 antibody titers. Arch Neurol 2010; 67(8):1016–7.
42. Uzawa A, Mori M, Hayakawa S, et al. Different responses to interferon beta-1b treatment in patients with neuromyelitis optica and multiple sclerosis. Eur J Neurol 2010;17(5):672–6.
43. Warabi Y, Matsumoto Y, Hayashi H. Interferon beta-1b exacerbates multiple sclerosis with severe optic nerve and spinal cord demyelination. J Neurol Sci 2007;252(1):57–61.
44. Bomprezzi R, Powers JM, Shimizu J, et al. IFNbeta-1b may severely exacerbate Japanese opticspinal MS in neuromyelitis optica spectrum: Japanese opticspinal MS: is it MS or neuromyelitis optica and does the answer dictate treatment? Neurology 2011;77(2):195 [discussion: 195–6].

45. Papeix C, Vidal JS, de Seze J, et al. Immunosuppressive therapy is more effective than interferon in neuromyelitis optica. Mult Scler 2007;13(2):256–9.
46. Costanzi C, Matiello M, Lucchinetti CF, et al. Azathioprine: tolerability, efficacy, and predictors of benefit in neuromyelitis optica. Neurology 2011;77(7):659–66.
47. Mandler RN, Ahmed W, Dencoff JE. Devic's neuromyelitis optica: a prospective study of seven patients treated with prednisone and azathioprine. Neurology 1998;51(4):1219–20.
48. Bichuetti DB, Lobato de Oliveira EM, Oliveira DM, et al. Neuromyelitis optica treatment: analysis of 36 patients. Arch Neurol 2010;67(9):1131–6.
49. Collongues N, de Seze J. Current and future treatment approaches for neuromyelitis optica. Ther Adv Neurol Disord 2011;4(2):111–21.
50. Jacob A, Matiello M, Weinshenker BG, et al. Treatment of neuromyelitis optica with mycophenolate mofetil: retrospective analysis of 24 patients. Arch Neurol 2009;66(9):1128–33.
51. Cree BA, Lamb S, Morgan K, et al. An open label study of the effects of rituximab in neuromyelitis optica. Neurology 2005;64(7):1270–2.
52. Jacob A, Weinshenker BG, Violich I, et al. Treatment of neuromyelitis optica with rituximab: retrospective analysis of 25 patients. Arch Neurol 2008;65(11):1443–8.
53. Weinstock-Guttman B, Ramanathan M, Lincoff N, et al. Study of mitoxantrone for the treatment of recurrent neuromyelitis optica (Devic disease). Arch Neurol 2006;63(7):957–63.
54. Kim SH, Kim W, Park MS, et al. Efficacy and safety of mitoxantrone in patients with highly relapsing neuromyelitis optica. Arch Neurol 2011;68(4):473–9.
55. Birnbaum J, Kerr D. Optic neuritis and recurrent myelitis in a woman with systemic lupus erythematosus. Nat Clin Pract Rheumatol 2008;4(7):381–6.
56. Arabshahi B, Pollock AN, Sherry DD, et al. Devic disease in a child with primary Sjogren syndrome. J Child Neurol 2006;21(4):285–6.
57. Mok CC, To CH, Mak A, et al. Immunoablative cyclophosphamide for refractory lupus-related neuromyelitis optica. J Rheumatol 2008;35(1):172–4.
58. Gajdos P, Chevret S, Toyka K. Intravenous immunoglobulin for myasthenia gravis. Cochrane Database Syst Rev 2008;1:CD002277.
59. Batocchi AP, Evoli A, Di Schino C, et al. Therapeutic apheresis in myasthenia gravis. Ther Apher 2000;4(4):275–9.
60. Zinman L, Ng E, Bril V. IV immunoglobulin in patients with myasthenia gravis: a randomized controlled trial. Neurology 2007;68(11):837–41.
61. Iodice V, Kimpinski K, Vernino S, et al. Immunotherapy for autoimmune autonomic ganglionopathy. Auton Neurosci 2009;146(1-2):22–5.
62. Schroeder C, Vernino S, Birkenfeld AL, et al. Plasma exchange for primary autoimmune autonomic failure. N Engl J Med 2005;353(15):1585–90.
63. Maddison P, Newsom-Davis J. Treatment for Lambert-Eaton myasthenic syndrome [update of Cochrane Database Syst Rev 2003;2:CD003279]. Cochrane Database Syst Rev 2005;2:CD003279.
64. Vernino S. Autoimmune and paraneoplastic channelopathies. Neurotherapeutics 2007;4(2):305–14.
65. Gibbons CH, Vernino SA, Freeman R. Combined immunomodulatory therapy in autoimmune autonomic ganglionopathy. Arch Neurol 2008;65(2):213–7.
66. Verschuuren JJ, Wirtz PW, Titulaer MJ, et al. Available treatment options for the management of Lambert-Eaton myasthenic syndrome. Expert Opin Pharmacother 2006;7(10):1323–36.
67. Seybold ME, Drachman DB. Gradually increasing doses of prednisone in myasthenia gravis. Reducing the hazards of treatment. N Engl J Med 1974;290(2):81–4.

68. Sghirlanzoni A, Peluchetti D, Mantegazza R, et al. Myasthenia gravis: prolonged treatment with steroids. Neurology 1984;34(2):170–4.
69. Hughes BW, Moro De Casillas ML, Kaminski HJ. Pathophysiology of myasthenia gravis. Semin Neurol 2004;24(1):21–30.
70. Palace J, Newsom-Davis J, Lecky B. A randomized double-blind trial of prednisolone alone or with azathioprine in myasthenia gravis. Myasthenia Gravis Study Group. Neurology 1998;50(6):1778–83.
71. Sathasivam S. Steroids and immunosuppressant drugs in myasthenia gravis. Nat Clin Pract Neurol 2008;4(6):317–27.
72. Schneider-Gold C, Hartung HP, Gold R. Mycophenolate mofetil and tacrolimus: new therapeutic options in neuroimmunological diseases. Muscle Nerve 2006; 34(3):284–91.
73. Mowzoon N, Sussman A, Bradley WG. Mycophenolate (CellCept) treatment of myasthenia gravis, chronic inflammatory polyneuropathy and inclusion body myositis. J Neurol Sci 2001;185(2):119–22.
74. Chaudhry V, Cornblath DR, Griffin JW, et al. Mycophenolate mofetil: a safe and promising immunosuppressant in neuromuscular diseases. Neurology 2001; 56(1):94–6.
75. O'Neill BP, Vernino S, Dogan A, et al. EBV-associated lymphoproliferative disorder of CNS associated with the use of mycophenolate mofetil. Neuro Oncol 2007;9(3):364–9.
76. Sanders DB, Hart IK, Mantegazza R, et al. An international, phase III, randomized trial of mycophenolate mofetil in myasthenia gravis. Neurology 2008;71(6):400–6.
77. Muscle Study Group. A trial of mycophenolate mofetil with prednisone as initial immunotherapy in myasthenia gravis. Neurology 2008;71(6):394–9.
78. Hehir MK, Burns TM, Alpers J, et al. Mycophenolate mofetil in AChR-antibody-positive myasthenia gravis: outcomes in 102 patients. Muscle Nerve 2010;41(5):593–8.
79. Meriggioli MN, Ciafaloni E, Al-Hayk KA, et al. Mycophenolate mofetil for myasthenia gravis: an analysis of efficacy, safety, and tolerability. Neurology 2003; 61(10):1438–40.
80. Tindall RS, Phillips JT, Rollins JA, et al. A clinical therapeutic trial of cyclosporine in myasthenia gravis. Ann N Y Acad Sci 1993;681:539–51.
81. Tindall RS, Rollins JA, Phillips JT, et al. Preliminary results of a double-blind, randomized, placebo-controlled trial of cyclosporine in myasthenia gravis. N Engl J Med 1987;316(12):719–24.
82. Ciafaloni E, Nikhar NK, Massey JM, et al. Retrospective analysis of the use of cyclosporine in myasthenia gravis. Neurology 2000;55(3):448–50.
83. Ponseti JM, Gamez J, Azem J, et al. Tacrolimus for myasthenia gravis: a clinical study of 212 patients. Ann N Y Acad Sci 2008;1132:254–63.
84. Nagaishi A, Yukitake M, Kuroda Y. Long-term treatment of steroid-dependent myasthenia gravis patients with low-dose tacrolimus. Intern Med 2008;47(8):731–6.
85. Minami N, Fujiki N, Doi S, et al. Five-year follow-up with low-dose tacrolimus in patients with myasthenia gravis. J Neurol Sci 2011;300(1-2):59–62.
86. Yoshikawa H, Kiuchi T, Saida T, et al. Randomised, double-blind, placebo-controlled study of tacrolimus in myasthenia gravis. J Neurol Neurosurg Psychiatry 2011;82(9):970–7.
87. De Feo LG, Schottlender J, Martelli NA, et al. Use of intravenous pulsed cyclophosphamide in severe, generalized myasthenia gravis. Muscle Nerve 2002; 26(1):31–6.
88. Drachman DB, Jones RJ, Brodsky RA. Treatment of refractory myasthenia: "rebooting" with high-dose cyclophosphamide. Ann Neurol 2003;53(1):29–34.

89. Maddison P, McConville J, Farrugia ME, et al. The use of rituximab in myasthenia gravis and Lambert-Eaton myasthenic syndrome. J Neurol Neurosurg Psychiatry 2011;82(6):671–3.

90. Zebardast N, Patwa HS, Novella SP, et al. Rituximab in the management of refractory myasthenia gravis. Muscle Nerve 2010;41(3):375–8.

91. Lebrun C, Bourg V, Tieulie N, et al. Successful treatment of refractory generalized myasthenia gravis with rituximab. Eur J Neurol 2009;16(2):246–50.

92. Imrich R, Vernino S, Eldadah BA, et al. Autoimmune autonomic ganglionopathy: treatment by plasma exchanges and rituximab. Clin Auton Res 2009;19(4):259–62.

93. Dalakas MC, Illa I, Dambrosia JM, et al. A controlled trial of high-dose intravenous immune globulin infusions as treatment for dermatomyositis. N Engl J Med 1993;329(27):1993–2000.

94. Mastaglia FL, Phillips BA, Zilko PJ. Immunoglobulin therapy in inflammatory myopathies. J Neurol Neurosurg Psychiatry 1998;65(1):107–10.

95. Soueidan SA, Dalakas MC. Treatment of inclusion-body myositis with high-dose intravenous immunoglobulin. Neurology 1993;43(5):876–9.

96. Walter MC, Lochmuller H, Toepfer M, et al. High-dose immunoglobulin therapy in sporadic inclusion body myositis: a double-blind, placebo-controlled study. J Neurol 2000;247(1):22–8.

97. Dyck PJ, Kurtzke JF. Plasmapheresis in Guillain-Barré syndrome. Neurology 1985;35(8):1105–7.

98. Dyck PJ, Litchy WJ, Kratz KM, et al. A plasma exchange versus immune globulin infusion trial in chronic inflammatory demyelinating polyradiculoneuropathy. Ann Neurol 1994;36(6):838–45.

99. Dyck PJ, Daube J, O'Brien P, et al. Plasma exchange in chronic inflammatory demyelinating polyradiculoneuropathy. N Engl J Med 1986;314(8):461–5.

100. Mendell JR, Barohn RJ, Freimer ML, et al. Randomized controlled trial of IVIg in untreated chronic inflammatory demyelinating polyradiculoneuropathy. Neurology 2001;56(4):445–9.

101. Kothbauer-Margreiter I, Sturzenegger M, Komor J, et al. Encephalopathy associated with Hashimoto thyroiditis: diagnosis and treatment. J Neurol 1996;243:585–93.

102. Castillo P, Boeve B, Schäuble B, et al. Steroid-responsive encephalopathy associated with thyroid autoimmunity: clinical and laboratory findings [abstract]. Neurology 2002;58(Suppl 3):A248.

103. Castillo P, Woodruff B, Caselli R, et al. Steroid-responsive encephalopathy associated with autoimmune thyroiditis. Arch Neurol 2006;63(2):197–202.

104. Hussain NS, Rumbaugh J, Kerr D, et al. Effects of prednisone and plasma exchange on cognitive impairment in Hashimoto encephalopathy. Neurology 2005;64(1):165–6.

105. Darnell RB, Posner JB. Paraneoplastic syndromes involving the nervous system. N Engl J Med 2003;349(16):1543–54.

106. Vedeler CA, Antoine JC, Giometto B, et al. Management of paraneoplastic neurological syndromes: report of an EFNS Task Force. Eur J Neurol 2006;13(7):682–90.

107. Grisold W, Drlicek M, Liszka-Setinek U, et al. Anti-tumour therapy in paraneoplastic neurological disease. Clin Neurol Neurosurg 1995;97(1):106–11.

108. Posner JB, Dalmau JO. Paraneoplastic syndromes affecting the central nervous system. Annu Rev Med 1997;48:157–66.

109. Shams'ili S, Grefkens J, de Leeuw B, et al. Paraneoplastic cerebellar degeneration associated with antineuronal antibodies: analysis of 50 patients. Brain 2003;126(Pt 6):1409–18.

110. Dalmau J, Tuzun E, Wu HY, et al. Paraneoplastic anti-N-methyl-D-aspartate receptor encephalitis associated with ovarian teratoma. Ann Neurol 2007; 61(1):25–36.
111. Rosenfeld MR, Dalmau J. Current therapies for neuromuscular manifestations of paraneoplastic syndromes. Curr Neurol Neurosci Rep 2006;6(1):77–84.
112. Keime-Guibert F, Graus F, Fleury A, et al. Treatment of paraneoplastic neurological syndromes with antineuronal antibodies (Anti-Hu, anti-Yo) with a combination of immunoglobulins, cyclophosphamide, and methylprednisolone. J Neurol Neurosurg Psychiatry 2000;68(4):479–82.
113. Uchuya M, Graus F, Vega F, et al. Intravenous immunoglobulin treatment in paraneoplastic neurological syndromes with antineuronal autoantibodies. J Neurol Neurosurg Psychiatry 1996;60(4):388–92.
114. Vernino S, O'Neill BP, Marks RS, et al. Immunomodulatory treatment trial for paraneoplastic neurological disorders. Neuro Oncol 2004;6:55–62.
115. Albert ML, Austin LM, Darnell RB. Detection and treatment of activated T cells in the cerebrospinal fluid of patients with paraneoplastic cerebellar degeneration. Ann Neurol 2000;47(1):9–17.
116. Bell J, Moran C, Blatt J. Response to rituximab in a child with neuroblastoma and opsoclonus-myoclonus. Pediatr Blood Cancer 2008;50(2):370–1.
117. Esposito M, Penza P, Orefice G, et al. Successful treatment of paraneoplastic cerebellar degeneration with rituximab. J Neurooncol 2008;86(3):363–4.
118. Shams'ili S, de Beukelaar J, Gratama JW, et al. An uncontrolled trial of rituximab for antibody associated paraneoplastic neurological syndromes. J Neurol 2006; 253(1):16–20.
119. Dalakas MC. The role of IVIg in the treatment of patients with stiff person syndrome and other neurological diseases associated with anti-GAD antibodies. J Neurol 2005;252(Suppl 1):I19–25.
120. Baker MR, Das M, Isaacs J, et al. Treatment of stiff person syndrome with rituximab. J Neurol Neurosurg Psychiatry 2005;76(7):999–1001.

Immunotherapy in Inflammatory Bowel Disease

Jatinder P. Ahluwalia, MD[a,b],*

KEYWORDS

- Crohn disease • Ulcerative colitis
- Anti-tumor necrosis factor-α • Infliximab • Adalimumab
- Certolizumab • Anti-α₄-integrin therapy • Natalizumab
- Biologics

Key Points

- Inflammatory bowel disease (IBD) is one of the most prevalent gastrointestinal diseases.

- The dysregulation of the immune system with the increased expression of proinflammatory cytokines, such as tumor necrosis factor (TNF)-α, and increased mucosal expression of vascular adhesion molecules play an important role in the pathogenesis of IBD.

- The availability of anti-TNF-α agents has revolutionized the treatment of patients with IBD.

- Anti-TNF-α agents are effective in inducing and maintaining remission in patients with Crohn disease and ulcerative colitis.

- Loss of response to biologics is not uncommon and may be related to immunogenicity to the immunologic agent used for IBD treatment.

- Side effects include serious infections, reactivation of latent tuberculosis and fungal infections in the case of anti-TNF-α therapy, and an increased risk of progressive multifocal leukoencephalopathy in the case of natalizumab.

- Additional therapies are needed for the treatment of patients who are primary nonresponders and those who lose response during scheduled maintenance therapy.

- Based on the therapeutic efficacy of antibodies to cytokines, such as anti-interleukin (IL)-12 and IL-23, immunotherapy and biologic therapy hold a considerable promise in the treatment of IBD.

Disclosure: There is no financial interest to declare.
a Gastroenterology Clinic of Acadiana and Lafayette General Medical Center, Lafayette, LA, USA
b Gastroenterology and Hepatology, Department of Medicine, Tulane University, New Orleans, LA, USA
* 1211 Coolidge Boulevard, Suite 303, Lafayette, LA 70503.
E-mail address: jpahluwalia@yahoo.com

Med Clin N Am 96 (2012) 525–544
doi:10.1016/j.mcna.2012.04.009   **medical.theclinics.com**
0025-7125/12/$ – see front matter © 2012 Elsevier Inc. All rights reserved.

INTRODUCTION

Inflammatory bowel disease (IBD), which includes Crohn disease (CD) and ulcerative colitis (UC), represents a group of chronic diseases that usually starts early in life, with 10% to 15% of the patients presenting with the disease later in life. Its incidence and prevalence seems to have increased, and it is considered to be one of the most prevalent gastrointestinal diseases.[1–3] Although the highest incidence and prevalence of IBD is reported to be in Europe, it is estimated that there are more than 1 million people with IBD in the United States.[3,4]

IBD is characterized by inflammation of the gastrointestinal tract and a relapsing and remitting or progressive clinical course resulting in significant morbidity and health care cost. Clinically, IBD is characterized by abdominal pain associated with diarrhea, rectal bleeding, and malnutrition. Although CD may affect any part of the gastrointestinal tract, UC is limited to the colon. IBD is also associated with an increased risk of colon cancer.[5]

Although the exact cause still remains unclear, IBD has been appreciated to have a genetic basis,[6] and environmental factors are thought to play a role in the pathogenesis of IBD as highlighted by the development of IBD in immigrants to high-prevalence areas[7] and discordance of IBD among monozygotic twins.[8] The importance of environmental factors is also underscored by a rising trend in the incidence and prevalence of IBD in countries undergoing rapid westernization.[9] In addition, the dysregulation of immune responses to intestinal bacterial antigens is hypothesized to play an important role in the development of IBD in genetically susceptible hosts.[10]

Standard nonsurgical treatment of IBD includes topical 5-aminosalicyclic acid agents, antimicrobials, steroids, and immunomodulators, such as azathioprine and 6-mercaptopurine. Patients with both CD and UC experience disease flares despite maintenance therapy with these agents used singly as monotherapy or in combination. Although these flares have been treated with short courses of corticosteroids, 20% to 40% of patients with IBD seem to become dependent on corticosteroids to maintain remission of the disease or become resistant to corticosteroids.[11–13] Of course, long-term use of corticosteroids is undesirable to avoid the known protean serious complications.

This article reviews the currently available immunologic agents for the treatment of patients with IBD and focuses on the efficacy of immunologic agents currently approved for the treatment of patients with CD and UC.

TUMOR NECROSIS FACTOR AND OTHER CYTOKINES IN IBD

Inflammation in UC and CD is regulated by increased secretion of proinflammatory cytokines.[14] Although an extensive review of cytokines involved in the development of IBD is beyond the scope of this article, it is noteworthy to mention that concentrations of cytokine tumor necrosis factor-α (TNF-α) are elevated in the blood,[15] mucosa,[16,17] and stool[18] of patients with IBD. In addition to TNF-α, the increased secretion of other proinflammatory cytokines in stools and rectal dialysates of patients with IBD was also seen in patients with both UC and CD.[19,20]

An increasing understanding of the involvement of the cytokines combined with the lack of adequate response and sustained remission of disease with standard medical treatment of IBD has allowed immunotherapy to emerge as an important modality in the treatment of patients with IBD. Several anti-TNF-α antibodies and other agents directed against cytokines or adhesion molecules involved in the pathogenesis of IBD have been developed and used in the treatment of IBD in clinical trials (**Table 1**). Thus far, 4 agents are approved for the treatment of IBD (see **Table 1**).

Table 1
Immunologic agents in IBD

Targeted Molecules	Antibody	Mode of Administration	Disease	FDA Approved	References
TNF	Infliximab	IV	CD, UC	+	Targan et al,[21] Hanauer et al,[22] Rutgeerts et al [23]
TNF	Adalimumab	SQ	CD, UC	+ (CD only)	Hanauer et al[24]
TNF	Certolizumab	SQ	CD	+	Schreiber et al,[25] Sandborn et al, [26] Sandborn et al [27]
CD3	Visilizumab	IV	UC	−	Baumgart et al,[28] Plevy et al [29]
CD40	Ch5D12	IV	CD	−	Kasran et al[30]
CD25	Daclizumab	IV	UC	−	Van Assche et al[31]
IL-6R	Tocilizumab (MRA)	IV	CD	−	Ito et al[32]
p40 of IL-12/IL-23	Briakinumab (ABT-874) & Ustekinumab	IV or SQ	CD	−	Elliott et al,[33] Mannon et al,[34] Toedter et al,[35] Sandborn et al[36]
Integrin α4	Natalizumab	IV	CD	+	Ghosh et al,[37] Sandborn et al[38]
Integrin α4β7	MLN-02	IV	UC	−	Feagan et al[39]

Abbreviations: IV, intravenous; SQ, subcutaneous.

ANTI-TNF-α THERAPY IN IBD
Infliximab

Infliximab (Remicade) is a chimeric murine monoclonal antibody against TNF-α that was released in 1998. It has shown significant benefits in patients with refractory luminal and fistulizing CD. It is approved by the US Food and Drug Administration (FDA) in IBD for the treatment of moderately to severely active CD and fistulizing CD and for the treatment of moderately to severely active UC. It is given intravenously as an induction dose of 5 mg/kg at weeks 0, 2, and 6 followed by a maintenance dose of 5 mg/kg every 8 weeks.

Infliximab in Luminal CD

Treatment of CD with cA2 (infliximab) was originally shown to be effective in normalizing the Crohn Disease Activity Index (CDAI) and the healing of colonic ulcerations in an open label study of 10 patients with active CD unresponsive to steroid treatment at a single center.[40]

This was followed by a 12-week multicenter, double-blind, placebo-controlled trial of cA2 (infliximab) in 108 patients with moderate-to-severe CD that was resistant to treatment (CDAI between 220–400).[21] Patients were randomly assigned to receive a single infusion of placebo or cA2 given in doses of 5 mg/kg, 10 mg/kg, or 20 mg/kg of body weight. The primary end point was the clinical response defined as a reduction of 70 or more points in the CDAI score at 4 weeks. At 4 weeks, 81% of the patients in the 5 mg/kg arm, 50% in the 10 mg/kg arm, and 64% in the 20 mg/kg arm had a clinical response compared with 17% of patients in the placebo group ($P<.001$ for the comparison of the cA2 group as a whole vs placebo). Among patients given cA2, 33% went into remission as defined by a CDAI score less than 150 compared with 4% of patients given placebo (P = .005). At 12 weeks, a significantly higher number of cA2-treated patients had a clinical response compared with placebo (41% vs 12%; P = .008), indicating that a single infusion of cA2 was an effective short-term treatment in many patients with moderate-to-severe treatment-resistant CD.

The benefit of maintenance therapy with infliximab in those who respond to the initial dose was assessed in a large international, randomized, double-blind trial termed A Crohn's Disease Clinical Trial Evaluating Infliximab in a New Long-Term Treatment Regimen (ACCENT I).[22] In total, 573 patients with a CDAI greater than or equal to 220 were given 5 mg/kg infliximab infusion at week 0 and the response was assessed at week 2 when patients were randomized to receive infusions of placebo at weeks 2 and 6 and then every 8 weeks until week 46 (group I), infusion of 5 mg/kg infliximab at the same time points (group II), or 5 mg/kg infliximab at weeks 2 and 6 followed by 10 mg/kg every 8 weeks (group III). Of the 573 patients entered into the study, 335 (58%) had a clinical response to infliximab at week 2. At week 30, 39% of the patients in group II and 45% of the patients in group III were in remission compared with only 21% in the placebo group. After 54 weeks, the median time to loss of response was 38 weeks in group II and more than 54 weeks in group III compared with 19 weeks in the placebo group (P = .002 and P = .002, respectively). A significantly higher percentage of patients receiving infliximab maintenance therapy on a scheduled basis had discontinued glucocorticoids and were in clinical remission with CDAI less than 150 (31.0% and 36.8% vs 10.7% for the 5 mg/kg and 10 mg/kg doses vs placebo, respectively). A post hoc analysis of C-reactive protein (CRP) in patients with a clinical response or in remission after induction therapy at week 14 in the ACCENT I trial showed a significant association between baseline CRP levels and maintenance of remission.[41] Forty-five percent of patients with a baseline CRP greater than or equal to 0.7 mg/dL versus 22% with CRP less than 0.7 mg/dL maintained remission (P = .012). Moreover, normalization of CRP at week 14 (decrease to <0.5 mg/dL) resulted in a higher probability of maintaining response or remission.

The long-term efficacy of treatment with infliximab was assessed in a large cohort of 614 patients with CD with a median follow-up of almost 5 years.[42] The primary analysis in this observational study looked at the proportion of patients with an initial response to infliximab who had sustained clinical benefit at the end of the 55-month follow-up. The analysis showed persistent improvement in symptoms in 63.4% of the patients receiving long-term infliximab treatment, indicating that infliximab is effective in maintaining improvement of symptoms in patients with CD not only during 1 year as published in randomized trials but also during a median follow-up of almost 5 years.

Infliximab in Fistulizing CD

Infliximab was shown initially to be an effective treatment of fistulas in patients with CD in 1999.[43] The study randomly assigned 94 patients with draining abdominal or perianal fistulas of at least 3 months' duration as a complication of CD to receive placebo, 5 mg/kg infliximab, or 10 mg/kg infliximab at weeks 0, 2, and 6. A reduction of greater than or equal to 50% from baseline in number of draining fistulas was observed in 68% of patients who received 5 mg/kg infliximab and 56% of those who received 10 mg/kg infliximab compared with 20% of patients in the placebo group (P = .002 and P = .02, respectively).

The pivotal maintenance trial that evaluated the efficacy and safety of infliximab in patients with fistulizing CD was the ACCENT II study.[44] This multicenter, double-blind, randomized, placebo-controlled trial included 306 adult patients with CD and 1 or more draining abdominal or perianal fistulas of at least a 3-month duration. Patients received 5 mg/kg infliximab on weeks 0, 2, and 6. The 195 patients who had a response at weeks 10 and 14 and the 87 nonresponders were then randomized to receive placebo or 5 mg/kg infliximab every 8 weeks to week 46 with a follow-up to week 54. Response was defined as a reduction of at least 50% from baseline in the number of draining fistulas at consecutive visits 4 weeks apart. The median time to a loss of response was greater than 40 weeks in patients who received infliximab maintenance therapy compared with 14 weeks in those who received placebo ($P<.001$). Complete absence of draining fistulas was also significantly better in the infliximab maintenance group versus the placebo group (36% vs 19%; $P = .009$).[44] A post hoc analysis of patients in the ACCENT II study also revealed a longer median duration of recto-vaginal fistula closure in the 5-mg/kg infliximab maintenance group compared with placebo (46 weeks vs 33 weeks) with an average follow-up of 53 and 48 weeks respectively.[45]

Thus, patients with fistulizing CD who respond to induction therapy with infliximab have an increased likelihood of a sustained response over 54 weeks if infliximab is continued as maintenance therapy every 8 weeks.

Infliximab in UC

The efficacy of infliximab for induction and maintenance therapy in adults with UC was evaluated in the randomized, double-blind, placebo-controlled trial termed Active Ulcerative Colitis Trials 1 and 2 (ACT-1 and ACT-2, respectively).[23] A total of 364 patients with moderate-to-severe active UC despite concurrent treatment with conventional therapy (ACT-1: corticosteroids alone or in combination with azathioprine or mercaptopurine; ACT-2: corticosteroids alone or in combination with azathioprine or mercaptopurine and medications containing 5-aminosalicylates) were randomly assigned in a 1:1:1 ratio to receive infusion of infliximab 5 mg/kg, 10 mg/kg, or placebo at weeks 0, 2, and 6 and then every 8 weeks through week 22 in ACT-2 or week 46 in the ACT-1. The primary end point was a clinical response at week 8. In the ACT-1 trial, 69% of patients given 5 mg/kg infliximab and 61% of those given 10 mg/kg had a clinical response at week 8 compared with 37% in the placebo group ($P<.001$ for both comparisons with placebo). In the ACT-2 trial, 64% of patients given 5 mg/kg infliximab and 69% of those given 10 mg/kg had a clinical response at week 8 compared with 29% given placebo ($P<.001$ for both comparisons with placebo). Response was defined as a decrease in the Mayo score greater than or equal to 3 and at least 30%, with an accompanying decrease in the subscore for rectal bleeding of at least 1 point or an absolute rectal bleeding subscore of 0 or 1). Patients who received infliximab were significantly more likely to have a clinical response at week 30 in both studies and at week 54 in the ACT-1 trial.

Thus, treatment with infliximab is effective in inducing a clinical response in patients with moderate-to-severe active UC and maintaining response if treatment is continued at 8-week intervals after the induction period.

ADALIMUMAB

Adalimumab (ADA) (Humira) is a fully humanized recombinant monoclonal antibody against TNF-α. It consists of humanized heavy- and light-chain variable regions and human IgG1 constant region. It binds specifically to TNF-α and blocks its interaction with p55 and p75 cell surface TNF receptors.[46] Unlike infliximab, it is administered subcutaneously with an induction dose of 160 mg at week 0 followed by 80 mg at

2 weeks. Subsequently, it is given as a maintenance dosage of 40 mg every other week.

ADA in Luminal CD

ADA has been shown to be effective in inducing and maintaining remission in patients with moderate-to-severe CD both in those naïve to infliximab and those with a loss of response to infliximab.

In a randomized, double-blind, placebo-controlled, dose-ranging study termed Clinical Assessment of Adalimumab Safety and Efficacy Studied in Induction Therapy in Crohn's Disease (CLASSIC-I), 299 patients with moderate-to-severe CD naïve to anti-TNF-α therapy were randomized to receive ADA 40 mg/20 mg, 80 mg/40 mg, or 160 mg/80 mg or placebo at weeks 0 and 2.[24] The primary end point was remission at week 4 defined by a CDAI score less than 150 points. Although the remission rate at 4 weeks was not significantly different in the 40 mg/20 mg and 80 mg/40 mg ADA groups versus placebo (18%, 24%, and 12%, respectively), it was significantly higher in the group that received ADA 160 mg/80 mg compared with placebo (36% vs 12%; $P = .001$).

To evaluate long-term efficacy and safety of ADA maintenance therapy in CD, 55 patients in clinical remission at week 4 in the CLASSIC-I trial were randomized to receive ADA 40 mg every other week, 40 mg weekly, or placebo in the CLASSIC-II trial.[47] Patients in the randomized arm with continued nonresponse or disease flare could switch to open label at ADA 40 mg every other week and again to 40 mg weekly. Of these 55 randomized patients, 79% who received ADA 40 mg every other week and 83% who received ADA 40 mg weekly were in remission at week 56 versus 44% for placebo ($P<.05$).

These findings were extended to the maintenance of remission in a larger study involving 854 patients with moderate-to-severe CD.[48] This study, termed the Crohn's Trial of the Fully Human Antibody Adalimumab for Remission Maintenance (CHARM) trial, was a phase 3, randomized, double-blind, placebo-controlled, 56-week study in patients with CD who may or may not have previously received anti-TNF-α therapy. In this trial, after an open-label induction therapy with ADA 80 mg at week 0 followed by 40 mg at week 2, patients were stratified by response (decrease in CDAI $\geq$70 points) at week 4 and randomized to double-blind treatment with placebo, ADA 40 mg every other week, or ADA 40 mg weekly through week 56. A significantly greater percentage of patients were in remission in ADA 40 mg every other week and 40 mg weekly versus placebo at week 26 (40%, 47%, and 17%, respectively; $P<.001$) and also at week 56 (36%, 41%, and 12%, respectively; $P<.001$). No significant difference in efficacy between ADA 40 mg every other week and 40 mg weekly was observed.

Recently, the steroid-sparing effect of ADA in the 1-year CHARM study and an additional 2 years in its open-label extension were published.[49] In the 206 patients randomized to ADA, modest steroid-free remission was noted after 1 year and 3 years of treatment (26% and 23%, respectively).

ADA in Patients with CD not Responding to Infliximab

ADA was first reported to induce remission (CDAI score <150 points) more frequently than placebo in patients with moderate-to-severe CD (CDAI score 220 to 450 points) who could not tolerate infliximab or had symptoms despite receiving infliximab therapy by Sandborn and colleagues.[50] In this 4-week, randomized, double-blind, placebo-controlled trial, 325 patients were randomized to receive induction with ADA 160 mg at weeks 0 and 80 mg at week 2 or placebo at the same time points. At week 4, 21% of the patients in the ADA group versus 7% in the placebo group achieved remission (P<.001). A systematic review that included patients in randomized control trials or open label cohorts evaluated the short-term or long-term efficacy of ADA in infliximab failures.[51] In a total of 1810 patients with CD identified in 15 studies, the short-term clinical response at 4 weeks ranged from 41% to 83%, whereas the long-term clinical remission at 12 months ranged from 19% to 68%.

ADA in Fistulizing CD

ADA was shown to result in complete fistula closure in a greater percentage of ADA-treated patients versus those receiving placebo in the randomized population at both week 26 (30% and 13%, P = .043) and week 56 (33% and 13%, P = .16) in the CHARM trial.[48] Among patients with complete fistula closure at week 26, 100% continued to have complete fistula closure at week 56.

ADA was also reported to be effective in fistula closure in patients who failed infliximab in an open-label, single-arm Crohn Disease WHO Failed Prior Infliximab to Collect Safety Data and Efficacy via Patient-Reported Measures (CHOICE) trial.[52] A total of 673 patients, 17% of whom were infliximab primary nonresponders and 83% were initial responders, were enrolled and treated with ADA (induction dose of 160 mg at weeks 0 and 80 mg at week 2 followed by a maintenance dose of 40 mg every other week) after a minimum of 8 weeks of an infliximab washout period. Complete fistula healing was achieved in 39% (34/88) of patients with baseline fistulas, indicating that ADA is an effective first-line therapy for anti-TNF-naïve patients and also an important option for infliximab-refractory or infliximab-intolerant patients.

ADA in UC

ADA is not approved for treatment of UC. However, open-label trials showed ADA to be effective in inducing and maintaining remission in active UC in patients intolerant of or refractory to standard therapy.[53–56]

One double-blind, randomized, placebo-controlled, multicenter study assessed the efficacy and safety of ADA for the induction of clinical remission in anti-TNF naïve patients with moderately to severely active UC.[57] Patients with a Mayo score ≥ 6 and endoscopic subscore ≥ 2 despite treatment with corticosteroids or immunosuppressants were included. The primary end point was clinical remission at week 8 (Mayo score ≤ 2). Initially, 160 patients were randomized 1:1 to treatment with ADA with an induction dose of 160 mg/80 mg (160 mg at weeks 0, 80 mg at week 2, 40 mg at weeks 4 and 6) or placebo. Subsequently, the protocol was amended to include a second induction group: ADA 80 mg/40 mg (80 mg at weeks 0, 40 mg at weeks 2 , 4, and 6). At week 8, clinical remission was noted in 18.5% of patients in the ADA 160 mg/80 mg group versus 9.2% in the placebo group (P = .031). A 10.0% remission rate was found in the ADA 80 mg/40 mg group compared with 9.2% in the placebo group (P = .833). Additional post hoc analyses showed that extensive disease, more active disease, and high CRP (CRP ≥ 10 mg/L) were associated with low rates of clinical remission, possibly reflecting a greater efficacy of ADA in less severe disease. After 8 weeks, 390 patients originally randomized to all 3 arms entered an open-label study and received ADA 40 mg every other week as maintenance therapy through 52 weeks. At the end of 52 weeks, 25.6% of the patients were in clinical remission with a maintenance therapy of 40 mg every other week.[58]

More recently, the Ulcerative Colitis Long-term Remission and Maintenance with Adalimumab 2 (ULTRA 2) study evaluating the induction and maintenance of clinical remission was published.[59] This randomized, double-blind, placebo-controlled trial assessed the efficacy of ADA in 494 patients with moderate-to-severe UC who received concurrent treatment with oral corticosteroids or an immunosuppressant.

The study stratified the patients based on prior exposure to TNF-α antagonists and randomly assigned them to groups given ADA 160 mg at weeks 0, 80 mg at week 2 and then 40 mg every other week, or placebo. Primary end points were remission at weeks 8 and 52. Significantly more patients treated with ADA achieved clinical remission at week 8 (16.5% on ADA vs 9.3% on placebo; $P = .019$) and week 52 (17.3% on ADA vs 8.5% on placebo; $P = .004$). Rates of remission were higher in anti-TNF-α naïve patients. At week 8, 21.3% of anti-TNF-α naïve patients treated with ADA versus 11.0% on placebo ($P = .017$) achieved remission. At week 52, the corresponding values were 22.0% on ADA versus 12.4% on placebo ($P = .029$). Among those previously exposed to anti-TNF agents, the rate of remission was 9.2% on ADA versus 6.9% on placebo at week 8 ($P = .559$) compared with 10.2% on ADA versus 3.0% on placebo at week 52 ($P = .039$).

Thus, ADA seems to be more effective than placebo in inducing and maintaining clinical remission in patients with moderate-to-severe UC without an adequate response to conventional therapy with steroids or immunosuppressants; the clinical remission may be better in those not previously exposed to an anti-TNF agent.

CERTOLIZUMAB PEGOL (CDP870)

Certolizumab pegol (CZP) (Cimzia; UCB Pharma, Brussels, Belgium) is a pegylated Fab fragment of an anti-TNF-α antibody. It is a humanized antibody that binds TNF-α with a high affinity. Unlike infliximab and ADA, it lacks the Fc portion and, thus, does not induce in vitro complement activation, antibody-dependent cellular cytotoxicity, or apoptosis.[60] Attachment of a 40-kDa polyethylene glycol moiety to the Fab fragment markedly increases the half-life of CZP to be comparable to that of the whole antibody product. It is administered subcutaneously and, like infliximab and ADA, has been approved by the US FDA for the treatment of CD. CZP is approved for CD only in the United States, Switzerland, and Russia.

The CZP dose for induction of remission is 400 mg subcutaneously at weeks 0, 2, and 4. The maintenance dose for admission is 400 mg subcutaneously administered every 4 weeks.

CZP in CD

A randomized placebo-controlled trial investigated the efficacy and safety of CZP in patients with active CD.[61] In this phase II study, 292 patients with moderate-to-severe CD were randomized to receive subcutaneous CZP 100, 200, or 400 mg or placebo at weeks 4 and 8.[61] A significant clinical benefit over placebo was noted for all CZP doses at week 2 (placebo, 15.1%; CZP 100 mg, 29.7%, $P = .33$; 200 mg, 30.6%, $P = .026$; 400 mg, 33.3%, $P = .010$). Clinical response rates were highest for CZP 400 mg at all time points and greatest at week 10 (placebo, 30.1% and CZP 400 mg, 52.8%, $P = .006$) but not significant at week 12 (placebo, 35.6% and CZP 400 mg, 44.4%, $P = .278$). Post hoc analysis showed that patients with a baseline CRP greater than or equal to 10 mg/L (n = 119) showed a clearer separation between active treatment and placebo at week 12 (placebo, 17.9% vs CZP 400 mg, 53.1%; $P = .005$) because of a lower placebo response rate than patients with a CRP less than 10 mg/L. Another randomized, double-blind, placebo-controlled trial published in 2007 involved 662 adult patients with moderate-to-severe CD.[26] Patients were stratified according to a baseline CRP level and were randomized to receive either CZP 400 mg (n = 331) or placebo (n = 329) subcutaneously at weeks 0, 2, and 4 and then every 4 weeks, with patients followed through week 26. In patients with a CRP greater than or equal to 10 mg/L, 37% of patients in the CZP group had a response at week 6 compared with

26% in the placebo group (P = .04). The response rate at both weeks 6 and 26 was 22% (31/144) in the CZA group versus 12% (19/154) in the placebo group (P = .05). Without stratification according to CRP, the response rate was 35% in the CZP group and 27% in the placebo group (P = .02) in the overall population at week 6, and 23% and 16%, respectively, at both weeks 6 and 26 (P = .02). However, the rate of remission (defined as a CDAI score of 150 points or less) at weeks 6 and 26 in the treated or placebo groups were not significantly different (P = .17).

Both of the 2 previously mentioned randomized control trials were affected by higher-than-expected placebo response and remission rates.[25,26] A more recent placebo-controlled randomized trial evaluated the efficacy of CZP therapy in 439 patients with moderate-to-severe CD naïve to anti-TNF therapy.[27] Patients were randomized to receive CZP 400 mg subcutaneously (n = 215) or placebo (n = 215) at weeks 0, 2, and 4. The clinical response (defined as ≥100-point decrease in base-line CDAI score) at weeks 2, 4, and 6 in the CZP and placebo groups were 33% and 20% (P = .001), 35% and 26% (P = .024), and 41% and 34% (P = .179), respectively. The clinical remission (defined as CDAI score of 150 or less) rates at weeks 2 and 4 in the CZP and placebo groups were 23% and 16% (P = .33), and 27% and 19% (P = .063), respectively. However, at the 6-week time point, a remission rate of 36% in the CZP group was also not significantly different from that of 35% in the placebo group (P = .174).

Thus, CZP treatment may have a modest improvement in response but no improvement in remission rate, compared with placebo, in patients with moderate-to-severe CD.

CZP in UC

Studies are currently underway to test if CZP is efficacious in patients with UC.

ANTI-TNF-α THERAPY AND MUCOSAL HEALING IN IBD

Mucosal healing has emerged as an important clinical outcome in patients with IBD and has been shown to be associated with improved clinical outcome.[62–64] Mucosal healing also predicts a better chance of sustained clinical remission in patients with early stage CD.[65]

The endoscopic substudy of the ACCENT I (see earlier discussion) CD trial examined the effects of infliximab on mucosal inflammation and mucosal healing.[66] Ileocolonic examinations were performed at weeks 0, 10, and 54. Complete mucosal healing was defined as the absence of all mucosal ulcerations. The principal end point was the proportion of patients randomized as responders with mucosal healing at week 10. Complete mucosal healing by week 10 occurred in more week-2 responders who received 3 doses of infliximab compared with a single dose (31% vs 0%, P = .01). Compared with the episodic group, a significantly higher proportion of week-2 responders in the combined scheduled maintenance group had complete mucosal healing (7% vs 50%, P = .007). Thus, scheduled infliximab maintenance therapy resulted in more improvement in mucosal ulceration and high rates of mucosal healing.

In the ACT-1 and ACT-2 trials, patients with UC treated with infliximab were more likely to undergo remission and mucosal healing compared with those given placebo.[23] Findings of these trials also showed that early mucosal healing with infliximab is associated with an improved long-term clinical outcome in UC.[67] In these trials, patients underwent endoscopic evaluations at weeks 0, 8, 30, and 54 (ACT-I only) and were categorized into 4 subgroups by week 8 based on Mayo endoscopy subscores: 0, normal or inactive disease; 1, mild disease with erythema, decreased vascular pattern, mild friability; 2, moderate disease with marked erythema, absent vascular pattern, friability, erosions; and 3, severe disease with spontaneous bleeding, ulceration. Infliximab-treated patients with lower week-8 endoscopy subscores were less likely to progress to colectomy through week 54 ($P = .0004$) and achieved better corticosteroid-free symptomatic remission at week 30 (46.0% [subscore 0]; 34.0% [subscore 1]; 11.0% [subscore 2]; and 6.5% [subscore 3]; $P<.0001$) and week 54 (47.0% [subscore 0]; 35.0% [subscore 1]; 5.3% [subscore 2]; and 5.3% [subscore 3]; $P<.0001$).

In a recent report of data from the EXTEND (Extend the Safety and Efficacy of Adalimumab through Endoscopic Healing) trial, adalimumab was also shown to induce and maintain mucosal healing in patients with moderately to severely active ileocolonic CD.[68]

ANTI-TNF-α THERAPY AND REDUCTION IN HOSPITALIZATION AND SURGERY

Treatment with anti-TNF agents has been shown to reduce disease-related hospitalization rates and surgery in patients with both CD and UC.

In the ACCENT I trial, patients receiving scheduled therapy with infliximab had significantly fewer hospitalizations (23% vs 38%) and surgeries (3% vs 7%) related to CD.[22] In the ACCENT II study, of the 282 patients given 5 mg/kg infliximab induction therapy at weeks 0, 2, and 6, 195 patients showed a greater than 50% reduction in the baseline number of draining fistulas at both weeks 10 and 14.[69] Among these responders, those randomized at week 14 to continue receiving 5 mg/kg infliximab maintenance therapy every 8 weeks had significantly fewer mean hospitalization days compared to those who received placebo maintenance (0.5 vs 2.5 days; $P<.05$).[69] ADA maintenance therapy also decreased the risk of hospitalization and surgery in patients with CD.[70] Data from the CHARM trial of a total of 778 patients randomized to ADA 40 mg every other week or ADA 40 mg weekly after an 80 mg/40 mg induction regimen, as outlined earlier, showed 52% and 60% relative reductions in all-cause hospitalization risk at 12 months and a 48% and 64% reduction in risk of CD-related hospitalization at 12 months, respectively, compared with placebo.[70] The 12-month estimated hospitalization risk for both the all-cause and CD-related hospitalizations was reduced by 56% in the combined ADA treatment group compared with placebo.[70] In comparison to placebo, anti-TNF-α therapy with infliximab was also effective in reducing UC-related hospitalizations (40 vs 20; $P = .003$) and surgeries per 100 patient-years of treatment (34 vs 21; $P = .03$) in the ACT-1 and ACT-2 randomized, double-blind, placebo-controlled studies.[71] Patients receiving infliximab for treatment of CD were also found to have a lower risk for hospitalization (hazard ratio = 0.73; 95% confidence interval [CI] 0.63–0.85) and lower rates of hospitalized days (rate ratio = 0.69; 95% CI 0.49–0.97) in a retrospective Canadian study that assessed health claims between 1996 and 2007 processed by the provincial health care insurer in Québec.[72]

Anti-TNF-α therapy with both infliximab and ADA has been shown to reduce the requirement for CD-related surgery.[69,70,72] In the ACCENT II study, the 5 mg/kg infliximab maintenance group had an approximately 50% reduction in the mean number of all surgeries and procedures compared with the placebo maintenance group for all randomized patients (60 vs 118 surgeries per 100 patients; $P<.01$).[69] In the CHARM study, fewer CD-related surgeries occurred in the ADA 40 mg every other week, 40 mg weekly, and combined ADA groups compared with placebo (0.4, 0.8, and 0.6 vs 3.8 per 100 patients; all $P<.05$).[70] Patients with CD treated with infliximab were also found to have a significantly lower risk of having CD-related intraabdominal surgery (hazard ratio = 0.64; 95% CI space 0.51–0.81).[72] Similarly, the colectomy rate after the treatment of patients with moderately to severely active UC with infliximab was lower at 17% compared with 10% in those receiving placebo ($P = .02$) through week 54.[71]

ANTI-α_4-INTEGRIN THERAPY IN IBD

Effective immune surveillance requires the recruitment and positioning of immune cells in specific tissue compartments,[73] which is accomplished by the selective expression of adhesion molecules and chemokine receptors on lymphocytes that allows them to bind to their endothelial ligands in vascular beds. Mucosa in patients with IBD is known to have a high expression of vascular adhesion molecules resulting in recruitment of inflammatory cells.[74] Thus, interfering with the interaction of adhesion molecules found on vascular beds and lymphocytes offers a novel tool for treatment of patients with IBD.

Natalizumab

Natalizumab (NZA) (Tysabri, Elan Pharmaceuticals and Biogen Idec) is a humanized monoclonal immunoglobulin G4 (IgG4) antibody against α_4-integrin that inhibits the adhesion and migration of leukocytes into inflamed tissue by binding α_4-integrin.[73] It is given as an intravenous infusion of 300 mg at weeks 0 and 4 and then every 4 weeks. Because of the increased risk of progressive multifocal leukoencephalopathy (PML),[38,75–77] it is only available now through a restricted prescribing program called the TYSABRI TOUCH Prescribing Program.[78]

NZA has been used in clinical trials of patients with CD. In one double-blind placebo-controlled trial, NZA produced a significant improvement in response rates (defined by a reduction of $\geq$70 points in the CDAI score).[37] The highest response rate was 71% and the highest remission rate (defined as a CDAI score $\leq$150) was 44% in the group given 2 infusions of 3 mg/kg 4 weeks apart.

The results of 2 controlled trials that evaluated NZA as induction and maintenance therapy in patients with active CD were also published in 2005.[38] In the first trial, 905 patients were randomized to receive either 300 mg NZA or placebo at weeks 0, 4, and 8; the primary outcome was response (decrease in the CDAI score $\geq$70 points) at week 10. In the second trial, 339 patients with a response to NZA in the first trial were randomly assigned to receive 300 mg NZA or placebo every 4 weeks through week 56; the primary outcome was a sustained response through week 36. Although NZA and placebo groups had similar rates of response (56% vs 49%, $P = .05$) and remission (37% vs 30%, $P = .12$) in the first trial at 10 weeks, a subgroup analysis of patients with elevated CRP as a marker for active inflammation demonstrated significantly greater response and remission rates for NZA than for placebo. The continuation of NZA in the second trial resulted in a higher rate of sustained response (61% vs 28%, $P<.001$) and remission (44% vs 26%, $P = .003$) through week 36 than did switching to placebo. Another randomized placebo-controlled trial confirmed superior early and sustained efficacy of NZA as an induction therapy in patients with moderate to severe CD and elevated CRP.[79]

Although NZA may be beneficial in patients with CD, it is important to risk stratify patients based on their exposure to the John Cunningham (JC) virus before starting treatment with NZA. A recent US FDA warning identifies positivity for anti-JC virus antibodies in patients treated with NZA longer than 2 years and a prior history of treatment with an immunosuppressant (eg, azathioprine, methotrexate, cyclophosphamide or mycophenolate mofetil) to increase the relative risk of PML to 11/1000 users.[77]

IMMUNOGENICITY

Because infliximab is a chimeric monoclonal antibody, it is not surprising that treatment with infliximab can result in the formation of antibodies against infliximab. In an earlier study assessing the influence of immunogenicity on long-term efficacy of infliximab in patients with CD, serum concentrations of infliximab and that of antibodies against infliximab were evaluated in a cohort of 125 consecutive patients with CD treated with infliximab.[80] A mean of 3.9 infliximab infusions (range 1–17) were administered per patient over a mean period of 10 months. In this study of patients with CD treated episodically (on demand) with infliximab, antibodies against infliximab were detected in 61% of the patients. Moreover, a serum antibody concentration of 8 mcg/mL or greater was associated with a shorter duration of response (35 days compared with 71 days in patients with concentration <8 mcg/mL; $P<.001$) and a higher risk of infusion reactions (relative risk, 2.40; 95% CI, 1.65 to 3.66; $P<.001$). Data from the ACCENT I trial also indicated a higher rate of anti-infliximab antibodies through week 72 in patients with CD given infliximab episodically as monotherapy versus those given infliximab maintenance therapy at a dose of 5 mg/kg or 10 mg/kg dose every 8 weeks (30% vs 8%, respectively; $P<.0001$).[81] However, there was a lower incidence of antibodies in patients receiving combined therapy with infliximab and immunomodulators compared with patients receiving infliximab alone (10% vs 18%, respectively; $P = .02$). Although the clinical response was similar in antibody-positive and antibody-negative patients in the overall population (64% vs 62%), fewer antibody-positive patients in the episodically treated group obtained clinical remission compared with those who were antibody negative (31% vs 37%, respectively). Thus, studies suggest that scheduled dosing of infliximab and the concomitant use of immunosuppressive therapy are more likely to yield a corticosteroid-free clinical remission.

Although ADA is a fully humanized antibody, its use does not totally eliminate the risk of developing anti-drug antibodies. In the recent ULTRA 2 study assessing the efficacy of ADA in the induction and maintenance of clinical remission in patients with moderate-to-severe UC, antibodies to ADA were detected in 2.9% of the patients in the ADA group.[59] Interestingly, all 7 of the 245 patients who developed antibodies to ADA received ADA monotherapy, suggesting that the use of immunomodulators along with anti-TNF-α therapy decreases the rate of the development of antibodies to anti-TNF agents, as noted previously in the Study of Biologic and Immunomodulator Naive Patients in Crohn Disease (SONIC) comparing efficacy of infliximab and azathioprine therapy alone or in combination for moderate-to-severe CD.[82]

In one CZP study, detectable anti-CZP antibodies developed in 8% of patients (26 of 331) in the CZP group.[26] In those receiving concomitant immunosuppressive therapy, only 4% of patients (4 of 126) developed anti-CZP antibodies, similar to the findings reported for infliximab in analysis of the data from the ACCENT I trial.[81]

Antibodies against NZA were found in 8% of the patients in the Efficacy of Natalizumab as Active Crohn Therapy (ENACT-1) study and 9% of the patients in the Evaluation of Natalizumab as Continuous Therapy (ENACT-2) study.[38] As seen for anti-TNF agents, concomitant immunosuppressive and corticosteroid therapy seemed to be moderately protective against the formation of antibodies against NZA.[38]

The development of antibodies to all available biologic agents is associated with an increased risk of infusion reactions and decreased clinical remission in patients with IBD (see later discussion). Although concomitant immunosuppressive and corticosteroid therapy may reduce the magnitude of the immunogenic response to the therapeutic agent used in the treatment of patients with CD or UC, immunogenicity to anti-TNF-α agents and anti-α_4-integrin contributes to a loss of response to treatment with these agents.

SIDE EFFECTS AND OTHER CHALLENGES LINKED TO ANTI-TNF-α THERAPY AND OTHER BIOLOGICS

Anti-TNF agents and other biologics are indicated as induction therapy in patients with moderate-to-severe CD or active UC not responding to conventional treatment with 5-aminosalicylates, glucocorticoids, or immunosuppressive agents, unremitting fistulizing CD despite standard therapy and maintenance of treatment in patients responding to induction therapy. As the use of biologic therapies for the treatment of IBD and other diseases has risen since the introduction of anti-TNF-α therapy in late 1990s, several important side effects related to the use of antibodies directed against TNF and other biologic agents have been appreciated. Hence, patients with IBD treated with anti-TNF-α or other biologic agents need to be monitored carefully during therapy.

Infusion Reactions

The overall incidence of infusion reactions to infliximab, including burning sensation, erythema, and pain, was 6.1% of infusions in 9.7% of the patients in a retrospective study of 165 consecutive patients with CD who received a total of 479 infliximab infusions.[83] Fifteen of 29 (51.7%) infusion reactions occurred after one of the first 3 infusions. Patients who were off treatment for more than 4 months were more susceptible to developing infusion reactions. All mild and moderate infusion reactions resolved rapidly after the administration of acetaminophen, antihistamines, steroids, or epinephrine. Genuine allergic reactions characterized by shortness of breath and urticaria, mediated by IgE and involving mast cell and basophil degranulation, were rare. Thus, most of the acute infusion reactions may not be IgE mediated.

Delayed reactions occur 3 to 14 days after anti-TNF-α therapy and commonly present with arthralgia and myalgia.[83] They are thought to be caused by the deposition of immune complexes and develop more often in patients with a large interval between the first administration of anti-TNF-α therapy and the subsequent adminstration.[84]

Because ADA and CZA are given subcutaneously, injection-site reactions have been reported in 3% to 4% of the patients treated with these agents.[26,48]

Infections

Although infections of the upper respiratory tract and urinary tract are most common, fatal sepsis has been reported in patients treated with infliximab.[85] In the CHARM study, infectious adverse events occurred in 15.2% and serious infectious adverse events occurred in 1.2% of the patients treated with ADA during the open-label induction period.[48] Serious infections occurred in 2% of the patients treated with CZA compared with less than 1% in the placebo group.[26]

Serious infections related to anti-TNF-α therapy include reactivation of latent tuberculosis, and the most important risk factor for reactivation was concomitant immunosuppressive therapy.[85,86] Adherence to guidelines for tuberculosis screening before initiating anti-TNF therapy is associated with a decrease in tuberculosis in this patient population. Because tuberculosis has been reported in patients with a negative tuberculin skin test before starting anti-TNF-α therapy, the T-cell–based interferon-γ assay may be a more reliable screening test for tuberculosis before starting anti-TNF-α therapy.[85,86]

Fungal infections in patients treated with infliximab include histoplasmosis (30%), candidiasis (23%), and aspergillosis (23%).[87] Listeriosis and pneumocystosis have also been reported. The risk of opportunistic infections in patients with IBD treated with infliximab has been reported to be between 0.3% and 0.9%, and the risk of opportunistic infection increases dramatically when anti-TNF-α therapy is combined with additional immunosuppressive therapy with corticosteroids or thiopurines.[85,88]

Because reactivation of hepatitis B has been documented in patients treated with anti-TNF-α therapy, screening for hepatitis B with hepatitis B surface antigen and vaccination of those not immune to hepatitis B is advocated before starting anti-TNF-α therapy.[89]

Malignancies

The most important concern with prolonged use of biologics is the risk of developing cancer, such as lymphoma.[85] Although a single-center cohort study of 734 patients with IBD treated with infliximab and 666 control patients followed for a median time of 58 and 144 months, respectively, found no difference in malignancies or mortality in the 2 groups,[86] cases of PML have been reported in patients given NZA.[38,75,76] As of January 4, 2012, there have been 201 confirmed cases of PML documented in patients treated with NZA since it became available in July 2006.[77] Although cases of often-fatal hepatosplenic T-cell lymphoma have also been linked to the use of infliximab, ADA and azathioprine/6-mercaptopurine,[90] the pros and cons of using biologics have to be weighed against the rarity of these cancers and the benefit of treating patients to avoid multiple complications related to IBD.

Loss of Response to Anti-TNF-α Therapy and Strategies for Management of Patients with Loss of Response

Patients who initially respond to an anti-TNF-α therapy may lose the response during scheduled maintenance treatment. Although the underlying reasons are not completely understood, several factors, including the development of neutralizing antibodies, genetic factors, individual differences in drug metabolism and elimination, concomitant medications, and smoking in patients with CD, seem to play a role.[91,92]

In addition to the reassessment of disease activity by checking inflammatory markers, such as CRP, and endoscopic or radiological studies to confirm ongoing inflammation, the measurement of the anti-TNF agent trough level and antibodies to the anti-TNF agent has been proposed as part of a strategy to determine the cause of loss of response.[91,92] In cases whereby trough levels are low or undetectable, the measurement of an antidrug antibody helps differentiate immunogenicity from rapid drug clearance. Those with a low or undetectable trough level can be treated with dose intensification either by increasing the dose or shortening the dosing interval, and those with antidrug antibody can be switched to another anti-TNF agent.[91,92] A recent multicenter retrospective study of patients with CD losing response to infliximab reported sustained clinical response at 12 months after dose escalation in 50% of the patients in the dose-doubling group compared with 39% in the interval-halving group (odds ratio 1.5, 95% CI 0.8–2.9, $P = .02$).[93]

Because commercial assays are not available for ADA and CZA, the management of patients with IBD losing response to these 2 agents is empiric.

SUMMARY

A growing understanding of the molecules involved in the pathogenesis of IBD has led to the development of treatment modalities that interfere with these molecules in the pathogenesis of CD and UC. Starting with the introduction of infliximab, several anti-TNF agents and antibodies that interfere with the interaction of lymphocytes with adhesion molecules in vascular beds have emerged as important tools in the treatment of patients with IBD with factors associated with poor prognosis[94] and those who fail to respond to conventional therapy. However, about one-third of the patients with IBD do not respond to an induction regimen with an anti-TNF agent.[22,24,47,48,61] In addition, several randomized control trials showed that between 25% and 40% of patients who initially benefit from treatment with an anti-TNF-α go on to develop intolerable adverse effects or lose the response during scheduled maintenance treatment.[44,48,61,80] Thus, additional therapies are needed for the treatment of patients with IBD. Based on the therapeutic efficacy of antibodies to cytokines, such as anti-IL-12p40, in clinical trials and other strategies targeting cytokine pathways to decrease inflammation in the bowel,[34,36,95] immunotherapy and biologic therapy hold a considerable promise in providing newer agents for the treatment of patients with IBD.

ACKNOWLEDGMENTS

The author thanks Dr Stephen Abshire for reviewing the article.

REFERENCES

1. Korzenik JR, Podolsky DK. Evolving knowledge and therapy of inflammatory bowel disease. Nat Rev Drug Discov 2006;5:197–209.
2. Loftus EV Jr. Clinical epidemiology of inflammatory bowel disease: incidence, prevalence, and environmental influences. Gastroenterology 2004;126:1504–17.
3. Molodecky NA, Soon IS, Rabi DM, et al. Increasing incidence and prevalence of the inflammatory bowel diseases with time, based on systematic review. Gastroenterology 2012;142:46–54.
4. Loftus CG, Loftus EV Jr, Harmsen WS, et al. Update on the incidence and prevalence of Crohn's disease and ulcerative colitis in Olmstead County, Minnesota, 1940–2000. Inflamm Bowel Dis 2007;13:254–61.
5. Bernstein CN, Blanchard JF, Kliewer E, et al. Cancer risk in patients with inflammatory bowel disease: a population-based study. Cancer 2001;91:854–62.
6. Cho J, Brant SR. Recent insights into the genetics of inflammatory bowel disease. Gastroenterology 2011;140:1704–12.
7. Tsironi E, Feakins RM, Probert CS, et al. Incidence of inflammatory bowel disease is rising and abdominal tuberculosis is following in Bangladeshis and East London, United Kingdom. Am J Gastroenterol 2004;99:1749–55.
8. Halme L, Paavola-Sakki P, Turunen U, et al. Family and twin studies in inflammatory bowel disease. World J Gastroenterol 2006;12:3668–72.
9. Thia KT, Loftus EV Jr, Sandborn WJ, et al. An update on the epidemiology of inflammatory bowel disease in Asia. Am J Gastroenterol 2008;103:3167–82.
10. Kaser A, Zeissig S, Blumberg RS. Inflammatory bowel disease. Ann Rev Immunol 2010;28:573–621.
11. Faubion WA Jr, Loftus E Jr, Harmsen WS, et al. The natural history of corticosteroid therapy for inflammatory bowel disease: a population-based study. Gastroenterology 2001;121:255–60.
12. Ho GT, Chiam P, Drummond H, et al. The efficacy of corticosteroid therapy in inflammatory bowel disease: analysis of a 5-year UK inception cohort. Aliment Pharmacol Ther 2006;24:319–30.
13. Munkholm P, Langholz E, Davidsen M, et al. Frequency of glucocorticoid resistance and dependency in Crohn's disease. Gut 1994;35:360–2.
14. Strober W, Fuss IJ. Proinflammatory cytokines in the pathogenesis of inflammatory bowel diseases. Gastroenterology 2011;140:1756–67.

15. Murch SH, Lamkin VA, Savage MO, et al. Serum concentrations of tumor necrosis factor alpha in childhood chronic inflammatory bowel disease. Gut 1991;32: 913–7.
16. Breese EJ, Michie CA, Nicholls SW, et al. Tumor necrosis factor alpha-producing cells in the intestinal mucosa of children with inflammatory bowel disease. Gastroenterology 1994;106:1455–66.
17. MacDonald TT, Hutchings P, Choy MY, et al. Tumor necrosis factor-alpha and interferon-gamma production measured at the single cell level in normal and inflamed human intestine. Clin Exp Immunol 1990;81:301–5.
18. Braegger CP, Nicholls S, Murch SH, et al. Tumor necrosis factor alpha in stool as a marker of intestinal inflammation. Lancet 1992;339:89–91.
19. Nielsen OH, Gionchetti P, Ainsworth M, et al. Rectal dialysate and fecal concentrations of neutrophil gelatinase-associated lipocalin, interleukin-8, and tumor necrosis factor-alpha in ulcerative colitis. Am J Gastroenterol 1999;94:2923–8.
20. Saiki T, Mitsuyama K, Toyonaga A, et al. Detection of pro- and anti-inflammatory cytokines in stools of patients with inflammatory bowel disease. Scand J Gastroenterol 1998;33:616–22.
21. Targan SR, Hanauer SB, van Deventer SJ, et al. A short-term study of chimeric monoclonal antibody cA2 to tumor necrosis factor alpha for Crohn's disease. N Engl J Med 1997;337:1029–35.
22. Hanauer SB, Feagan BG, Lichtenstein GR, et al. Maintenance infliximab for Crohn's disease: the ACCENT I randomized trial. Lancet 2002;359:1541–9.
23. Rutgeerts P, Sandborn WJ, Feagan BG, et al. Infliximab for induction and maintenance therapy for ulcerative colitis. N Engl J Med 2005;353:2462–76.
24. Hanauer SB, Sandborn WJ, Rutgeerts P, et al. Human anti-tumor necrosis factor monoclonal antibody (adalimumab) in Crohn's disease: the CLASSIC-I trial. Gastroenterology 2006;130:323–33.
25. Schreiber S, Rutgeerts P, Fedorak RN, et al. A randomized, placebo-controlled trial of certolizumab pegol (CDP870) for treatment of Crohn's disease. Gastroenterology 2005;129:807–18.
26. Sandborn WJ, Feagan BG, Stoinov S, et al. Certolizumab pegol for the treatment of Crohn's disease. N Engl J Med 2007;357:228–38.
27. Sandborn WJ, Schreiber S, Feagan BG, et al. Certolizumab pegol for active Crohn's disease: a placebo-controlled, randomized trial. Clin Gastroenterol Hepatol 2011;9:670–8.
28. Baumgart DC, Targan SR, Dignass AU, et al. Prospective randomized open-labile multicenter phase I/II dose escalation trial of visilizumab (HuM291) in severe steroid-refractory ulcerative colitis. Inflamm Bowel Dis 2010;16:620–9.
29. Plevy S, Salzberg B, Van Assche G, et al. A phase I study of visilizumab, a humanized anti-CD 3 monoclonal antibody, in severe steroid-refractory ulcerative colitis. Gastroenterology 2007;133:1414–22.
30. Kasran A, Boon L, Wortel CH, et al. Safety and tolerability of antagonist anti-human CD40 Mab ch5D12 in patients with moderate to severe Crohn's disease. Aliment Pharmacol Ther 2005;22:111–22.
31. Van Assche G, Sandborn WJ, Feagan BG, et al. Daclizumab, a humanized monoclonal antibody to the interleukin 2 receptor (CD25), for the treatment of moderately to severely active ulcerative colitis: a randomized, double blind, placebo controlled, and dose ranging trial. Gut 2006;55:1568–74.
32. Ito H, Takazoe M, Fukuda Y, et al. A pilot randomized trial of a human anti-interleukin-6 receptor monoclonal antibody in active Crohn's disease. Gastroenterology 2004;126:989–96.

33. Elliott M, Benson J, Blank M, et al. Ustekinumab: lessons learned from targeting interleukin-12/23p40 in immune-mediated diseases. Ann N Y Acad Sci 2009; 1182:97–110.
34. Mannon PJ, Fuss IJ, Elson CO, et al. Anti-interleukin-12 antibody for active Crohn's disease. N Engl J Med 2004;351:2069–79.
35. Toedter GP, Blank M, Lang Y, et al. Relationship of C-reactive protein with clinical response after therapy with ustekinumab in Crohn's disease. Am J Gastroenterol 2009;104:2768–73.
36. Sandborn WJ, Feagan BG, Fedorak RN, et al. A randomized trial of Ustekinumab, a human interleukin-12/23 monoclonal antibody, in patients with moderate-to-severe Crohn's disease. Gastroenterology 2008;135:1130–41.
37. Ghosh S, Gordin E, Gordon FH, et al. Natalizumab for active Crohn's disease. N Engl J Med 2003;348:24–32.
38. Sandborn WJ, Colombel JF, Enns R, et al. Natalizumab induction and maintenance therapy for Crohn's disease. N Engl J Med 2005;353:1912–25.
39. Feagan BG, Greenberg FR, Wild G, et al. Treatment of ulcerative colitis with a humanized antibody to the alpha4beta7 integrin. N Engl J Med 2005;352: 2499–507.
40. Van Dullemen HM, van Deventer SJ, Hommes DW, et al. Treatment of Crohn's disease with anti-tumor necrosis factor chimeric monoclonal antibody (cA2). Gastroenterology 1995;109:129–35.
41. Reinisch W, Wang Y, Oddens BJ, et al. C-reactive protein, an indicator for maintained response or remission to infliximab in patients with Crohn's disease: a post-hoc analysis from ACCENT I. Aliment Pharmacol Ther 2012;35:568–76.
42. Schnitzler F, Fidder H, Ferrante M, et al. Long term outcome of treatment with infliximab in 614 patients with Crohn's disease: results from a single-center cohort. Gut 2009;58:492–500.
43. Present DH, Rutgeerts P, Targan S, et al. Infliximab for the treatment of fistulas in patients with Crohn's disease. N Engl J Med 1999;340:1398–405.
44. Sands BE, Anderson FH, Bernstein CN, et al. Infliximab maintenance therapy for fistulizing Crohn's disease. N Engl J Med 2004;350:876–85.
45. Sands BE, Blank MA, Patel K, et al. Long-term treatment of rectovaginal fistulas in Crohn's disease: response to infliximab in the ACCENT II study. Clin Gastroenterol Hepatol 2004;2:912–20.
46. Guidi L, Pugliese D, Armuzzi A. Update on the management of inflammatory bowel disease: specific role of adalimumab. Clin Exp Gastroenterol 2011;4: 163–72.
47. Sandborn WJ, Hanauer SB, Rutgeerts P, et al. Adalimumab for maintenance treatment of Crohn's disease: results of the CLASSIC II trial. Gut 2007;56:1232–9.
48. Colombel JF, Sandborn WJ, Rutgeerts P, et al. Adalimumab for maintenance of clinical response and remission in patients with Crohn's disease: the CHARM trial. Gastroenterology 2007;132:52–65.
49. Kamm MA, Hanauer SB, Panaccione R, et al. Adalimumab sustains steroid-free remission after 3 years of therapy for Crohn's disease. Aliment Pharmacol Ther 2011;34:306–17.
50. Sandborn WJ, Rutgeerts P, Enns R, et al. Adalimumab induction therapy for Crohn's disease previously treated with infliximab: a randomized trial. Ann Intern Med 2007;146:829–38.
51. Ma C, Panaccione R, Heitman SJ, et al. Systematic review: the short-term and long-term efficacy of adalimumab following discontinuation of infliximab. Aliment Pharmacol Ther 2009;30:977–86.

52. Lichtiger S, Binion DG, Wolf DC, et al. The CHOICE trial: adalimumab demonstrates safety, fistula healing, improved quality of life and increased work productivity in patients with Crohn's disease who failed prior infliximab therapy. Aliment Pharmacol Ther 2010;32:1228–39.

53. Afif W, Leighton JA, Hanauer SB, et al. Open-label study of adalimumab in patients with ulcerative colitis including those with prior loss of response or intolerance to infliximab. Inflamm Bowel Dis 2009;15:1302–7.

54. Gies N, Krocker KI, Wong K, et al. Treatment of ulcerative colitis with adalimumab or infliximab: long-term follow-up of a single-center cohort. Aliment Pharmacol Ther 2010;32:522–8.

55. Oussalah A, Laclotte C, Chevaux JB, et al. Long-term outcome of adalimumab therapy for ulcerative colitis with intolerance or lost response to infliximab: a single-center experience. Aliment Pharmacol Ther 2008;28:966–72.

56. Peyrin-Biroulet L, Laclotte C, Roblin X, et al. Adalimumab induction therapy for ulcerative colitis with intolerance or lost response to infliximab: an open-label study. World J Gastroenterol 2007;13:2328–32.

57. Reinisch W, Sandborn WJ, Hommes DW, et al. Adalimumab for induction of clinical remission in moderately to severely active ulcerative colitis: results of a randomised controlled trial. Gut 2011;60:780–7.

58. Reinisch W, Sandborn WJ, Kumar A, et al. 52-week clinical efficacy with adalimumab in patients with moderately to severely active ulcerative colitis who failed corticosteroids and/or immunosuppressants [abstract]. J Crohns Colitis 2011;5: S87.

59. Sandborn WJ, van Assche G, Reinisch W, et al. Adalimumab induces and maintains clinical remission in patients with moderate-to-severe ulcerative colitis. Gastroenterology 2012;142:257–65.

60. Nesbitt A, Fossati G, Bergin M, et al. Mechanism of action of certolizumab pegol (CDP870): in vitro comparison with other anti-tumor necrosis factor alpha agents. Inflamm Bowel Dis 2007;13:1323–32.

61. Schreiber S, Khaliq-Kareemi M, Lawrance IC, et al. Maintenance therapy with certolizumab pegol for Crohn's disease. N Engl J Med 2007;357:239–50.

62. Froslie KF, Jahnsen J, Moum BA, et al. Mucosal healing in inflammatory bowel disease: results from a Norwegian population-based cohort. Gastroenterology 2007;133:412–22.

63. Ha C, Kornbluth A. Mucosal healing in inflammatory bowel disease: where do we stand? Curr Gastroenterol Rep 2010;12:471–8.

64. Vant MH. Mucosal healing: impact on the natural course or therapeutic strategies. Dig Dis 2009;27:470–5.

65. Baert F, Moortgat L, Van Assche G, et al. Mucosal healing predicts sustained clinical remission in patients with early-stage Crohn's disease. Gastroenterology 2010;138:463–8.

66. Rutgeerts P, Diamond RH, Bala M, et al. Scheduled maintenance treatment with infliximab is superior to episodic treatment for the healing of mucosal ulceration associated with Crohn's disease. Gastrointest Endosc 2006;63:433–42.

67. Colombel JF, Rutgeerts P, Reinisch W, et al. Early mucosal healing with infliximab is associated with improved long-term clinical outcomes in ulcerative colitis. Gastroenterology 2011;141:1194–201.

68. Rutgeerts P, Van Assche G, Sandborn WJ, et al. Adalimumab induces and maintains mucosal healing in patients with Crohn's disease: data from the EXTEND trial. Gastroenterology 2012;142:1102–11.

69. Lichtenstein GR, Yan S, Bala M, et al. Infliximab maintenance treatment reduces hospitalizations, surgeries, and procedures in fistulizing Crohn's disease. Gastroenterology 2005;128:862–9.
70. Feagan BG, Panaccione R, Sandborn WJ, et al. Effects of adalimumab therapy on the incidence of hospitalization and surgery in Crohn's disease: results from the CHARM study. Gastroenterology 2008;135:1493–9.
71. Sandborn WJ, Rutgeerts P, Feagan BG, et al. Colectomy rate comparison after treatment of ulcerative colitis with placebo or infliximab. Gastroenterology 2009;137:1250–60.
72. Leombruno JP, Nguyen GC, Grootendorst P, et al. Hospitalization and surgical rates in patients with Crohn's disease treated with infliximab: a matched analysis. Pharmacoepidemiol Drug Saf 2011;20:838–48.
73. Eksteen B, Liaskou E, Adams DH. Lymphocyte homing and its role in the pathogenesis of IBD. Inflamm Bowel Dis 2008;14:1298–312.
74. Koizumi M, King N, Lobb R, et al. Expression of vascular adhesion molecules in inflammatory bowel disease. Gastroenterology 1992;103:840–7.
75. Van Assche G, Van Ranst M, Sciot R, et al. Progressive multifocal leukoencephalopathy after natalizumab therapy for Crohn's disease. N Engl J Med 2005;353:362–8.
76. Yousry TA, Major EO, Ryschkewitsch C, et al. Evaluation of patients treated with natalizumab for progressive multifocal leukoencephalopathy. N Engl J Med 2006;354:924–33.
77. Update on Tysabri and PML. National Multiple Sclerosis Society Web site. Available at: http://www.nationalmssociety.org/news/news-detail/index.aspx?nid=2308. Published April 11, 2011. Updated January 20, 2012. Accessed March 10, 2012.
78. The TYSABRI TOUCH® Prescribing Program. Tysabri (natalizumab) web site. Available at: http://www.tysabri.com/tysbProject/tysb.portal/_baseurl/threeColLayout/SCSRepository/en_US/tysb/home/treatment-withtysabri/touch-prescribing-program.xml. Accessed March 15, 2012.
79. Targan SR, Feagan BG, Fedorak RN, et al. Natalizumab for the treatment of active Crohn's disease: results of the ENCORE trial. Gastroenterology 2007;132:1672–83.
80. Baert F, Noman M, Vermeire S, et al. Influence of immunogenicity on the long-term efficacy of infliximab in Crohn's disease. N Engl J Med 2003;348:601–8.
81. Hanauer SB, Wagner CL, Bala M, et al. Incidence and importance of antibody responses to infliximab after maintenance or episodic treatment in Crohn's disease. Clin Gastroenterol Hepatol 2004;2:542–53.
82. Colombel JF, Sandborn WJ, Reinisch W, et al. Infliximab, azathioprine, or combination therapy for Crohn's disease. N Engl J Med 2010;362:1383–95.
83. Cheifetz A, Smedley M, Martin S, et al. The incidence and management of infusion reactions to infliximab: a large center experience. Am J Gastroenterol 2003;98:1315–24.
84. Mayer L, Young Y. Infusion reactions and their management. Gastroenterol Clin North Am 2006;35:857–66.
85. Hoentjen F, van Bodegraven AA. Safety of anti-tumor necrosis factor therapy in inflammatory bowel disease. World J Gastroenterol 2009;15:2067–73.
86. Fidder H, Schnitzler F, Ferrante M, et al. Long-term safety of infliximab for the treatment of inflammatory bowel disease: a single-centre cohort study. Gut 2009;58:501–8.
87. Tsiodras S, Samonis G, Boumpas DT, et al. Fungal infections complicating tumor necrosis factor alpha blockade therapy. Mayo Clin Proc 2008;83:181–94.

88. Toruner M, Loftus EV Jr, Harmsen WS, et al. Risk factors for opportunistic infections in patients with inflammatory bowel disease. Gastroenterology 2008;134: 929–36.

89. Hou JK, Velayos F, Terrault N, et al. Viral hepatitis and inflammatory bowel disease. Inflamm Bowel Dis 2010;16:925–32.

90. Thai A, Prindiville T. Hepatosplenic T-cell lymphoma and inflammatory bowel disease. J Crohns Colitis 2010;4:511–22.

91. Yanai H, Hanauer SB. Assessing response and loss of response to biological therapies in IBD. Am J Gastroenterol 2011;106:685–98.

92. Danese S, Fiorino G, Reinisch W. Review article: causative factors and the clinical management of patients with Crohn's disease who lose response to anti-TNF-α therapy. Aliment Pharmacol Ther 2011;34:1–10.

93. Katz L, Gisbert JP, Manoogian B, et al. Doubling the infliximab dose versus halving the infusion intervals in Crohn's disease patients with loss of response. Inflamm Bowel Dis 2012. [Epub ahead of print].

94. Loly C, Belaiche J, Louis E. Predictors of severe Crohn's disease. Scand J Gastroenterol 2008;43:948–54.

95. Perrier C, Rutgeerts P. Cytokine blockade in inflammatory bowel diseases. Immunotherapy 2011;3:1341–52.

Immunotherapy in Renal Diseases

Ajay Kher, MBBS[a],*, Vijay Kher, MD, DM[b]

KEYWORDS

- Glomerulonephritis • Nephrotic syndrome
- Immunosuppression • Crescentic glomerulonephritis

Key Points

- Immunotherapy for renal disease over the last 50 years has resulted in significant improvement in outcomes.
- Corticosteroids are the mainstay of treatment of minimal change disease.
- Evaluation of the risk of progression to end-stage renal disease is required before treating membranous and immunoglobulin-A nephropathy.
- Corticosteroids with cyclosporin are used to treat focal segmental glomerulosclerosis, many novel therapies are under investigation.
- Lupus nephritis is a classic immune-mediated disease, treated with corticosteroids, cyclophosphamide or mycophenolate mofetil.
- Crescentic glomerulonephritis (antineutrophil cytoplasmic antibody vasculitis or anti–glomerular basement membrane) is usually treated with combination therapy of cyclophosphamide, corticosteroids, and plasmapheresis.
- The role of novel targeted therapies such as rituximab, belimumab, and ecluzimab is being established.

Among renal diseases immunotherapy is used for treatment of glomerulonephritis, kidney transplantation, renal cell carcinoma, and occasionally acute interstitial nephritis. Immunotherapy in renal disease has evolved with the development and availability of various drugs during different eras. Such therapy consisted initially of corticosteroids in the 1950s, and progressively came to include cyclophosphamide, nitrogen mustard, and azathioprine (AZA) in the 1960s and 1970s. Cyclosporine and later tacrolimus, mycophenolate mofetil (MMF), immunoglobulins with or without

---

[a] The Transplant Institute, Beth Israel Deaconess Medical Center, 110 Francis Street, 7th Floor, Boston, MA 02215, USA
[b] Division of Nephrology and Renal Transplant Medicine, Kidney and Urology Institute, Medanta-The Medicity, Gurgaon, India
* Corresponding author.
E-mail address: akher@bidmc.harvard.edu

Med Clin N Am 96 (2012) 545–564
doi:10.1016/j.mcna.2012.04.007   **medical.theclinics.com**

plasmapheresis, anti–B-cell mediated therapies such as rituximab or belimumab, and other novel targeted therapies have now become available. This review focuses on the use of these agents for the treatment of various forms of glomerulonephritis. The reader is referred to recent reviews for more information on immunotherapy for renal transplantation,[1,2] renal cell cancer,[3] and acute interstitial nephritis.[4]

Glomerular diseases are immunologically mediated disorders, which manifest as:

1. Acute nephritis syndrome
2. Nephrotic syndrome
3. Rapidly progressive glomerulonephritis
4. Chronic glomerulonephritis
5. Asymptomatic urinary manifestations.

The diagnosis of different glomerular diseases is based on clinical features and syndromes, laboratory characteristics, and renal histology, usually including immuno-fluorescence, light microscopy, and electron microscopy. The differential diagnosis of nephritic syndrome, nephrotic syndrome, and rapidly progressive glomerulonephritis is presented in **Box 1**.

Box 1
Differential diagnosis of nephrotic or nephritic syndrome

Nephrotic syndrome

    Minimal change disease

    Membranous nephropathy

    Focal segmental glomerulosclerosis

    Amyloidosis

    Light chain deposition disease

    Diabetes mellitus

    Preeclampsia

Nephritic syndrome

    Postinfectious glomerulonephritis

    Membranoproliferative glomerulonephritis

    Lupus nephritis

    Immunoglobulin-A (IgA) nephropathy

    Fibrillary glomerulonephritis

    Cryoglobulinemia

    Hereditary nephritis

    Pauci-immune glomerulonephritis (granulomatosis with polyangiitis, microscopic polyarteritis nodosa)

    Anti–glomerular basement membrane (GBM) disease (Goodpasture syndrome)

Rapidly progressive glomerulonephritis

    Pauci-immune glomerulonephritis (granulomatosis with polyangiitis, microscopic polyarteritis nodosa)

    Anti-GBM disease (Goodpasture syndrome)

    Immune complex glomerulonephritis (Lupus, IgA, postinfectious, and so forth)

NONIMMUNOSUPPRESSIVE TREATMENTS

The rate of progression of kidney disease varies with the activity of the original disease and the efficacy of the treatment. After a substantial loss of nephrons has occurred, even if the original disease is not active, the adaptive hyperfiltration leads to a common pathway to progression of chronic kidney disease (CKD). Treatment of hypertension and use of angiotensin-converting enzyme inhibitors or angiotensin receptor blockers for reduction of proteinuria should be used to slow the progression of CKD. These interventions and other treatments for the management of associated conditions of anemia, bone and mineral disorders, and cardiovascular disease are not discussed here, and the reader is referred to other reviews on this issue.[5]

MINIMAL CHANGE DISEASE

Minimal change disease (MCD) is the most common cause of nephrotic syndrome in children. Historical studies before the advent of antibiotics and steroids show that 40% of children with nephrotic syndrome died of infections, renal failure, or thromboembolism.[6]

Initial Treatment

Corticosteroids are the treatment of choice for MCD (**Box 2**), and this is based on large trials in children and smaller ones in adults that show benefit.[7–11] The early study of corticosteroids in the 1970s found that prednisone led to a rapid decrease in proteinuria compared with controls. However, it also noted that a significant proportion (>50%) of the control group also had resolution of the proteinuria, although it took more than 2 years.[8] Since then many studies have shown that in comparison with the quick response to steroids in children (within 8 weeks), adults need to be treated for longer, although the response rates are similar.[11] Studies have used different doses of steroids; most recommend using prednisone 1 mg/kg of body weight daily for at least 8 weeks. For those who have attained complete remission by 8 weeks, the prednisone dose can be tapered. Slow tapering is recommended to sustain the remission. For those who have not attained remission, prednisone is continued at full dose until 1 to 2 weeks after remission is attained. Most of those who will respond

---

Box 2
Treatment of minimal change disease

Initial treatment

    Prednisone 1 mg/kg daily for at least 8 weeks

Relapse

    Prednisone 1 mg/kg daily

Frequently relapsing and steroid dependent

    Cyclosporine (4–6 mg/kg/d in divided doses)

    OR

    Cyclophosphamide (oral 2 mg/kg daily for 8–12 weeks)

Steroid-resistant disease

    Cyclosporine (4–6 mg/kg/d in divided doses)

    OR

    Cyclophosphamide (oral 2 mg/kg daily for 8–12 weeks)

usually do so by 16 weeks and those who do not are labeled as steroid resistant. There is a small number with spontaneous early remission (5%–10%), with up to 70% in remission by 3 years.[8,11,12] Hence, steroids help in inducing early remissions and to maintain it. Patients may have some decrease in renal function at the time of nephrotic syndrome but they return to normal once nephrosis resolves.[11–15] The outcome of treated MCD is good, and an important prognostic factor is the initial response to steroid therapy.[16] Most patients attain complete remission. Developing end-stage renal disease (ESRD) from MCD is rare and is seen only in steroid-resistant cases. On repeat biopsy all such cases have focal segmental glomerulosclerosis (FSGS), usually thought to be the result of mislabeling of FSGS as MCD on the original biopsy sample, although it could also be due to progression from MCD to FSGS.[11,17]

Treatment of Relapse

Relapse will occur in 50% to 75% of patients after stopping steroids, and 10% to 25% will have frequent relapses.[11,12,15] There are no trials to guide therapy for relapses, but a repeat course of steroids usually resolves the flare.[13,14] If the patient is having significant steroid toxicity or has frequent flares, it is reasonable to consider steroid-sparing strategies and use other immunosuppressive agents.

Steroid-Dependent Disease or Frequently Relapsing MCD

Continuous low-dose steroids,[13] cyclophosphamide,[13,15] or cyclosporine[18–21] may be used for patients who have either steroid-dependent or frequently relapsing disease. Treatment with these agents is begun after a remission has been induced by steroids.

Steroid-Resistant MCD

Five percent to 10% of adults with MCD will be steroid resistant. Some of them may have FSGS after being mislabeled because of sampling issues, as already mentioned. Cyclosporine is preferred for the treatment of steroid-resistant MCD because it is also effective for steroid-resistant FSGS.[19,20,22,23] Those who are unable to tolerate cyclosporine or are resistant to it may be treated with cyclophosphamide.[22,24]

MEMBRANOUS NEPHROPATHY

To understand the role of immunosuppressive therapy in membranous nephropathy, it is important to appreciate the natural history of the disease and the prognostic risk factors. Spontaneous complete remission occurs in up to 30% of patients at 5 years and partial remission occurs in 25% to 40%; progression to ESRD is approximately 14% at 5 years, 35% at 10 years, and 41% at 15 years.[25,26] Similarly, it has been noted that in those with penicillamine-associated or gold-associated membranous nephropathy it may take many months for the proteinuria to resolve, even after removal of the offending agent.[27,28]

A significant proportion of patients will have spontaneous remission, and the overall outcomes are benign. Hence, immunosuppressive therapy should only be used for those with substantial risk for progression to ESRD. Many studies have shown that older age at presentation, male gender, nephrotic-range proteinuria, and higher serum creatinine at presentation are associated with risk of progression to ESRD. Persistence of high levels of proteinuria has been shown to be predictive of progression to ESRD,[29] and has been validated in 2 separate cohorts.[30] Based on follow-up of 6 months, patients can be classified as low risk, moderate risk, or high risk for progression to ESRD. Immunosuppressive therapy would be recommended only for moderate and high risk of progression.

First-line therapy is cyclophosphamide with prednisone or cyclosporine with prednisone; those who fail on one regimen are treated with the other, and those who fail on both are treated with rituximab (**Box 3**). Trials have shown that cytotoxic therapy (cyclophosphamide or chlorambucil) with steroids are effective in preventing progression to ESRD and in inducing remission.[31,32] As cyclophosphamide is equally as effective as chlorambucil and is associated with fewer side effects, most clinicians prefer cyclophosphamide for cytotoxic treatment of membranous nephropathy.[33] Treatment is given for 6 months with alternating months of steroids and cyclophosphamide. Cyclosporine with low-dose prednisone has also been shown to be effective in inducing remission and preventing progression to ESRD.[34–36] Tacrolimus has also been effective, although most clinicians use cyclosporine, having had more experience with this drug in treating the condition. The duration of cyclosporine treatment is based on the response to initial therapy. Once complete remission is achieved therapy can be tapered and stopped, whereas for those in partial remission the therapy is continued for 1 to 2 years. High relapse rates have been noted after stopping treatment with either cyclophosphamide or cyclosporine. The treatment of the relapse depends on the initial regimen and the response, and can be another course of cyclophosphamide or cyclosporine or a switch to the other regimen. Those who do not respond to the first-choice therapy with a reduction in proteinuria in 6 months are considered to be resistant to it, and should be treated with the other regimen. Rituximab may be used for treatment of resistant patients, based on observational studies.[37,38]

Phospholipase A$_2$ receptor (PLA2R), a transmembrane receptor, is expressed on glomerular podocytes and has been shown to be a major antigen for idiopathic membranous nephropathy.[39] Anti-PLA2R antibodies were found in 70% of those with idiopathic membranous nephropathy, and a decline in it was noted to precede resolution of proteinuria in those treated with rituximab while a relapse was preceded by an increase in these antibodies.[40,41] In the future, these may provide additional monitoring parameters and may guide therapy based on their presence and levels.

PRIMARY FOCAL SEGMENTAL GLOMERULOSCLEROSIS

FSGS is a histologic pattern of injury, which may present in response to previous glomerular injury or hypertrophy (secondary) or without an identifiable cause (primary), or can be due to genetic mutations of podocyte proteins (mutations in nephrin, podocin, and α-actinin-4). The clinical presentation may aid in this distinction, as primary FSGS usually presents acutely with overt nephrotic syndrome (edema, hypoalbuminemia)

Box 3
Treatment of membranous nephropathy

Steroids (intravenous methylprednisolone 1 g/d for 3 days followed by prednisone 0.5 mg/kg/d during months 1, 3, and 5) AND cyclophosphamide (oral 2–2.5 mg/kg/d during months 2, 4, and 6)

OR

Cyclosporine (125–225 ng/mL) AND low-dose prednisone (0.15 mg/kg/d, maximum 15 mg/d)

Resistant disease

    Use the other agent (cyclophosphamide AND steroids OR cyclosporine AND prednisone)

    OR

    Rituximab (2 doses of 1 g given 2 weeks apart or 4 weekly doses of 375 mg/m^2)

whereas secondary FSGS presents with proteinuria but without edema or hypoalbuminemia. It is important to differentiate between these conditions because the treatment is different for each. Immunosuppressive therapy is the mainstay in the treatment of primary FSGS but is not of benefit for genetic or secondary FSGS. Nonimmunosuppressive therapy, as already mentioned, should be used in all types of FSGS. The following discussion concerns patients with primary FSGS.

Prognostic Factors and Risk Factors for Progression

The natural history of FSGS in untreated patients is a progressive course toward ESRD. Factors that influence prognosis are the degree of proteinuria, renal function at presentation, pathologic findings, and response to treatment. Those with nephrotic syndrome have 5- and 10-year renal survival rates of 60% to 90% and 30% to 55%, respectively.[42–45] Those with massive proteinuria (>10 g/d) have a worse prognosis, with progression to ESRD within 5 years. In comparison, those with non-nephrotic proteinuria and normal renal function have a good prognosis, with >85% renal survival at 10 years. Worse renal function at presentation is associated with worse outcomes.[45,46] The presence of fibrosis on the biopsy is a poor prognostic sign.[44] Among the various histologic variants of FSGS, collapsing FSGS has the worst prognosis.[47] The response to treatment is a strong predictor of outcomes. Those who achieve partial or complete remission with treatment have much better outcomes than those who do not achieve remission.[42,43,46,47]

Treatment

The initial treatment is with prednisone (**Box 4**), although as there are no randomized studies the recommendation is based on observational experience. Prednisone has provided rates of 40% to 80% complete or partial response.[42,48,49] Prednisone is usually continued for 12 to 16 weeks. Dosing regimen for prednisone is 1 mg/kg daily or 2 mg/kg on alternate days. Those who respond will have some effect within 8 to 12 weeks. Duration for 6 to 8 months is required, and shorter courses lead to fewer remissions.[47,50] The management of the steroid course is based on the response. For those with complete remission, steroids may be tapered over another 3 months. For those with partial remission, steroids are tapered more slowly. Patients who do not respond within 3 to 4 months are considered steroid resistant and are treated with cyclosporine. Cyclosporine is also used for treatment of those who are steroid dependent. Treatment of relapses is based on previous response and the toxicity, and may comprise a repeat course of steroids or cyclosporine. Randomized trials and uncontrolled studies have shown that cyclosporine with low-dose prednisone is effective in reducing proteinuria; however, its impact on progression to ESRD is not known.[23,51,52]

Box 4
Treatment of primary FSGS

Initial treatment

    Prednisone (1 mg/kg daily or 2 mg/kg on alternate days) for 12–16 weeks

Steroid-resistant or -dependent disease

    Cyclosporine (100 mg twice a day or 2–4 mg/kg/d) with low-dose steroids (prednisone 15 mg/d or 0.15 mg/kg/d)

    OR

    MMF

Cyclosporine is used at a dose of 2 to 4 mg/kg/d in divided doses or 100 mg twice a day with target levels between 100 and 175 ng/mL, with low-dose prednisone 15 mg/d (0.15 mg/kg/d). Randomized and observational studies have suggested some benefit of MMF with or without steroids in FSGS.[53,54]

LUPUS NEPHRITIS

Renal involvement is common in lupus and can present with different pathologic lesions. Immunosuppressive therapy is warranted for patients with diffuse and focal proliferative lupus nephritis, which is discussed here. Immunosuppressive therapy for proliferative lupus, similar to antineutrophil cytoplasmic antibody (ANCA) disease and anti–glomerular basement membrane (anti-GBM) disease consists of 2 phases, first an induction phase and then a maintenance phase (**Box 5**). The induction phase consists of use of potent immunosuppression to induce remission, then once it is achieved a maintenance phase begins with use of less aggressive therapy. The duration of each of these phases is variable and has to be individualized based on the response of the disease, the risk for progression, and the side effects of the medications.

Induction

Landmark studies from the National Institutes of Health[55–58] demonstrated the benefit of cyclophosphamide (0.5–1.0 g/m^2, given monthly for 6 months and then quarterly for 2 years) with steroids over steroids alone, and also showed that prolonged administration at quarterly intervals decreased the relapses. Good overall outcomes were achieved with the combination of cyclophosphamide with steroids, but were

---

Box 5
Treatment of lupus nephritis

Induction phase

  Steroids (methylprednisolone intravenous pulse 500–1000 mg/d for 3 days followed by prednisone 1 mg/kg/d)

  AND

  Cyclophosphamide (intravenous 6 doses of 500 mg every 2 weeks OR intravenous 0.5–1 g/m^2 monthly for 4–7 months)

  OR

  MMF (1 g/d for 1 week, 2 g/d for 1 week, then 3 g/d until remission achieved)

Maintenance phase

  MMF (2 g/d) for 18 to 24 months

  OR

  Azathioprine (2 mg/kg/d)

Resistant disease

  Treat with other induction agent (cyclophosphamide or MMF with steroids)

  OR

  Rituximab (2 doses of 0.5–1 g 2 weeks apart or 4 weekly doses of 375 mg/m^2)

Lupus diffuse proliferative with membranous nephritis

  MMF AND tacrolimus AND steroids

associated with significant side effects. Hence, studies were conducted to assess less intense immunosuppressive regimens. The Euro-lupus trial showed that a shorter and lower-dose cyclophosphamide regimen (6 fixed doses of 500 mg given every fortnight, total 3 g) with prednisone followed by AZA provided similar short-term and long-term outcomes, with fewer adverse events. The trial also showed that early response to therapy was predictive of good outcomes long term[59–61]; however, this study had no African Americans. Another option for low-dose cyclophosphamide therapy is use of 4 to 7 doses of monthly intravenous cyclophosphamide with transition to AZA or MMF once remission is induced, allowing for lower doses for those who achieve remission earlier.[62] The majority of these patients were African Americans or Hispanics, who have worse outcomes, and hence the results may not be applicable to other populations.

Another option is induction with MMF as used in the ALMS trial.[63] The target dose here was 3 g daily, which was reached by a progressive increase in dose weekly from 1 g daily for the first week. There were no differences in the primary or secondary outcomes when compared with cyclophosphamide. In a subset analysis MMF was found to work better for African Americans,[64] this result being similar to those of other trials that have shown worse outcomes with cyclophosphamide in African Americans.[65] Long-term follow-up of a Chinese study comparing MMF with cyclophosphamide showed similar remission rates with lower rates of infections.[66,67] A meta-analysis also showed decreased remission rates and increased adverse events with cyclophosphamide.[68] It is noteworthy that the MMF trials have only a short-term follow-up and also that these studies were not powered to show safety benefits.

Maintenance

Following reduction or cessation of immunosuppression, up to 50% of patients may relapse.[66,69–72] Hence, after attainment of remission, immunosuppression is continued to maintain remission and reduce relapses. The ideal maintenance regimen is not defined. Most studies have used either AZA or MMF for 12 to 24 months. AZA and MMF have better efficacy and safety profiles than continued intravenous cyclophosphamide.[62] The MAINTAIN trial compared AZA (2 mg/kg/d) with MMF (2 g/d), and after 3 years no significant difference in the rate of renal relapse (25% vs 19%) was noted. Occurrence of adverse events was similar except for anemia and leukopenia, which were more common in the AZA arm.[73] The ALMS trial was a multinational trial that compared induction with MMF with cyclophosphamide, and those who achieved remission were then randomized to maintenance therapy with either MMF or AZA.[74] The investigators showed that renal outcomes were significantly better with MMF maintenance, independent of the induction agent used. This finding, combined with the trend toward benefit in the MAINTAIN trial, leads to a recommendation for the use of MMF rather than AZA. AZA may be preferred for those who do not tolerate MMF or for women who wish to become pregnant. The usual dose of MMF is 2 g/d, tapered over time in stable patients.

Resistant Lupus Nephritis

Patients who do not respond to the initial therapy (cyclophosphamide or MMF) and are considered resistant to the initial therapy are usually treated with the other agent. Patients who fail or cannot tolerate both regimens may be considered for treatment with rituximab. However, this protocol is based on small observational studies, and no long-term safety or efficacy data are available. Different regimens of rituximab have been used, and include 2 doses of 0.5 to 1 g on days 1 and 15,[75] or 4 weekly doses of 375 mg/m^2.[76]

Diffuse Proliferative Lupus with Membranous Nephritis

Patients with combined diffuse proliferative and membranous lupus have a worse prognosis than those with diffuse proliferative nephritis alone.[77] Moreover, those with combined lesions had a lower rate of achieving remission (27% vs 60%) and poorer renal survival at 10 years (50% vs 75%). Patients with combined lesions respond better to induction therapy with MMF (0.75–1 g/d) and tacrolimus (3–4 mg/d with trough 5–7 ng/mL) compared with intravenous cyclophosphamide, with higher complete remissions at 9 months (65% vs 15%) and similar partial response rates (30% vs 40%).[78] All patients also received steroids.

IMMUNOGLOBULIN-A NEPHROPATHY

Immunoglobulin A (IgA) nephropathy is the most common form of glomerulonephritis.[79] IgA nephropathy has a spectrum of disease ranging from persistent asymptomatic microscopic hematuria without proteinuria with normal renal function to severe nephritic presentation. The classic presentation is with gross hematuria in the setting of a recent upper respiratory infection. Patients with IgA nephropathy are generally thought to have good prognosis; however, long-term follow-up has shown that some of them will progress to ESRD. Those with no or little proteinuria have good outcomes, but a substantial proportion may develop proteinuria and renal insufficiency over the long term. Progression to ESRD is 15% to 25% in 10 years and 20% to 30% in 20 years.[80–83] Clinical predictors of progression to ESRD are elevated serum creatinine, hypertension, and persistent proteinuria greater than 1 g/d.[84–86] Histologic features predictive of progression include markers of inflammatory disease (crescent formation, immune deposits in the capillary loops) and markers of chronic fibrotic disease (interstitial fibrosis, tubular atrophy, glomerulosclerosis). A consensus on pathologic classification of IgA nephropathy has been developed. The Oxford classification has been validated in multiple different cohorts.[87–89] A prognostic scoring system has also been developed.[86]

The treatment of IgA nephropathy is uncertain and is difficult to assess because of its slow progression.[90,91] Nonimmunosuppressive therapies should be used in all patients, and immunosuppression limited to selected patients. Hence, immunosuppressive therapy is limited to those who are thought to be at high risk of progression to ESRD. Patients with isolated hematuria with no proteinuria and normal function usually are not biopsied and not treated, but should be monitored for signs of progression. Patients with more severe disease (nephrotic-range proteinuria, rising creatinine level, and severe histologic findings) may benefit from immunosuppressive therapy in addition to nonimmunosuppressive therapy. The benefits of steroids have been studied in uncontrolled and small randomized studies.[92–95] Steroids are associated with a reduction in proteinuria and may be associated with improved renal survival. A prospective study among patients with moderate proteinuria (1–3.5 g/d) who were randomly assigned to supportive care or steroids (1 g intravenous methylprednisolone for 3 days on months 1, 3, and 5 with alternate-day prednisone at 0.5 mg/kg for 6 months) showed that steroids were associated with reduced incidence of doubling of serum creatinine at 5 years (2% vs 21%) and 10 years (2% vs 30%).[93,94] Combined treatment with steroids and angiotensin inhibitors provides additional benefit in comparison with angiotensin inhibitors alone.[96,97]

Crescentic IgA Nephropathy

There are no randomized trials evaluating treatments for crescentic IgA nephropathy. Observational data suggest benefit through the use of aggressive treatment as used for other forms of rapidly progressive glomerulonephritis (crescentic glomerulone-phritis). This therapy includes pulse methylprednisolone followed by oral prednisone with cyclophosphamide, with or without plasmapheresis.[98–101]

GRANULOMATOSIS WITH POLYANGIITIS (WEGENER SYNDROME) AND MICROSCOPIC POLYANGIITIS

Renal presentation in these conditions is with nephritic syndrome or rapidly progressive glomerulonephritis, which are associated with ANCA. Kidney biopsies show segmental necrotizing glomerulonephritis with few or no immune deposits (pauci-immune), and crescents are commonly present.

Induction

Initial treatment is usually with cyclophosphamide and prednisone (**Box 6**). Recent studies have shown that short-term results are equally good with rituximab, hence it may be used for those unable to tolerate or who refuse treatment with cyclophospha-mide. Aggressive treatment is warranted, because if left untreated there is high mortality from this disease.[102] Steroids should not be used alone, as the remission rate is substantially lower than that of cyclophosphamide (56% vs 85%) and the relapse rates are higher.[103] Cyclophosphamide can be dosed as daily oral dose or monthly intrave-nous pulses. Trials have shown that both of these regimens induce remission at similar rates. Higher cumulative cyclophosphamide dose, lower rates of relapse, and more leukopenia and infection are associated with oral dosing of cyclophosphamide.[104–107] For steroids a 3-day course of methylprednisolone pulse (7–15 mg/kg, 500–1000 mg) is followed by prednisone (1 mg/kg, 60–80 mg/d). These regimens attain remission rates of 85% to 90%, with 75% attaining complete remission. Most patients achieve a remis-sion within 2 to 6 months.[105,108,109]

Box 6
Treatment of granulomatosis with polyangiitis (Wegener syndrome) and microscopic polyangiitis

Induction phase

Steroids (methylprednisolone intravenous 500–1000 mg daily for 3 days followed by prednisone 1 mg/kg)

AND

Plasmapheresis for those with pulmonary hemorrhage, severe renal disease, or combined ANCA and anti-GBM disease

AND

Cyclophosphamide (by mouth or intravenous)

OR

Rituximab

Maintenance phase

Azathioprine (12–18 months)

OR

Methotrexate (12–18 months)

Two randomized trials have shown the efficacy of rituximab in the initial treatment of ANCA vasculitis.[110,111] However, both only had short-term follow-up; hence, rituximab remains a treatment option for those who do not tolerate or refuse cyclophosphamide therapy or for those who fail treatment with cyclophosphamide. The RAVE trial randomly assigned rituximab or cyclophosphamide to 197 patients with granulomatosis with polyangiitis (75%) or microscopic polyangiitis (24%), of whom 49 were newly diagnosed while the rest had relapsing disease.[111] All patients received steroids. Rituximab was not inferior in inducing remission but was superior in doing so in those with relapsing disease. The other trial had 44 new patients assigned in 3:1 ratio to 4 doses of rituximab with 2 doses of cyclophosphamide versus cyclophosphamide for 3 to 6 months followed by AZA. No differences in sustained remission were noted.[110]

Plasmapheresis is recommended for selected patients with ANCA disease, combined ANCA and anti-GBM disease, pulmonary hemorrhage, or severe renal disease. An initial trial suggested that plasmapheresis was of benefit in those with severe renal failure requiring dialysis on presentation.[112] The MEPEX trial randomized 137 patients with pauci-immune glomerulonephritis and serum creatinine greater than 5.7 mg/dL to plasmapheresis or a methylprednisolone pulse. All patients received oral prednisone and cyclophosphamide (for 3 months) followed by maintenance with AZA. Plasmapheresis was noted to be associated with higher likelihood of being dialysis independent at 3 months and 1 year.[113] There have been no randomized trials of plasmapheresis in pulmonary hemorrhage in ANCA disease; however, its use is based on the benefit seen in anti-GBM disease and the possible benefit from rapid removal of ANCA, and the benefit seen in those treated with it in comparison with historical controls.[114]

Maintenance

After remission is attained, all patients are switched from cyclophosphamide to less toxic immunotherapy (AZA or methotrexate). Dialysis-dependent patients with no renal recovery after 2 to 3 months should not receive continued immunosuppression, unless required for extrarenal manifestations. Methotrexate in weekly oral doses has been shown to be effective in maintaining remission[115]; however, patients with serum creatinine levels persistently above 2.5 mg/dL were excluded. AZA has also been shown to be effective in maintaining remission after cyclophosphamide induction.[109] Methotrexate and AZA provide similar efficacy and are associated with similar relapse rates.[116] Azathioprine has also been compared with MMF.[117] Relapses were more frequent in the MMF group while the rates of adverse events were similar. Hence, either AZA or methotrexate may be used for maintenance, whereas MMF should not be used. AZA may be preferred for women desiring pregnancy or for those with a significantly reduced glomerular filtration rate.

Cyclophosphamide is continued for 1 to 2 months after remission is induced. The transition to AZA or methotrexate is initiated based on the last dose of cyclophosphamide and the white blood cell count. There are no studies to guide the duration of therapy, which is usually continued for 12 to 18 months after stable remission.

Treatment of Relapses

Relapses are common in ANCA disease, and may occur during maintenance therapy or after cessation of therapy. The rates of relapse vary widely from 11% to 57%.[108,109,117] Those with mild or non–organ-threatening relapses may be treated by increasing the dose of steroids and maintenance medications if already using such agents, or reinstitution of maintenance medications and a short course of steroids.

ANTI-GBM (GOODPASTURE) DISEASE

Anti-GBM disease presents clinically as rapidly progressive glomerulonephritis, and pathologically presents with crescentic glomerulonephritis; immunofluorescence shows linear deposits of immunoglobulin G. Anti-GBM can present as a renal limited disease or as a pulmonary-renal syndrome. Untreated it has extremely poor outcomes, with almost universal mortality from renal failure or pulmonary hemorrhage.[118] Early diagnosis and treatment is key.[119,120] A retrospective study[120] showed that patients with serum creatinine less than 5.7 mg/dL at presentation had 1-year patient and renal survival of 100% and 95%, respectively, whereas those who required immediate dialysis had a 1-year patient and renal survival of 65% and 8%. The first-line treatment is prednisone, cyclophosphamide, and plasmapheresis (**Box 7**).[120–123] The only randomized study of plasmapheresis showed that 2 of 8 patients who received pheresis versus 6 of 9 who received only immunosuppression became dialysis dependent.[124] However, these differences were not statistically significant. Most clinicians still recommend using pheresis, based on the improved outcomes seen in the pheresis era in comparison with historical controls and the biological plausibility of benefit from quicker removal of pathogenic anti-GBM antibodies by pheresis.

Pulse methylprednisone (15–20 mg/kg for a maximum of 1000 mg) is given daily for 3 days, followed by prednisone (1 mg/kg daily for maximum of 60–80 mg/d) accompanied by cyclophosphamide (2 mg/kg daily orally). There is a low risk of recurrence of this disease and anti-GBM antibody formation can spontaneously cease, although it may take many months. Hence the duration of therapy is unknown. Plasmapheresis is performed for 2 to 3 weeks, cyclophosphamide can be stopped after 2 to 3 months, and prednisone can be stopped after 6 months.[119,123] However, therapy can be individualized based on monitoring of anti-GBM antibody levels, and may be tapered earlier if they have been persistently negative or need to be extended or intensified if antibody levels are persistent or reappear.

There is a subset of patients who have combined ANCA and anti-GBM disease. In these cases the initial management is the same as that for anti-GBM disease, and long-term management is the same as for ANCA disease, as these patients have a substantial risk for relapse.

NOVEL IMMUNOTHERAPIES FOR GLOMERULONEPHRITIS

As newer mechanisms of pathogenic pathways of glomerulonephritis are unraveled, many novel designer drugs targeted to specific pathogenic molecules are being used.

- Rituximab (a chimeric monoclonal anti-CD20 antibody) has been used in resistant or steroid-dependent MCD and focal segmental glomerulosclerosis.[125–128]

Box 7
Treatment of anti-GBM disease

Steroids (intravenous methylprednisolone 15–20 mg/kg for 3 days followed by prednisone 1 mg/kg daily)

AND

Cyclophosphamide (by mouth 2 mg/kg daily)

AND

Plasmapheresis

It has also been used in membranous nephritis and in resistant or relapsing ANCA vasculitis, as already described.

- Belimumab (a humanized monoclonal anti–B-lymphocyte stimulator antibody) has been recently approved by the Food and Drug Administration for systemic lupus erythematosus.[129]
- Adalimumab is a humanized monoclonal anti–tumor necrosis factor (TNF)-α antibody. TNF-α is an inflammatory cytokine released by macrophages and renal tubular cells in glomerulonephritis, and has been incriminated for progressive sclerosis and for proteinuria in angiotensin II–induced renal injury. Phase I and II trials of adalimumab for the treatment of FSGS are currently ongoing as the FONT trials I and II.[130]
- Fresolimumab is a humanized monoclonal anti–transforming growth factor (TGF)-β antibody. TGF-β is a cytokine implicated as a modulator of extracellular matrix production and is associated with interstitial fibrosis. TGF-β is also a regulator of podocyte structure and function, and activates the Smad cascade. Fresolimumab is an engineered humanized G4 subclass monoclonal antibody to TGF-β (antagonizing all 3 isoforms of TGF-β) and is being tried in phase I and II trials on FSGS.[131]
- Eculizumab (a monoclonal antibody against complement protein C5) is approved for treatment of paroxysmal nocturnal hemoglobinuria and atypical hemolytic uremic syndrome. Trials are also under way for its use in dense deposit disease.

SUMMARY

Therapy for renal diseases has come a long way during the last 50 years as regards the use of immunosuppressive drugs. Clinicians are surely and steadily moving toward targeted therapies as the understanding of pathogenic mechanisms is improving. It is hoped that in the future more specific drugs are developed for the treatment of renal diseases.

REFERENCES

1. Marfo K, Lu A, Ling M, et al. Desensitization protocols and their outcome. Clin J Am Soc Nephrol 2011;6(4):922–36.
2. Webber A, Hirose R, Vincenti F. Novel strategies in immunosuppression: issues in perspective. Transplantation 2011;91(10):1057–64.
3. Rosenblatt J, McDermott DF. Immunotherapy for renal cell carcinoma. Hematol Oncol Clin North Am 2011;25(4):793–812.
4. Praga M, Gonzalez E. Acute interstitial nephritis. Kidney Int 2010;77(11):956–61.
5. Abboud H, Henrich WL. Clinical practice. Stage IV chronic kidney disease. N Engl J Med 2010;362(1):56–65.
6. Tune BM, Mendoza SA. Treatment of the idiopathic nephrotic syndrome: regimens and outcomes in children and adults. J Am Soc Nephrol 1997;8(5):824–32.
7. The primary nephrotic syndrome in children. Identification of patients with minimal change nephrotic syndrome from initial response to prednisone. A report of the International Study of Kidney Disease in Children. J Pediatr 1981;98(4):561–4.
8. Black DA, Rose G, Brewer DB. Controlled trial of prednisone in adult patients with the nephrotic syndrome. Br Med J 1970;3(5720):421–6.
9. Coggins CH. Adult minimal change nephropathy: experience of the collaborative study of glomerular disease. Trans Am Clin Climatol Assoc 1986;97:18–26.

10. Imbasciati E, Gusmano R, Edefonti A, et al. Controlled trial of methylprednisolone pulses and low dose oral prednisone for the minimal change nephrotic syndrome. Br Med J (Clin Res Ed) 1985;291(6505):1305–8.
11. Nakayama M, Katafuchi R, Yanase T, et al. Steroid responsiveness and frequency of relapse in adult-onset minimal change nephrotic syndrome. Am J Kidney Dis 2002;39(3):503–12.
12. Tse KC, Lam MF, Yip PS, et al. Idiopathic minimal change nephrotic syndrome in older adults: steroid responsiveness and pattern of relapses. Nephrol Dial Transplant 2003;18(7):1316–20.
13. Nolasco F, Cameron JS, Heywood EF, et al. Adult-onset minimal change nephrotic syndrome: a long-term follow-up. Kidney Int 1986;29(6):1215–23.
14. Fujimoto S, Yamamoto Y, Hisanaga S, et al. Minimal change nephrotic syndrome in adults: response to corticosteroid therapy and frequency of relapse. Am J Kidney Dis 1991;17(6):687–92.
15. Mak SK, Short CD, Mallick NP. Long-term outcome of adult-onset minimal-change nephropathy. Nephrol Dial Transplant 1996;11(11):2192–201.
16. Gulati S, Kher V, Sharma RK, et al. Steroid response pattern in Indian children with nephrotic syndrome. Acta Paediatr 1994;83(5):530–3.
17. Tarshish P, Tobin JN, Bernstein J, et al. Prognostic significance of the early course of minimal change nephrotic syndrome: report of the International Study of Kidney Disease in Children. J Am Soc Nephrol 1997;8(5):769–76.
18. Cattran DC, Alexopoulos E, Heering P, et al. Cyclosporin in idiopathic glomerular disease associated with the nephrotic syndrome: workshop recommendations. Kidney Int 2007;72(12):1429–47.
19. Meyrier A, Condamin MC, Broneer D. Treatment of adult idiopathic nephrotic syndrome with cyclosporin A: minimal-change disease and focal-segmental glomerulosclerosis. Collaborative Group of the French Society of Nephrology. Clin Nephrol 1991;35(Suppl 1):S37–42.
20. Meyrier A. Treatment of idiopathic nephrosis by immunophillin modulation. Nephrol Dial Transplant 2003;18(Suppl 6):vi79–86.
21. Bargman JM. Management of minimal lesion glomerulonephritis: evidence-based recommendations. Kidney Int Suppl 1999;70:S3–16.
22. Waldman M, Crew RJ, Valeri A, et al. Adult minimal-change disease: clinical characteristics, treatment, and outcomes. Clin J Am Soc Nephrol 2007;2(3):445–53.
23. Ponticelli C, Rizzoni G, Edefonti A, et al. A randomized trial of cyclosporine in steroid-resistant idiopathic nephrotic syndrome. Kidney Int 1993;43(6):1377–84.
24. Elhence R, Gulati S, Kher V, et al. Intravenous pulse cyclophosphamide–a new regime for steroid-resistant minimal change nephrotic syndrome. Pediatr Nephrol 1994;8(1):1–3.
25. Glassock RJ. Diagnosis and natural course of membranous nephropathy. Semin Nephrol 2003;23(4):324–32.
26. Schieppati A, Mosconi L, Perna A, et al. Prognosis of untreated patients with idiopathic membranous nephropathy. N Engl J Med 1993;329(2):85–9.
27. Hall CL, Fothergill NJ, Blackwell MM, et al. The natural course of gold nephropathy: long term study of 21 patients. Br Med J (Clin Res Ed) 1987;295(6601):745–8.
28. Hall CL, Jawad S, Harrison PR, et al. Natural course of penicillamine nephropathy: a long term study of 33 patients. Br Med J (Clin Res Ed) 1988;296(6629):1083–6.
29. Pei Y, Cattran D, Greenwood C. Predicting chronic renal insufficiency in idiopathic membranous glomerulonephritis. Kidney Int 1992;42(4):960–6.

30. Cattran DC, Pei Y, Greenwood CM, et al. Validation of a predictive model of idiopathic membranous nephropathy: its clinical and research implications. Kidney Int 1997;51(3):901–7.
31. Jha V, Ganguli A, Saha TK, et al. A randomized, controlled trial of steroids and cyclophosphamide in adults with nephrotic syndrome caused by idiopathic membranous nephropathy. J Am Soc Nephrol 2007;18(6):1899–904.
32. Ponticelli C, Zucchelli P, Passerini P, et al. A 10-year follow-up of a randomized study with methylprednisolone and chlorambucil in membranous nephropathy. Kidney Int 1995;48(5):1600–4.
33. Ponticelli C, Altieri P, Scolari F, et al. A randomized study comparing methylprednisolone plus chlorambucil versus methylprednisolone plus cyclophosphamide in idiopathic membranous nephropathy. J Am Soc Nephrol 1998;9(3):444–50.
34. Cattran DC, Appel GB, Hebert LA, et al. Cyclosporine in patients with steroid-resistant membranous nephropathy: a randomized trial. Kidney Int 2001;59(4): 1484–90.
35. Alexopoulos E, Papagianni A, Tsamelashvili M, et al. Induction and long-term treatment with cyclosporine in membranous nephropathy with the nephrotic syndrome. Nephrol Dial Transplant 2006;21(11):3127–32.
36. Cattran D. Management of membranous nephropathy: when and what for treatment. J Am Soc Nephrol 2005;16(5):1188–94.
37. Fervenza FC, Abraham RS, Erickson SB, et al. Rituximab therapy in idiopathic membranous nephropathy: a 2-year study. Clin J Am Soc Nephrol 2010;5(12): 2188–98.
38. Fervenza FC, Cosio FG, Erickson SB, et al. Rituximab treatment of idiopathic membranous nephropathy. Kidney Int 2008;73(1):117–25.
39. Beck LH Jr, Bonegio RG, Lambeau G, et al. M-type phospholipase A2 receptor as target antigen in idiopathic membranous nephropathy. N Engl J Med 2009; 361(1):11–21.
40. Hofstra JM, Beck LH Jr, Beck DM, et al. Anti-phospholipase A receptor antibodies correlate with clinical status in idiopathic membranous nephropathy. Clin J Am Soc Nephrol 2011;6(6):1286–91.
41. Beck LH Jr, Fervenza FC, Beck DM, et al. Rituximab-induced depletion of anti-PLA2R autoantibodies predicts response in membranous nephropathy. J Am Soc Nephrol 2011;22(8):1543–50.
42. Rydel JJ, Korbet SM, Borok RZ, et al. Focal segmental glomerular sclerosis in adults: presentation, course, and response to treatment. Am J Kidney Dis 1995;25(4):534–42.
43. Korbet SM, Schwartz MM, Lewis EJ. Primary focal segmental glomerulosclerosis: clinical course and response to therapy. Am J Kidney Dis 1994;23(6):773–83.
44. Wehrmann M, Bohle A, Held H, et al. Long-term prognosis of focal sclerosing glomerulonephritis. An analysis of 250 cases with particular regard to tubulointerstitial changes. Clin Nephrol 1990;33(3):115–22.
45. Korbet SM. Primary focal segmental glomerulosclerosis. J Am Soc Nephrol 1998;9(7):1333–40.
46. Troyanov S, Wall CA, Miller JA, et al. Focal and segmental glomerulosclerosis: definition and relevance of a partial remission. J Am Soc Nephrol 2005;16(4): 1061–8.
47. Banfi G, Moriggi M, Sabadini E, et al. The impact of prolonged immunosuppression on the outcome of idiopathic focal-segmental glomerulosclerosis with nephrotic syndrome in adults. A collaborative retrospective study. Clin Nephrol 1991;36(2):53–9.

48. Cattran DC, Rao P. Long-term outcome in children and adults with classic focal segmental glomerulosclerosis. Am J Kidney Dis 1998;32(1):72–9.
49. Chun MJ, Korbet SM, Schwartz MM, et al. Focal segmental glomerulosclerosis in nephrotic adults: presentation, prognosis, and response to therapy of the histologic variants. J Am Soc Nephrol 2004;15(8):2169–77.
50. Ponticelli C, Villa M, Banfi G, et al. Can prolonged treatment improve the prognosis in adults with focal segmental glomerulosclerosis? Am J Kidney Dis 1999; 34(4):618–25.
51. Cattran DC, Appel GB, Hebert LA, et al. A randomized trial of cyclosporine in patients with steroid-resistant focal segmental glomerulosclerosis. North America Nephrotic Syndrome Study Group. Kidney Int 1999;56(6):2220–6.
52. Heering P, Braun N, Mullejans R, et al. Cyclosporine A and chlorambucil in the treatment of idiopathic focal segmental glomerulosclerosis. Am J Kidney Dis 2004;43(1):10–8.
53. Cattran DC, Wang MM, Appel G, et al. Mycophenolate mofetil in the treatment of focal segmental glomerulosclerosis. Clin Nephrol 2004;62(6):405–11.
54. Gipson DS, Trachtman H, Kaskel FJ, et al. Clinical trial of focal segmental glomerulosclerosis in children and young adults. Kidney Int 2011;80(8):868–78.
55. Austin HA 3rd, Klippel JH, Balow JE, et al. Therapy of lupus nephritis. Controlled trial of prednisone and cytotoxic drugs. N Engl J Med 1986;314(10):614–9.
56. Boumpas DT, Austin HA 3rd, Vaughn EM, et al. Controlled trial of pulse methylprednisolone versus two regimens of pulse cyclophosphamide in severe lupus nephritis. Lancet 1992;340(8822):741–5.
57. Gourley MF, Austin HA 3rd, Scott D, et al. Methylprednisolone and cyclophosphamide, alone or in combination, in patients with lupus nephritis. A randomized, controlled trial. Ann Intern Med 1996;125(7):549–57.
58. Illei GG, Austin HA, Crane M, et al. Combination therapy with pulse cyclophosphamide plus pulse methylprednisolone improves long-term renal outcome without adding toxicity in patients with lupus nephritis. Ann Intern Med 2001; 135(4):248–57.
59. Houssiau FA, Vasconcelos C, D'Cruz D, et al. The 10-year follow-up data of the Euro-Lupus Nephritis Trial comparing low-dose and high-dose intravenous cyclophosphamide. Ann Rheum Dis 2010;69(1):61–4.
60. Houssiau FA, Vasconcelos C, D'Cruz D, et al. Early response to immunosuppressive therapy predicts good renal outcome in lupus nephritis: lessons from long-term followup of patients in the Euro-Lupus Nephritis Trial. Arthritis Rheum 2004;50(12):3934–40.
61. Houssiau FA, Vasconcelos C, D'Cruz D, et al. Immunosuppressive therapy in lupus nephritis: the Euro-Lupus Nephritis Trial, a randomized trial of low-dose versus high-dose intravenous cyclophosphamide. Arthritis Rheum 2002;46(8):2121–31.
62. Contreras G, Pardo V, Leclercq B, et al. Sequential therapies for proliferative lupus nephritis. N Engl J Med 2004;350(10):971–80.
63. Appel GB, Contreras G, Dooley MA, et al. Mycophenolate mofetil versus cyclophosphamide for induction treatment of lupus nephritis. J Am Soc Nephrol 2009; 20(5):1103–12.
64. Isenberg D, Appel GB, Contreras G, et al. Influence of race/ethnicity on response to lupus nephritis treatment: the ALMS study. Rheumatology (Oxford) 2010;49(1):128–40.
65. Dooley MA, Hogan S, Jennette C, et al. Cyclophosphamide therapy for lupus nephritis: poor renal survival in black Americans. Glomerular Disease Collaborative Network. Kidney Int 1997;51(4):1188–95.

66. Chan TM, Tse KC, Tang CS, et al. Long-term study of mycophenolate mofetil as continuous induction and maintenance treatment for diffuse proliferative lupus nephritis. J Am Soc Nephrol 2005;16(4):1076–84.
67. Chan TM, Li FK, Tang CS, et al. Efficacy of mycophenolate mofetil in patients with diffuse proliferative lupus nephritis. Hong Kong-Guangzhou Nephrology Study Group. N Engl J Med 2000;343(16):1156–62.
68. Walsh M, James M, Jayne D, et al. Mycophenolate mofetil for induction therapy of lupus nephritis: a systematic review and meta-analysis. Clin J Am Soc Nephrol 2007;2(5):968–75.
69. Ioannidis JP, Boki KA, Katsorida ME, et al. Remission, relapse, and re-remission of proliferative lupus nephritis treated with cyclophosphamide. Kidney Int 2000; 57(1):258–64.
70. Mosca M, Bencivelli W, Neri R, et al. Renal flares in 91 SLE patients with diffuse proliferative glomerulonephritis. Kidney Int 2002;61(4):1502–9.
71. Moroni G, Gallelli B, Quaglini S, et al. Withdrawal of therapy in patients with proliferative lupus nephritis: long-term follow-up. Nephrol Dial Transplant 2006;21(6):1541–8.
72. Grootscholten C, Berden JH. Discontinuation of immunosuppression in proliferative lupus nephritis: is it possible? Nephrol Dial Transplant 2006;21(6):1465–9.
73. Houssiau FA, D'Cruz D, Sangle S, et al. Azathioprine versus mycophenolate mofetil for long-term immunosuppression in lupus nephritis: results from the MAINTAIN nephritis trial. Ann Rheum Dis 2010;69(12):2083–9.
74. Dooley MA, Jayne D, Ginzler EM, et al. Mycophenolate versus azathioprine as maintenance therapy for lupus nephritis. N Engl J Med 2011;365(20):1886–95.
75. Vigna-Perez M, Hernandez-Castro B, Paredes-Saharopulos O, et al. Clinical and immunological effects of rituximab in patients with lupus nephritis refractory to conventional therapy: a pilot study. Arthritis Res Ther 2006;8(3):R83.
76. Melander C, Sallee M, Trolliet P, et al. Rituximab in severe lupus nephritis: early B-cell depletion affects long-term renal outcome. Clin J Am Soc Nephrol 2009; 4(3):579–87.
77. Najafi CC, Korbet SM, Lewis EJ, et al. Significance of histologic patterns of glomerular injury upon long-term prognosis in severe lupus glomerulonephritis. Kidney Int 2001;59(6):2156–63.
78. Bao H, Liu ZH, Xie HL, et al. Successful treatment of class V+IV lupus nephritis with multitarget therapy. J Am Soc Nephrol 2008;19(10):2001–10.
79. Donadio JV, Grande JP. IgA nephropathy. N Engl J Med 2002;347(10):738–48.
80. Alamartine E, Sabatier JC, Guerin C, et al. Prognostic factors in mesangial IgA glomerulonephritis: an extensive study with univariate and multivariate analyses. Am J Kidney Dis 1991;18(1):12–9.
81. Rekola S, Bergstrand A, Bucht H. Deterioration of GFR in IgA nephropathy as measured by ^{51}Cr-EDTA clearance. Kidney Int 1991;40(6):1050–4.
82. Geddes CC, Rauta V, Gronhagen-Riska C, et al. A tricontinental view of IgA nephropathy. Nephrol Dial Transplant 2003;18(8):1541–8.
83. D'Amico G. Natural history of idiopathic IgA nephropathy: role of clinical and histological prognostic factors. Am J Kidney Dis 2000;36(2):227–37.
84. Wakai K, Kawamura T, Endoh M, et al. A scoring system to predict renal outcome in IgA nephropathy: from a nationwide prospective study. Nephrol Dial Transplant 2006;21(10):2800–8.
85. Reich HN, Troyanov S, Scholey JW, et al. Remission of proteinuria improves prognosis in IgA nephropathy. J Am Soc Nephrol 2007;18(12):3177–83.
86. Berthoux F, Mohey H, Laurent B, et al. Predicting the risk for dialysis or death in IgA nephropathy. J Am Soc Nephrol 2011;22(4):752–61.

87. El Karoui K, Hill GS, Karras A, et al. Focal segmental glomerulosclerosis plays a major role in the progression of IgA nephropathy. II. Light microscopic and clinical studies. Kidney Int 2011;79(6):643–54.
88. Herzenberg AM, Fogo AB, Reich HN, et al. Validation of the Oxford classification of IgA nephropathy. Kidney Int 2011;80(3):310–7.
89. Shi SF, Wang SX, Jiang L, et al. Pathologic predictors of renal outcome and therapeutic efficacy in IgA nephropathy: validation of the oxford classification. Clin J Am Soc Nephrol 2011;6(9):2175–84.
90. Appel GB, Waldman M. The IgA nephropathy treatment dilemma. Kidney Int 2006;69(11):1939–44.
91. Barratt J, Feehally J. Treatment of IgA nephropathy. Kidney Int 2006;69(11):1934–8.
92. Nolin L, Courteau M. Management of IgA nephropathy: evidence-based recommendations. Kidney Int Suppl 1999;70:S56–62.
93. Pozzi C, Bolasco PG, Fogazzi GB, et al. Corticosteroids in IgA nephropathy: a randomised controlled trial. Lancet 1999;353(9156):883–7.
94. Pozzi C, Andrulli S, Del Vecchio L, et al. Corticosteroid effectiveness in IgA nephropathy: long-term results of a randomized, controlled trial. J Am Soc Nephrol 2004;15(1):157–63.
95. Katafuchi R, Ikeda K, Mizumasa T, et al. Controlled, prospective trial of steroid treatment in IgA nephropathy: a limitation of low-dose prednisolone therapy. Am J Kidney Dis 2003;41(5):972–83.
96. Manno C, Torres DD, Rossini M, et al. Randomized controlled clinical trial of corticosteroids plus ACE-inhibitors with long-term follow-up in proteinuric IgA nephropathy. Nephrol Dial Transplant 2009;24(12):3694–701.
97. Lv J, Zhang H, Chen Y, et al. Combination therapy of prednisone and ACE inhibitor versus ACE-inhibitor therapy alone in patients with IgA nephropathy: a randomized controlled trial. Am J Kidney Dis 2009;53(1):26–32.
98. Lai KN, Lai FM, Leung AC, et al. Plasma exchange in patients with rapidly progressive idiopathic IgA nephropathy: a report of two cases and review of literature. Am J Kidney Dis 1987;10(1):66–70.
99. Roccatello D, Ferro M, Coppo R, et al. Report on intensive treatment of extracapillary glomerulonephritis with focus on crescentic IgA nephropathy. Nephrol Dial Transplant 1995;10(11):2054–9.
100. McIntyre CW, Fluck RJ, Lambie SH. Steroid and cyclophosphamide therapy for IgA nephropathy associated with crescenteric change: an effective treatment. Clin Nephrol 2001;56(3):193–8.
101. Tumlin JA, Lohavichan V, Hennigar R. Crescentic, proliferative IgA nephropathy: clinical and histological response to methylprednisolone and intravenous cyclophosphamide. Nephrol Dial Transplant 2003;18(7):1321–9.
102. Hoffman GS, Kerr GS, Leavitt RY, et al. Wegener granulomatosis: an analysis of 158 patients. Ann Intern Med 1992;116(6):488–98.
103. Nachman PH, Hogan SL, Jennette JC, et al. Treatment response and relapse in antineutrophil cytoplasmic autoantibody-associated microscopic polyangiitis and glomerulonephritis. J Am Soc Nephrol 1996;7(1):33–9.
104. de Groot K, Adu D, Savage CO. The value of pulse cyclophosphamide in ANCA-associated vasculitis: meta-analysis and critical review. Nephrol Dial Transplant 2001;16(10):2018–27.
105. de Groot K, Harper L, Jayne DR, et al. Pulse versus daily oral cyclophosphamide for induction of remission in antineutrophil cytoplasmic antibody-associated vasculitis: a randomized trial. Ann Intern Med 2009;150(10):670–80.

106. Guillevin L, Cordier JF, Lhote F, et al. A prospective, multicenter, randomized trial comparing steroids and pulse cyclophosphamide versus steroids and oral cyclophosphamide in the treatment of generalized Wegener's granulomatosis. Arthritis Rheum 1997;40(12):2187–98.

107. Haubitz M, Schellong S, Gobel U, et al. Intravenous pulse administration of cyclophosphamide versus daily oral treatment in patients with antineutrophil cytoplasmic antibody-associated vasculitis and renal involvement: a prospective, randomized study. Arthritis Rheum 1998;41(10):1835–44.

108. Wegener's Granulomatosis Etanercept Trial (WGET) Research Group. Etanercept plus standard therapy for Wegener's granulomatosis. N Engl J Med 2005;352(4):351–61.

109. Jayne D, Rasmussen N, Andrassy K, et al. A randomized trial of maintenance therapy for vasculitis associated with antineutrophil cytoplasmic autoantibodies. N Engl J Med 2003;349(1):36–44.

110. Jones RB, Tervaert JW, Hauser T, et al. Rituximab versus cyclophosphamide in ANCA-associated renal vasculitis. N Engl J Med 2010;363(3):211–20.

111. Stone JH, Merkel PA, Spiera R, et al. Rituximab versus cyclophosphamide for ANCA-associated vasculitis. N Engl J Med 2010;363(3):221–32.

112. Pusey CD, Rees AJ, Evans DJ, et al. Plasma exchange in focal necrotizing glomerulonephritis without anti-GBM antibodies. Kidney Int 1991;40(4): 757–63.

113. Jayne DR, Gaskin G, Rasmussen N, et al. Randomized trial of plasma exchange or high-dosage methylprednisolone as adjunctive therapy for severe renal vasculitis. J Am Soc Nephrol 2007;18(7):2180–8.

114. Klemmer PJ, Chalermskulrat W, Reif MS, et al. Plasmapheresis therapy for diffuse alveolar hemorrhage in patients with small-vessel vasculitis. Am J Kidney Dis 2003;42(6):1149–53.

115. Langford CA, Talar-Williams C, Barron KS, et al. Use of a cyclophosphamide-induction methotrexate-maintenance regimen for the treatment of Wegener's granulomatosis: extended follow-up and rate of relapse. Am J Med 2003; 114(6):463–9.

116. Pagnoux C, Mahr A, Hamidou MA, et al. Azathioprine or methotrexate maintenance for ANCA-associated vasculitis. N Engl J Med 2008;359(26):2790–803.

117. Hiemstra TF, Walsh M, Mahr A, et al. Mycophenolate mofetil vs azathioprine for remission maintenance in antineutrophil cytoplasmic antibody-associated vasculitis: a randomized controlled trial. JAMA 2010;304(21):2381–8.

118. Wilson CB, Dixon FJ. Anti-glomerular basement membrane antibody-induced glomerulonephritis. Kidney Int 1973;3(2):74–89.

119. Pusey CD. Anti-glomerular basement membrane disease. Kidney Int 2003; 64(4):1535–50.

120. Levy JB, Turner AN, Rees AJ, et al. Long-term outcome of anti-glomerular basement membrane antibody disease treated with plasma exchange and immunosuppression. Ann Intern Med 2001;134(11):1033–42.

121. Savage CO, Pusey CD, Bowman C, et al. Antiglomerular basement membrane antibody mediated disease in the British Isles 1980-4. Br Med J (Clin Res Ed) 1986;292(6516):301–4.

122. Madore F, Lazarus JM, Brady HR. Therapeutic plasma exchange in renal diseases. J Am Soc Nephrol 1996;7(3):367–86.

123. Jindal KK. Management of idiopathic crescentic and diffuse proliferative glomerulonephritis: evidence-based recommendations. Kidney Int Suppl 1999;70:S33–40.

124. Johnson JP, Moore J Jr, Austin HA 3rd, et al. Therapy of anti-glomerular base-ment membrane antibody disease: analysis of prognostic significance of clin-ical, pathologic and treatment factors. Medicine (Baltimore) 1985;64(4):219–27.
125. Bagga A, Sinha A, Moudgil A. Rituximab in patients with the steroid-resistant nephrotic syndrome. N Engl J Med 2007;356(26):2751–2.
126. Fujinaga S, Hirano D, Nishizaki N, et al. Single infusion of rituximab for persistent steroid-dependent minimal-change nephrotic syndrome after long-term cyclo-sporine. Pediatr Nephrol 2010;25(3):539–44.
127. Guigonis V, Dallocchio A, Baudouin V, et al. Rituximab treatment for severe steroid- or cyclosporine-dependent nephrotic syndrome: a multicentric series of 22 cases. Pediatr Nephrol 2008;23(8):1269–79.
128. Haffner D, Fischer DC. Nephrotic syndrome and rituximab: facts and perspec-tives. Pediatr Nephrol 2009;24(8):1433–8.
129. Navarra SV, Guzman RM, Gallacher AE, et al. Efficacy and safety of belimumab in patients with active systemic lupus erythematosus: a randomised, placebo-controlled, phase 3 trial. Lancet 2011;377(9767):721–31.
130. Trachtman H, Vento S, Gipson D, et al. Novel therapies for resistant focal segmental glomerulosclerosis (FONT) phase II clinical trial: study design. BMC Nephrol 2011;12:8.
131. Trachtman H, Fervenza FC, Gipson DS, et al. A phase 1, single-dose study of fresolimumab, an anti-TGF-beta antibody, in treatment-resistant primary focal segmental glomerulosclerosis. Kidney Int 2011;79(11):1236–43.

Immunotherapies in Dermatologic Disorders

Robyn S. Fallen, BHSc[a], Collin R. Terpstra, MD[b],
Hermenio C. Lima, MD, PhD[c],*

KEYWORDS

- Biologics • Immunotherapy • Immunostimulants
- Immunosuppressants • Skin diseases

Key Points

- The skin is an immunologic organ and many dermatoses are characterized by inflammatory responses triggered by infections and environmental antigens or autoantigens.
- Immunotherapy in dermatologic disorders involves the use of immunomodulators, such as immunosuppressants or immunostimulants, to re-establish skin homeostasis.
- Biologics used for immunotherapy are not a homogeneous group. They are allergenic extracts, blood or blood components, cytokines, fusion proteins, monoclonal antibodies, and vaccines.
- Improved understanding of the mechanisms of skin disease will assist clinicians in counseling patients on available immunomodulators and in selecting appropriate therapy.

INTRODUCTION

In no other part of the body are inflammatory reactions more apparent than in the skin.[1] Human integument is an immunologic organ that has antigens for lymphocytes and produces many types of cytokines and inflammatory mediators.[2] Complex relationships between cells and inflammatory mediators in the skin have been unveiled. Many dermatoses are defined by immune responses developed after contact with infectious or environmental antigens.[3] Some may result from the triggering of antibodies and lymphocytes reactive to autoantigens of the epidermis or dermis.[4] Health disorders of this tissue may be caused by either an exacerbation or reduction of the immune response.

Many therapies exist to treat dermatoses. The treatment of disease arising from immune dysregulation is considered a form of immunotherapy.[5] Therapies that try

[a] Michael G. DeGroote School of Medicine, Waterloo Regional Campus, McMaster University, 10-B Victoria Street South, Kitchener, Ontario N2G 1C5, Canada
[b] Division of Allergy, Department of Medicine, Michael G. DeGroote School of Medicine, McMaster University, HSC Rm 3W11, 1280 Main Street West, Hamilton, ON L8S 4K1, Canada
[c] Division of Dermatology, Department of Medicine, Michael G. DeGroote School of Medicine, McMaster University, 10-B Victoria Street S-Office #3017, Kitchener, Ontario N2G 1C5, Canada
* Corresponding author.
E-mail address: hlima@mcmaster.ca

Med Clin N Am 96 (2012) 565–582
doi:10.1016/j.mcna.2012.04.004
0025-7125/12/$ – see front matter © 2012 Elsevier Inc. All rights reserved.
medical.theclinics.com

to modify the immune response to re-establish the skin homeostasis are also defined as immunotherapy. Immunotherapy involves the use of immunomodulators. By redirecting the orientation of the immune response, immunomodulators may have potential use as immunostimulants or immunosuppressants.

Definitions of immunotherapy are diverse and therefore immunotherapy can include many types of immunomodulators. Until recently, chemicals from diverse sources used to manipulate the immune system were known as immunosuppressants. These immunotherapeutic agents are now better considered immunomodulators and are used to reduce exaggerated activity of the immune system. Several publications on this group of drugs have shown the important role of these therapies as essential pharmacotherapy agents and as a type of immunotherapy in dermatology. This type of immunotherapy is not included in this review.

The modification of the antigen-specific IgE immune response profile by the repeated administration of an antigen to patients with a specific allergy is a type of immunotherapy.[6] There are examples of its application in dermatology, mainly for atopic dermatitis (AD).[7,8] The other group of immunomodulators is the biologics. Biologics are complex preparations of organic substances obtained from animals or modified organisms isolated by biotechnological methods or assays. Biologics are blood products, vaccines, protein extracts, recombinant protein, and monoclonal antibodies. These products usually must be injected or infused into the body to be effective. Its pharmacologic action depends on interactions with biochemical or immunologic processes in the body. With recent developments in the understanding of the pathophysiology of the immune system, new immunomodulatory therapies using cytokines and monoclonal antibodies have been developed. These novel agents are especially useful in the treatment of diseases caused by immune system dysregulation or the lack of immune response.[9]

From the basic science standpoint, immunomodulators are used to characterize immunologic events in a variety of biological processes. Studies have already led to important discoveries about the pathophysiology of skin diseases. From a clinical standpoint, there is no doubt about the important role of these therapies as essential components in the pharmacotherapy of clinicians in any field of medicine. Immunomodulators have high potential utility in the daily dermatologic clinic. The objective of this article is to discuss the immunomodulators most used by dermatologists.

In this review we sought to conduct a literature search on immunotherapies used to treat skin disease and summarize the most relevant data obtained. All studies, including reviews, clinical trials, editorials, letters, meta-analyses, practical guides, randomized clinical trials, and controlled clinical trials published up to January 2012 were included. There was no restriction on the language of the studies.

Articles and summaries were analyzed to identify relevant studies. Potentially relevant texts were obtained for evaluation. The authors decided on the publications that satisfied the inclusion criteria and methodological quality parameters and performed this appraisal without conflict of interest.

IMMUNOTHERAPIES USED IN DERMATOLOGY

Many immunomodulators are used to treat skin diseases. The following sections present procedures of immunomodulation used in dermatology.

Biologic Agents Used in Immunotherapies

Biologics have been in use for more than 100 years as vaccines.[10] However, they received renewed attention when they started to be used for the treatment of autoimmune diseases. Biologic agents used in immunotherapies are classified on the basis of origin. Allergenic extracts, blood or blood components, cytokines, fusion proteins, monoclonal antibodies, and vaccines are used as immunomodulators to treat or prevent diseases.

In a more strict definition, the word "biologics" is used to describe the new immunotherapies that emerged through the application of biotechnological engineering.[11] These medications are usually of 3 types: fusion proteins, signaling proteins, and monoclonal antibodies. Biologics are not a homogeneous group of drugs.

Fusion proteins are usually a combination of 2 different protein components that form a single active molecule. A portion is the site that recognizes a specific protein and it is connected to a second structure that can be a part of the Fc portion of human immunoglobulin that serves to stabilize the structure of this protein as a whole. This structure increases biological half-life, allowing less frequent administration of the active molecule. Fusion proteins are composed of products with human sequences and therefore they have low immunogenicity.[12]

Signaling proteins are recombinant proteins generated from sequences obtained from the genome of the organism itself. The first step is to obtain these biological drawings or get the "blueprint" that is the template DNA sequence encoding the desired molecule. These sequences are transfected into cells or microorganisms for synthesis. The purified protein is thus synthesized for use. They are identical to normal human proteins and capable of acting by interacting with cellular receptors.

Cytokines are signaling proteins. Cytokines are divided into the pro-inflammatory category that is the activator of lymphocytes and leukocytes, immunosuppressors, growth factors, and interferons. The use of these proteins is based on the biological function discovered for these proteins. IL-10 was one of the first cytokines used in dermatology, and it was used for its ability to divert the helper T cell (T_H) subtype 1 to subtype 2.[13]

Monoclonal antibodies were derived from the technological development of hybridomas created by J. Georges F. Köhler and César Milstein.[14] These biologics used in medical practice are usually derived from mice, which are modified by genetic engineering to appear more human. Thus, these monoclonal antibodies can be considered chimeric, humanized, or human. These processes progressively reduce the immunogenicity of monoclonal antibodies. Thus, the humanized antibodies retain less genomic sequences than murine chimeric antibodies.

Allergenic Extracts for Antigen-Specific Immunotherapy in Dermatology

Antigen-specific immunotherapy is the process of modification of the profile of immune response by repeated administration of an allergen to patients with a specific allergy, determined by the participation of IgE against this antigen. Subcutaneous doses with a progressive concentration sequence of the antigen are used. Immunotherapy has an average duration of 4 to 5 years, with dosages maintained at intervals of 2 to 4 weeks.[15]

Introduced in 1911, the details of the mechanisms of action of antigen-specific immunotherapy remain unknown. The main basis of the process is the suppression of allergen-specific IgE and the induction of IgG4 and IgA. The therapy results in reduction of allergic symptoms and inflammation induced by the activation of mast cells. Immunotherapies do not produce immune tolerance.[16]

This immunotherapy is effective in reducing the threat of anaphylaxis from insect bites.[17] The main application of this therapy in dermatology is its use in the treatment of AD. Systematic studies on the effectiveness of specific immunotherapy for patients with AD are scarce.[18] These studies must determine the success rates of therapies and the schedules with the lowest rate of side effects, and therefore, an effective immunotherapy for the treatment of AD is still controversial.[19]

Blood or Blood Components Used for Immunotherapy in Dermatology

The use of blood as autohemotherapy is not usual in dermatology. The main use of autologous blood injection is for chronic urticaria, although the occurrence of IgG anti-Fc(epsilon) RI alpha reactivity defines an autoimmune-mediated subtype of chronic urticaria.[20,21] The rationale is that patients can benefit from repeated low-dose applications of the circulating histamine-releasing factors responsible for their urticarial symptoms. A clinical study observed a reduction of urticarial symptoms in patients who tested positive to a skin test with autologous serum after 8 weekly intramuscular injections of their own blood.[22] Other studies confirmed the finding that these patients can benefit from autohemotherapy.[23]

The use of antibodies for the treatment of infections began in 1890 when von Behring and Kitasato used antibodies to treat tetanus and diphtheria. Kabat and Tiselius determined that most of the immunoglobulin was in the fraction of plasma globulins. Sequentially, Cohn produced almost pure IgG from plasma. The initial intravenous (IV) use of immunoglobulins was associated with several fatalities. However, the removal of aggregates by Hassig and Isliker allowed successful IV use.[24]

Treatment with IV immunoglobulin (IVIg) is used to restore the immune balance in patients with inflammatory or autoimmune disease.[25] It is not used to restore immunity. This only happens in situations of immunodeficiency caused by the absence of immunoglobulin. IVIg is useful for immunotherapy of immunoglobulin-mediated diseases. Therefore, it is used as primary immunosuppressant therapy in autoimmune diseases.

There are many indications for use of IVIg in dermatology.[26] IVIg may be helpful in treating pediatric and adult patients with AD.[27] There is absolute indication for IVIg therapy in Kawasaki disease. The morbidity and mortality of Kawasaki disease is decreased when IVIg therapy is given in the early phase of the disease.[28] There is some evidence that IVIg is beneficial as adjunct therapy for systemic lupus erythematosus flare-ups and lupus nephritis.[29] IVIg was justified for severe Churg-Strauss syndrome unresponsive to high dose of corticosteroids.[30] There is evidence of beneficial effect from IVIg therapy for Henoch-Schönlein purpura.[31] Data also suggest that IVIg has therapeutic and steroid-sparing effects in patients with severe pemphigus vulgaris. However, IVIg therapy has not had an important role as an adjunctive immunotherapy for the treatment of patients with refractory pemphigus foliaceus or bullous pempigoid.[32] IVIg seems to be useful to stabilize metastatic melanoma when added to standard therapy.[33] There are reports describing a beneficial effect of IVIg in severe chronic idiopathic and autoimmune urticarial.[34] Few reports suggest the possible effectiveness of IVIg in case of severe resistant psoriasis with psoriatic arthritis.[35] Similarly, cases of unresponsive pyoderma gangrenosum were successfully treated with IVIg.[36] The use of IVIg in toxic epidermal necrolysis (TEN) is surrounded by controversy despite evidence indicating therapeutic benefit. There is an absence of clinical randomized controlled studies.[37] Nonetheless, the early administration of high-dose immunoglobulin should be considered in the absence of any therapeutic alternative.[38]

THE NEW BIOLOGICS IN MEDICINE

The direct targeting of inflammatory cascades by blocking specific cytokines is a modern treatment option for autoimmune diseases.[39] The rationale for this therapy arises from pathophysiology; in different autoimmune diseases there is increase in the production of proinflammatory cytokines by the immune system. Inflammatory cytokines, like many other cytokines, have an important role both in maintaining health and in participating in disease manifestation.[40]

The treatment of these autoimmune diseases in some way affects the immune system, leading to reduction of activity in that specific immune system. Biologics also act to block the action of autoimmune cells or destroy malignant cells but are designed to have high specificity, potentially increasing their safety. Moreover, the biologics differ from other drugs because they can intervene in the development of diseases. However, the long-term effects of this interference with the immune system are yet to be known.[39,41]

The concept of biologic therapy for skin inflammatory diseases derived from their etiopathogenesis. As in a chess game, these new forms of treatment have evolved from an integration of the knowledge of interactions between the immune system cells (pieces) and their cytokines (movements) that initiate pathologic processes and ultimately lead to the development of the clinical features of the disease from the lack of homeostasis in the immune system.[42]

As a result, two logical biologic therapeutic approaches have been used: one is the administration of counter regulatory cytokines and the second is the blocking of cytokines. The use of monoclonal antibodies or fusion proteins to neutralize cytokines started to be used on a large scale because of their efficacy and practicality.[43] These studies have proved to be a useful biological model and test ground for evaluation of the skin immune system. Although some of these drugs were not initially developed in the treatment of patients with skin diseases but were eventually used resulting in a profound influenced the studies presented here.[43,44] In summary, the new biologics are proteins molecules that modulate the immune system by downregulating the inflammatory response or increases anti-tumoral specific defenses.

THE NEW BIOLOGICS FOR TREATMENT OF DERMATOLOGIC DISORDERS

Although clinical efficacy is important, concerns regarding optimal regimens, first line choices, when and how to combine drugs, and risks and benefits associated with different subgroups of patients remain.[45] This is especially true in dermatology as new biologics emerge because patients often feel frustrated with the ineffectiveness of current therapies.[46,47] The desire for more aggressive efficacy may sometimes affect safety but the recent data suggest improved safety over some older immunomodulatory agents.[48,49] Biologics are present in alphabetic order to avoid any induction of preference or orientation by the authors.

Adalimumab (Humira)

Adalimumab is a fully human monoclonal IgG1 antibody against tumor necrosis factor (TNF) α and is administered by subcutaneous injection. It blocks soluble and transmembrane TNF-α. It is also able to mediate complement-induced cytolysis.[50] As a humanized antibody, adalimumab was designed to induce lower rate and low-titer antibodies during therapy.[51] However, the long-term immunogenicity of adalimumab exists without adverse events.[52]

In immunomodulatory application, TNF-α antagonists are most useful in reducing TNF-α that is pathogenic. Theoretically, if calibrated correctly to pharmacokinetic and pharmacodynamic equilibrium, these antagonists should allow immune system stability without causing major immunosuppression.[53]

Adalimumab has been approved for the treatment of psoriatic arthritis and moderate to severe chronic psoriasis in dermatology. Case reports mention adalimumab in treating hidradenitis suppurativa, pyoderma gangrenosum, Sweet syndrome, cutaneous sarcoidosis, pemphigus, systemic vasculitides, multicentric reticulohistiocytosis, and stomatitis.[54,55]

Alefacept (Amevive)

Alefacept (Amevive) is a fully human lymphocyte function-associated antigen 3/immunoglobulin 1 fusion protein, which consists of the extracellular CD2-binding portion of leukocyte functioning antigen 3 and the Fc portion of human IgG1. It prevents T cell migration and activation. It also induces apoptosis of the T cells CD45RO.[56–59]

Alefacept is approved for the treatment of adult patients with moderate to severe chronic plaque psoriasis. Administered subcutaneously once a week, it improves the quality of life of patients with moderate to severe psoriasis, with the Psoriasis Area and Severity Index (PASI) score of 75 higher in the treated group than in the placebo group. Recurrence of the disease was observed within 60 to 70 days after discontinuation of treatment.[60]

Adverse effects with the first injection are more common and wane with subsequent doses. It can be administered safely for long periods. CS4$^+$ T lymphocyte counts should be monitored every 2 weeks throughout the 12-week course of alefacept.[57] There are published data regarding its use for nail,[61] palmoplantar,[62] and scalp psoriasis.[63] A patient with IgA pemphigus showed improvement with alefacept and mycophenolate mofetil (1 g/d). Other studies used alefacept for erythema nodosum, lichen planus, and pyoderma gangrenosum.[26,64]

Alemtuzumab (Campath, MabCampath, or Campath-1H)

Alemtuzumab is a humanized anti-CD52 monoclonal antibody. It belongs to the family of Campath-1 antibodies. It was developed to prevent graft-versus-host disease (GVHD) and graft rejection in stem cell transplantation.[65] A few studies have investigated the efficacy of alemtuzumab in the treatment of established, acute GVHD (aGVHD).[66] In patients with steroid-refractory aGVHD, alemtuzumab had an overall response rate of 70% and the overall survival rate was 50%.[67] Recent reports showed some efficacy of alemtuzumab in combination with other medications for selected patients with chronic GVHD.[68]

Alemtuzumab is also used in the dermatological field for the treatment of cutaneous T-cell lymphoma.[69] Alemtuzumab therapy is also suggested for mycosis fungoides or for Sézary syndrome refractory to treatment. Therapy using 30 mg, 3 times weekly for up to 12 weeks, improved erythroderma in 69% of patients, with complete resolution in 38%.[70]

Basiliximab (Simulect)

Basiliximab is a chimeric mouse-human monoclonal antibody to the α chain of the IL-2 receptor of T cells. Trials have been conducted to assess the efficacy and feasibility of basiliximab therapy in patients with steroid-refractory aGVHD.[71] A significant improvement of skin symptoms was observed in most cases, with some subjects showing a complete resolution. Basiliximab has been reported to be an efficient therapy in some cases of lichen planus with dosage of 20 mg every 4 days.[72]

Efalizumab (Raptiva)

Efalizumab is a recombinant humanized monoclonal IgG1 antibody against CD11a, the α subunit of leukocyte functioning antigen 1. It interferes with T-cell adhesion to the endothelial cells, its activation, reactivation in the skin, and its migration to sites of inflammation.[58,73]

Efalizumab is administered with a first dose of 0.7 mg/kg, then 1.0 mg/kg subcutaneous injection once weekly. The most common side effects include headaches, myalgia, pain, and fever. Safe studies described the occurrence of infections during efalizumab therapy, such as bacterial sepsis, viral meningitis, invasive fungal disease, progressive multifocal leukoencephalopathy (JC virus), and other opportunistic infections.[74] Efalizumab should be discontinued if hemolytic anemia or thrombocytopenia occurs. Live or attenuated vaccines should be avoided during efalizumab therapy.[75]

Efalizumab is approved for the treatment of patients with plaque psoriasis. It has been used with success in the treatment of disseminated granuloma annulare.[76] Efalizumab did not prove to be effective in the treatment of psoriatic arthritis.[77] Sequential therapy in plaque psoriasis after infliximab has been proposed with controversial results.[78,79] Efalizumab had been presented as an alternative therapy for discoid lupus erythematosus. However, some studies indicated successful results while others demonstrated induction of the disease.[80-82]

Etanercept (Enbrel)

Etanercept is a dimeric fusion protein of the p75 component of human TNF receptor fused to human IgG Fc. Etanercept acts as a competitive inhibitor of TNF-α by binding to this cytokine and preventing interactions with its cell surface receptors.[9] It does not fix complement, cause antibody-dependent cytotoxicity, or trigger T-cell apoptosis. Etanercept is administered for psoriasis as a self-administered subcutaneous injection at a dosage of 50 mg twice weekly for 3 months with a subsequent decrease to 50 mg weekly.[83] Overall, its safety profile may be more favorable than those of other biologics.[39]

Etanercept is indicated for psoriatic arthritis and moderate to severe psoriasis. Recent reports showed some efficacy of etanercept in selected patients with acute and chronic GVHD,[68,84] Behçet disease,[85] hidradenitis suppurativa,[86] pemphigus vulgaris,[87] pemphigus foliaceous,[88] pityriasis rubra pilaris,[89] and Sweet syndrome.[90]

Infliximab (Remicade)

Infliximab is a chimeric monoclonal IgG1 antibody with anti–TNF-α properties. Infliximab binds to and blocks both the monomeric and trimeric soluble TNF-α and transmembrane TNF-α. In addition, it also fixes complement and induces apoptosis of cells with TNF on its surface.[91]

Infliximab is administered by IV infusion in single doses ranging from 3 to 20 mg/kg based on disease type and severity.[92-95] It is usually well tolerated. Headache, nausea, and upper respiratory tract infections are the most common side effects seen. It should be avoided in patients with demyelinating disease, congestive heart failure, and tuberculosis. No direct toxic effect was demonstrated with increase in dose. However, the probability and intensity of adverse reactions tends to increase with higher dosage.[96]

Infliximab is approved for the treatment of psoriasis and psoriatic arthritis. Patients with psoriasis can achieve significant improvement with this immunotherapy. Other studies evaluated its use for aGVHD,[97] Behçet disease,[85] necrobiosis lipoidica diabectorum,[98] pityriasis rubra pilaris,[99] SAPHO syndrome,[100] scleroderma,[101] subcorneal pustular dermatosis,[102] and toxic epidermal necrolysis.[103]

Inolimomab

Inolimomab is a murine monoclonal antibody developed for the treatment of GVHD. Its target is the alpha chain of the IL-2 receptor.[104,105] In a recent study, inolimomab was used in 20 patients with aGVHD. The overall complete response rate for this second-line treatment was 35% with inolimomab.[84]

Ipilimumab

A monoclonal antibody directed against cytotoxic T lymphocyte–associated antigen-4 (CTLA4). CTLA4 is an antigen that is expressed on activated T cells and exhibits affinity for B7 costimulatory molecules. By binding CTLA4, ipilimumab enhances T-cell activation and blocks B7-1 and B7-2 T-cell costimulatory pathways.[106] Ipilimumab is recommended for treatment of melanoma that cannot be removed by surgery or has metastasized.[107] The recommended dose and schedule for ipilimumab is 3 mg/kg as an IV infusion every 3 weeks for a total of 4 doses. Other studies have evaluated its use for other types of cancer.[108]

Omalizumab (Xolair)

Omalizumab is a recombinant humanized monoclonal antibody directed against the constant $C\varepsilon3$ region of IgE, which blocks its interaction with both high- and low-affinity IgE receptors ($FC\varepsilon RI$ and $FC\varepsilon RII$) on mast cells, basophils, macrophages, dendritic cells, and B lymphocytes. Studies have shown omalizumab to be effective in reducing not only free IgE but also bound IgE and $FC\varepsilon RI$ expression.[109]

In patients with elevated IgE levels, omalizumab is effective for the treatment of asthma and allergic respiratory disease.[110] Dosing is based on weight on an IgE level between 30 to 1500 IU/mL and ranges from 75 to 600 g every 2 to 4 weeks. The efficacy of omalizumab has also been studied in other atopic diseases, such as allergic rhinitis, allergic bronchopulmonary aspergillosis, food allergy, and AD.[111]

AD acts as a precursor to future atopic diseases in more than 60% of patients.[112] IgE is commonly elevated in patients with AD with levels of IgE in the 1000 to 10,000 IU/mL range, with levels correlating to disease severity. Mast cells and basophils can drive inflammation in the skin. It is unclear however, whether chronic AD is itself driven by elevated IgE.

Many studies have investigated the efficacy of omalizumab in AD. However, most studies are small case series that used omalizumab in patients with IgE levels more than 700 IU/mL, which causes an inherent underdosing, or lack placebo controls, which is concerning because of the large placebo effect in AD. Despite these limitations, studies show promising improvements in AD severity on the Global Assessment (IGA) or Scoring Atopic Dermatitis (SCORAD) indices.[113–117] Improvement is also evident in patients with concomitant atopic asthma.[118–120] Although studies may demonstrate reduction in the levels of free IgE and even expression of $FC\varepsilon RI$ with omalizumab therapy, this may not correlate to clinical improvement.[121,122] Another mechanism has been raised that allows for improvement in AD despite partial neutralization of free IgE from underdosing. Negative trials raise the question of the overall efficacy of omalizumab for patients with AD.[123]

Heil and colleagues[124] recently published the first randomized double-blind 2:1 placebo-controlled trial conducted on 20 chronic patients with AD during a 20-week period. The patient population was larger than most previous studies, and the average IgE level was approximately 300 IU/mL and thus amenable to standard omalizumab dosing. They found significant reductions in free IgE levels within 1 week in addition to bound IgE to $FC\varepsilon RI$ as previous studies had indicated. Further, immunohistologic examination showed marked reductions in IgE-positive cells within the dermis and epidermis, predominantly in dendritic cells. Whereas immunologic changes were evidenced, the reported incidence of pruritus actually went up in the treatment group and IGA scores were not significantly different. This again raises several questions. What is the role of IgE in chronic AD? Is omalizumab titrated to adequately bind free IgE in AD? Is there a subset of patients with AD for whom omalizumab could be used, such as young asthmatic patients with known atopy? Although omalizumab can reduce free IgE and FCεRI saturation, it does not necessarily correlate with mitigating disease activity in chronic AD.

Omalizumab therapy has also been studied in several other cutaneous diseases. Omalizumab has shown promising results in patients with chronic idiopathic urticaria.[125–127] A recent randomized clinical trial showed beneficial effects within 1 week of omalizumab being administered in appropriate IgE level-based dosages.[128] Omalizumab therapy seems to have mixed results in the treatment of cholinergic urticaria.[129,130] Cutaneous mastocytosis has fewer trials but did show positive results.[131] Overall, many trials were small case series involving 1 to 3 patients but showed promising results with complete resolution in most patients.

Rituximab (MabThera, Rituxan)

Rituximab is a chimeric murine/human IgG monoclonal antibody with anti-CD20 activity. CD20 antigen is expressed on B lymphocytes, either malignant or benign. It induces B-cell lysis by several mechanisms of cytolysis, including complement-dependent cytotoxicity, antibody-dependent cellular cytotoxicity, and induction of apoptosis. The effect on B cells has encouraged its use in the treatment of many autoimmune disorders.

Rituximab is administered as 375 mg/m^2 IV per week for 4 weeks ± monthly follow-up doses. It has been on the market for more than 10 years and is relatively safe, given that it does not affect T cells. However, it carries a potential risk of cytopenias (particularly neutropenia) and severe infections, especially when combined with other immunosuppressors.[132,133]

Many studies report successful treatment of pemphigus with rituximab.[134] Rituximab can induce complete remission of pemphigus vulgaris in combination with immunosuppressors or without them.[135,136] Although many patients treated with rituximab did not achieve complete remission, there was still the benefit of tapered corticosteroid treatment. Pemphigus foliaceus has a pathogenesis similar to pemphigus vulgaris, and this has encouraged the use of rituximab in the treatment of this condition. However, there are fewer successes.[137,138] Patients with paraneoplastic pemphigus treated with rituximab for 4 weeks had varied responses.[139–141] Schmidt and colleagues analyzed the efficacy of rituximab in patients with bullous pemphigoid and achieved full clinical remission.[142–144] With a pathogenesis similar to the other bullous autoimmune skin diseases, several studies have tried rituximab for epidermolysis bullosa acquisita. Some patients achieved partial remission and enhanced/improved quality of life and were able to decrease their corticosteroid dosages when using rituximab.[145–147] Dermatomyositis is an idiopathic inflammatory disease with B-cell perivascular infiltrates; rituximab has been used for treatment of refractory cases. Patients with dermatomyositis demonstrated improvement when treated with rituximab. The skin rash and alopecia were reduced, but there were varying responses in regaining muscle strength.[148–151]

Ustekinumab (Stelara)

Although clinical response to anti-TNF suggested a role for T$_H$1 cells in psoriasis, evidence coming from other studies demonstrated that the T$_H$1/T$_H$2 paradigm and key role of TNF were not sufficient to explain the full pathogenesis of psoriasis. At this point some academic resistance was raised to an immunologic pathogenesis for psoriasis.[152] However, the main interpretation was that an important piece of the immunologic cytokine puzzle was missing. Researchers first noted that IL-12 is crucial for T$_H$1 cell differentiation.[153] Interferon-γ mediates many of the proinflammatory activities of IL-12. The use of anti-IL-12 monoclonal antibody in an experimental model of psoriasis also suggested the therapeutic value of blocking IL-12 in humans.[154] IL-23 favors the proliferation of the T$_H$17 subtype and the consequent production of IL-22 and IL-6 that stimulate the proliferation of keratinocytes. IL-17 favors infiltration of neutrophils into the skin, forming the typical Munro microabscess with some participation of IL-22 in psoriasis.[155] II-23 could also mediate and sustain late-stage chronic inflammation by the production of IL-17 by T$_H$17.[156] These findings confirm the centrality of this pathway for the induction of autoimmunity.[157]

Ustekinumab is a human monoclonal antibody that blocks the activity of the cytokines IL-12 and IL-23. Immune dysregulation involving IL-12/IL-23 has been implicated in many inflammatory disorders.[157] Ustekinumab is injected subcutaneously in the following protocol based on weight. Patients weighing less than 100 kg (220 lbs) should receive 45 mg initially, 45 mg 4 weeks later, and then 45 mg every 12 weeks. Patients weighing more than 100 kg (220 lbs) should receive 90 mg initially, 90 mg 4 weeks later, and then 90 mg every 12 weeks. Patients treated with 45 or 90 mg of ustekinumab achieved a significant improvement on PASI at 12 weeks.[158–160]

Ustekinumab is approved for the treatment of psoriasis and psoriatic arthritis in the field of dermatology.[161] Patients with psoriasis can achieve significant improvement with this immunotherapy.[162] Other studies evaluated its use for aGVHD,[163] hidradenitis suppurativa,[164] subacute lupus,[165] pityriasis rubra pilaris,[166] and pyoderma gangrenosum.[167]

SUMMARY

In medicine, the gold standard is the intervention believed to be the best available option. Given the proven role of the immune system in skin diseases, substantial interest exists in targeting them with immunotherapy. Many pathways operate in the development of different dermatoses. This fact places biologics as the standard-setting paradigm for the therapy and understanding of the pathogenesis of many skin diseases. However, large studies are needed to provide information on therapeutic effects, adverse events, and the place in treatment for each biologic. The challenge for the future is in combining biologic therapies to improve the quality and duration of responses while diminishing side effects. The ultimate goal is to broaden the understanding of the mechanisms of skin diseases and to achieve the proper application of immunomodulators for each clinical challenge. The ability to manipulate the regulatory function of the immune system according to the desired therapeutic effect is the ideal. An integrated immunologic approach to therapy holds great promise in reducing the burden of skin diseases.

REFERENCES

1. Lima HC. Papel das células T reguladoras no desenvolvimento de dermatoses. An Bras Dermatol 2006;81(3):269–81 [in Portuguese].
2. Bos JD. The skin as an organ of immunity. Clin Exp Immunol 1997;107(Suppl 1):3–5.
3. Hertl M, Riechers R. Autoreactive T cells as potential targets for immunotherapy of autoimmune bullous skin diseases. Clin Dermatol 2001;19(5):592–7.
4. Novak N, Bieber T. The skin as a target for allergic diseases. Allergy 2000;55(2):103–7.
5. Lima XT, Abuabara K, Kimball AB, et al. Briakinumab. Expert Opin Biol Ther 2009;9(8):1107–13.
6. Fitzsimons T, Grammer LC. Immunotherapy—definition and mechanism. Allergy Proc 1990;11(4):156.
7. Werfel T, Breuer K, Rueff F, et al. Usefulness of specific immunotherapy in patients with atopic dermatitis and allergic sensitization to house dust mites: a multi-centre, randomized, dose-response study. Allergy 2006;61(2):202–5.

8. Novak N, Thaci D, Hoffmann M, et al. Subcutaneous immunotherapy with a de-pigmented polymerized birch pollen extract-a new therapeutic option for patients with atopic dermatitis. Int Arch allergy Immunol 2011;155(3):252–6.
9. Singri P, West DP, Gordon KB. Biologic therapy for psoriasis: the new thera-peutic frontier. Arch Dermatol 2002;138(5):657–63.
10. Bliss M. The history of insulin. Diabetes Care 1993;16(Suppl 3):4–7.
11. Osborne R. Fresh from the biologic pipeline. Nat Biotechnol 2009;27(3):222–5.
12. Mehlis SL, Gordon KB. The immunology of psoriasis and biologic immuno-therapy. J Am Acad Dermatol 2003;49(Suppl 2):S44–50.
13. Reich K, Bruck M, Grafe A, et al. Treatment of psoriasis with interleukin-10. J Invest Dermatol 1998;111(6):1235–6.
14. dos Santos RV, de Lima PM, Nitsche A, et al. Aplicações terapêuticas dos anticor-pos monoclonais. Rev Bras Alerg Imunopatol 2006;29(2):77–85 [in Portuguese].
15. Kundig TM. Immunotherapy concepts under investigation. Allergy 2011; 66(Suppl 95):60–2.
16. Soyer OU, Akdis M, Akdis CA. Mechanisms of subcutaneous allergen immuno-therapy. Immunol Allergy Clin North Am 2011;31(2):175–90, vii–viii.
17. Nelson HS. Subcutaneous injection immunotherapy for optimal effectiveness. Immunol Allergy Clin North Am 2011;31(2):211–26, viii.
18. Bussmann C, Bockenhoff A, Henke H, et al. Does allergen-specific immuno-therapy represent a therapeutic option for patients with atopic dermatitis? J Allergy Clin Immunol 2006;118(6):1292–8.
19. Williams HC, Grindlay DJ. What's new in atopic eczema? An analysis of system-atic reviews published in 2007 and 2008. Part 2. Disease prevention and treat-ment. Clin Exp Dermatol 2010;35(3):223–7.
20. Fiebiger E, Maurer D, Holub H, et al. Serum IgG autoantibodies directed against the alpha chain of Fc epsilon RI: a selective marker and pathogenetic factor for a distinct subset of chronic urticaria patients? J Clin Invest 1995;96(6):2606–12.
21. Hide M, Francis DM, Grattan CE, et al. Autoantibodies against the high-affinity IgE receptor as a cause of histamine release in chronic urticaria. N Engl J Med 1993;328(22):1599–604.
22. Staubach P, Onnen K, Vonend A, et al. Autologous whole blood injections to patients with chronic urticaria and a positive autologous serum skin test: a placebo-controlled trial. Dermatology 2006;212(2):150–9.
23. Kocaturk E, Aktas S, Turkoglu Z, et al. Autologous whole blood and autologous serum injections are equally effective as placebo injections in reducing disease activity in patients with chronic spontaneous urticaria: a placebo controlled, randomized, single-blind study. J Dermatolog Treat 2011. [Epub ahead of print].
24. Austen KF. Therapeutic immunology. 2nd edition. Malden (MA): Blackwell Science; 2001.
25. Lee SJ, Chinen J, Kavanaugh A. Immunomodulator therapy: monoclonal antibodies, fusion proteins, cytokines, and immunoglobulins. J Allergy Clin Immunol 2010;125(2 Suppl 2):S314–23.
26. Smith DI, Swamy PM, Heffernan MP. Off-label uses of biologics in dermatology: interferon and intravenous immunoglobulin (part 1 of 2). J Am Acad Dermatol 2007;56(1):e1–54.
27. Simon D. Systemic therapy of atopic dermatitis in children and adults. Curr Probl Dermatol 2011;41:156–64.
28. Bayry J, Negi VS, Kaveri SV. Intravenous immunoglobulin therapy in rheumatic diseases. Nat Rev Rheumatol 2011;7(6):349–59.

29. Karim MY, Pisoni CN, Khamashta MA. Update on immunotherapy for systemic lupus erythematosus—what's hot and what's not! Rheumatology (Oxford) 2009;48(4):332–41.
30. Hot A, Perard L, Coppers B, et al. Marked improvement of Churg-Strauss vasculitis with intravenous gamma globulins during pregnancy. Clin Rheumatol 2007; 26(12):2149–51.
31. Aries PM, Hellmich B, Gross WL. Intravenous immunoglobulin therapy in vasculitis: speculation or evidence? Clin Rev Allergy Immunol 2005;29(3):237–45.
32. Gurcan HM, Jeph S, Ahmed AR. Intravenous immunoglobulin therapy in autoimmune mucocutaneous blistering diseases: a review of the evidence for its efficacy and safety. Am J Clin Dermatol 2010;11(5):315–26.
33. Schachter J, Katz U, Mahrer A, et al. Efficacy and safety of intravenous immunoglobulin in patients with metastatic melanoma. Ann N Y Acad Sci 2007;1110:305–14.
34. Morgan M, Khan DA. Therapeutic alternatives for chronic urticaria: an evidence-based review, part 2. Ann Allergy Asthma Immunol 2008;100(6):517–26 [quiz: 526–8, 544].
35. Jolles S, Hughes J. Use of IGIV in the treatment of atopic dermatitis, urticaria, scleromyxedema, pyoderma gangrenosum, psoriasis, and pretibial myxedema. Int Immunopharmacol 2006;6(4):579–91.
36. De Zwaan SE, Iland HJ, Damian DL. Treatment of refractory pyoderma gangrenosum with intravenous immunoglobulin. Australas J Dermatol 2009;50(1):56–9.
37. Wootton CI, Patel AN, Williams HC. In a patient with toxic epidermal necrolysis, does intravenous immunoglobulin improve survival compared with supportive care? Arch Dermatol 2011;147(12):1437–40.
38. Enk A. Guidelines on the use of high-dose intravenous immunoglobulin in dermatology. Eur J Dermatol 2009;19(1):90–8.
39. Lima XT, Seidler EM, Lima HC, et al. Long-term safety of biologics in dermatology. Dermatol Ther 2009;22(1):2–21.
40. Feldmann M, Brennan FM, Maini R. Cytokines in autoimmune disorders. Int Rev Immunol 1998;17(1–4):217–28.
41. Krueger JG. The immunologic basis for the treatment of psoriasis with new biologic agents. J Am Acad Dermatol 2002;46(1):1–23 [quiz: 23–6].
42. Lima HC, Kimball AB. Targeting IL-23: insights into the pathogenesis and the treatment of psoriasis. Indian J Dermatol 2010;55(2):171–5.
43. Fallen R, Mitra A, Lima H. Insights into the pathogenesis and treatment of psoriasis. In: O'Daly J, editor. Psoriasis/book 3. Rijeka (Croatia): In Tech–Open Access Publisher; 2011. p. 133–58.
44. Schon MP, Boehncke WH. Psoriasis. N Engl J Med 2005;352(18):1899–912.
45. Kimball AB, Gladman D, Gelfand JM, et al. National Psoriasis Foundation clinical consensus on psoriasis comorbidities and recommendations for screening. J Am Acad Dermatol 2008;58(6):1031–42.
46. Seston EM, Ashcroft DM, Griffiths CE. Balancing the benefits and risks of drug treatment: a stated-preference, discrete choice experiment with patients with psoriasis. Arch Dermatol 2007;143(9):1175–9.
47. Reich K, Burden AD, Eaton JN, et al. Efficacy of biologics in the treatment of moderate to severe psoriasis: a network meta-analysis of randomized controlled trials. Br J Dermatol 2012;166(1):179–88.
48. Lebwohl M. Psoriasis. Lancet 2003;361(9364):1197–204.
49. Black LE, Green JD, Rener J, et al. Safety evaluation of immunomodulatory biopharmaceuticals: can we improve the predictive value of preclinical studies? Hum Exp Toxicol 2000;19(4):205–7.

50. Furst DE, Wallis R, Broder M, et al. Tumor necrosis factor antagonists: different kinetics and/or mechanisms of action may explain differences in the risk for developing granulomatous infection. Semin Arthritis Rheum 2006;36(3): 159–67.

51. Baidoo L, Lichtenstein GR. What next after infliximab? Am J Gastroenterol 2005; 100(1):80–3.

52. Bender NK, Heilig CE, Droll B, et al. Immunogenicity, efficacy and adverse events of adalimumab in RA patients. Rheumatol Int 2007;27(3):269–74.

53. Lima HC. Fatos e mitos sobre imunomoduladores. An Bras Dermatol 2007; 82(3):207–21 [in Portuguese].

54. Howell SM, Bessinger GT, Altman CE, et al. Rapid response of IgA pemphigus of the subcorneal pustular dermatosis subtype to treatment with adalimumab and mycophenolate mofetil. J Am Dermatol 2005;53(3):541–3.

55. Traczewski P, Rudnicka L. Adalimumab in dermatology. Br J Clin Pharmacol 2008;66(5):618–25.

56. Ellis CN, Krueger GG. Treatment of chronic plaque psoriasis by selective targeting of memory effector T lymphocytes. N Engl J Med 2001;345(4):248–55.

57. Alefacept (Amevive) [package insert], Biogen, Inc. FDA; 2008. Available at: http://www.fda.gov/CDER/foi/label/2003/alefbio013003LB.htm. Accessed October 22, 2008.

58. Menter A, Gottlieb A, Feldman SR, et al. Guidelines of care for the management of psoriasis and psoriatic arthritis: section 1. Overview of psoriasis and guidelines of care for the treatment of psoriasis with biologics. J Am Acad Dermatol 2008;58(5):826–50.

59. Strober BE, Menon K. Alefacept for the treatment of psoriasis and other dermatologic diseases. Dermatol Ther 2007;20(4):270–6.

60. Wexler D, Searles G, Landells I, et al. Update on alefacept safety. J Cutan Med Surg 2009;13(Suppl 3):S139–47.

61. Ayroldi E, Bastianelli A, Cannarile L, et al. A pathogenetic approach to autoimmune skin disease therapy: psoriasis and biological drugs, unresolved issues, and future directions. Curr Pharm Des 2011;17(29):3176–90.

62. Carr D, Tusa MG, Carroll CL, et al. Open label trial of alefacept in palmoplantar pustular psoriasis. J Dermatolog Treat 2008;19(2):97–100.

63. Krell J, Nelson C, Spencer L, et al. An open-label study evaluating the efficacy and tolerability of alefacept for the treatment of scalp psoriasis. J Am Acad Dermatol 2008;58(4):609–16.

64. Wollina U, Haroske G. Pyoderma gangraenosum. Curr Opin Rheumatol 2011; 23(1):50–6.

65. Pangalis GA, Dimopoulou MN, Angelopoulou MK, et al. Campath-1H (anti-CD52) monoclonal antibody therapy in lymphoproliferative disorders. Med Oncol 2001; 18(2):99–107.

66. Kanda J, Lopez RD, Rizzieri DA. Alemtuzumab for the prevention and treatment of graft-versus-host disease. Int J Hematol 2011;93(5):586–93.

67. Schnitzler M, Hasskarl J, Egger M, et al. Successful treatment of severe acute intestinal graft-versus-host resistant to systemic and topical steroids with alemtuzumab. Biol Blood Marrow Transplant 2009;15(8):910–8.

68. Wolff D, Schleuning M, von Harsdorf S, et al. Consensus conference on clinical practice in chronic GVHD: second-line treatment of chronic graft-versus-host disease. Biol Blood Marrow Transplant 2011;17(1):1–17.

69. Hui D, Lam W, Toze C, et al. Alemtuzumab in clinical practice: a British Columbia experience. Leuk Lymphoma 2008;49(2):218–26.

70. Gribben JG, Hallek M. Rediscovering alemtuzumab: current and emerging therapeutic roles. Br J Haematol 2009;144(6):818–31.
71. Funke VA, de Medeiros CR, Setubal DC, et al. Therapy for severe refractory acute graft-versus-host disease with basiliximab, a selective interleukin-2 receptor antagonist. Bone Marrow Transplant 2006;37(10):961–5.
72. Rebora A, Parodi A, Murialdo G. Basiliximab is effective for erosive lichen planus. Arch Dermatol 2002;138(8):1100–1.
73. Lebwohl M, Tyring SK, Hamilton TK, et al. A novel targeted T-cell modulator, efalizumab, for plaque psoriasis. N Engl J Med 2003;349(21):2004–13.
74. Raptiva-prescribing. FDA; 2008. Available at: http://www.gene.com/gene/products/information/pdf/raptiva-prescribing.pdf. Accessed October 24, 2008.
75. Raptiva PI. FDA; 2008. Available at: http://www.fda.gov/medWatch/SAFETY/2005/Raptiva_PI.pdf. Accessed October 24, 2008.
76. Goffe BS. Disseminated granuloma annulare resolved with the T-cell modulator efalizumab. Arch Dermatol 2004;140(10):1287–8.
77. Papp KA, Caro I, Leung HM, et al. Efalizumab for the treatment of psoriatic arthritis. J Cutan Med Surg 2007;11(2):57–66.
78. Barde C, Thielen AM, Saurat JH. Infliximab then efalizumab, the 'hit and run' approach does not work. Dermatology 2008;216(2):171–2.
79. Penz S, Pelletier F, Riou-Gotta MO, et al. Sequential therapy in plaque psoriasis using the "Hit and Run" approach: infliximab followed by efalizumab. Int J Dermatol 2012;51(2):236–7.
80. Rodriguez-Lojo R, Paradela S, Martinez-Gomez W, et al. Refractory discoid lupus erythematosus: response to efalizumab. J Eur Acad Dermatol Venereol 2009;23(10):1203–5.
81. Durox H, Sparsa A, Loustaud-Ratti V, et al. Efalizumab-induced lupus-like syndrome. Acta Derm Venereol 2008;88(3):270–1.
82. Bentley DD, Graves JE, Smith DI, et al. Efalizumab-induced subacute cutaneous lupus erythematosus. J Am Acad Dermatol 2006;54(Suppl 5):S242–3.
83. Brown BC, Warren RB, Griindlay DJ, et al. What's new in psoriasis? Analysis of the clinical significance of systematic reviews on psoriasis published in 2007 and 2008. Clin Exp Dermatol 2009;34(6):664–7.
84. Xhaard A, Rocha V, Bueno B, et al. Steroid-refractory acute GVHD: lack of long-term improved survival using new generation anticytokine treatment. Biol Blood Marrow Transplant 2012;18(3):406–13.
85. Ramos-Casals M, Brito-Zeron P, Munoz S, et al. A systematic review of the off-label use of biological therapies in systemic autoimmune diseases. Medicine (Baltimore) 2008;87(6):345–64.
86. Pelekanou A, Kanni T, Savva A, et al. Long-term efficacy of etanercept in hidradenitis suppurativa: results from an open-label phase II prospective trial. Exp Dermatol 2010;19(6):538–40.
87. Shetty A, Marcum CB, Glass LF, et al. Successful treatment of pemphigus vulgaris with etanercept in four patients. J Drugs Dermatol 2009;8(10):940–3.
88. Gubinelli E, Bergamo F, Didona B, et al. Pemphigus foliaceus treated with etanercept. J Am Acad Dermatol 2006;55(6):1107–8.
89. Guedes R, Leite L. Therapeutic hotline. Treatment of pityriasis rubra pilaris with etanercept. Dermatol Ther 2011;24(2):285–6.
90. Ambrose NL, Tobin AM, Howard D. Etanercept treatment in Sweet's syndrome with inflammatory arthritis. J Rheumatol 2009;36(6):1348–9.

91. Gardam MA, Keystone EC, Menzies R, et al. Anti-tumour necrosis factor agents and tuberculosis risk: mechanisms of action and clinical management. Lancet Infect Dis 2003;3(3):148–55.
92. Baert FJ, D'Haens GR, Peeters M, et al. Tumor necrosis factor alpha antibody (infliximab) therapy profoundly down-regulates the inflammation in Crohn's ileocolitis. Gastroenterology 1999;116(1):22–8.
93. Kahn P, Weiss M, Imundo LF, et al. Favorable response to high-dose infliximab for refractory childhood uveitis. Ophthalmology 2006;113(5):860–4 e862.
94. Gottlieb AB, Masud S, Ramamurthi R, et al. Pharmacodynamic and pharmacokinetic response to anti-tumor necrosis factor-alpha monoclonal antibody (infliximab) treatment of moderate to severe psoriasis vulgaris. J Am Acad Dermatol 2003;48(1):68–75.
95. Kobbe G, Schneider P, Rohr U, et al. Treatment of severe steroid refractory acute graft-versus-host disease with infliximab, a chimeric human/mouse antiTNF alpha antibody. Bone Marrow Transplant 2001;28(1):47–9.
96. Vultaggio A, Matucci A, Parronchi P, et al. Safety and tolerability of infliximab therapy: suggestions and criticisms based on wide clinical experience. Int J Immunopathol Pharmacol 2008;21(2):367–74.
97. Pidala J, Kim J, Field T, et al. Infliximab for managing steroid-refractory acute graft-versus-host disease. Biol Blood Marrow Transplant 2009;15(9):1116–21.
98. Suarez-Amor O, Perez-Bustillo A, Ruiz-Gonzalez I, et al. Necrobiosis lipoidica therapy with biologicals: an ulcerated case responding to etanercept and a review of the literature. Dermatology 2010;221(2):117–21.
99. Garcovich S, Di Giampetruzzi AR, Antonelli G, et al. Treatment of refractory adult-onset pityriasis rubra pilaris with TNF-alpha antagonists: a case series. J Eur Acad Dermatol Venereol 2010;24(8):881–4.
100. Ben Abdelghani K, Dran DG, Gottenberg JE, et al. Tumor necrosis factor-alpha blockers in SAPHO syndrome. J Rheumatol 2010;37(8):1699–704.
101. Phumethum V, Jamal S, Johnson SR. Biologic therapy for systemic sclerosis: a systematic review. J Rheumatol 2011;38(2):289–96.
102. Gupta AK, Skinner AR. A review of the use of infliximab to manage cutaneous dermatoses. J Cutan Med Surg 2004;8(2):77–89.
103. Wojtkiewicz A, Wysocki M, Fortuna J, et al. Beneficial and raid effect of infliximab on the course of toxic epidermal necrolysis. Acta Derm Venereol 2008;88(4):420–1.
104. Bay JO, Dhedin N, Goerner M, et al. Inolimomab in steroid-refractory acute graft-versus-host disease following allogeneic hematopoietic stem cell transplantation: retrospective analysis and comparison with other interleukin-2 receptor antibodies. Transplantation 2005;80(6):782–8.
105. Bayes M, Rabasseda X, Proud JR. Gateways to clinical trials. Methods Find Exp Clin Pharmacol 2006;28(4):233–77.
106. Adams GP, Weiner LM. Monoclonal antibody therapy of cancer. Nat Biotechnol 2005;23(9):1147–57.
107. Hodi FS, O'Day SJ, McDermott DF, et al. Improved survival with ipilimumab in patients with metastatic melanoma. N Engl J Med 2010;363(8):711–23.
108. Calabro L, Danielli R, Sigalotti L, et al. Clinical studies with anti-CTLA-4 antibodies in non-melanoma indications. Semin Oncol 2010;37(5):460–7.
109. Vichyanond P. Omalizumab in allergic diseases, a recent review. Asian Pac J Allergy Immunol 2011;29(3):209–19.
110. D'Amato G. Role of anti-IgE monoclonal antibody (omalizumab) in the treatment of bronchial asthma and allergic respiratory diseases. Eur J Pharmacol 2006; 533(1–3):302–7.

111. Morjaria JB, Polosa R. Off-label use of omalizumab in non-asthma conditions: new opportunities. Expert Rev Respir Med 2009;3(3):299–308.
112. Bieber T. Atopic dermatitis. N Engl J Med 2008;358(14):1483–94.
113. Amrol D. Anti-immunoglobulin E in the treatment of refractory atopic dermatitis. South Med J 2010;103(6):554–8.
114. Park SY, Choi MR, Na JI, et al. Recalcitrant atopic dermatitis treated with omalizumab. Ann Dermatol 2010;22(3):349–52.
115. Vigo PG, Girgis KR, Pfuetze BL, et al. Efficacy of anti-IgE therapy in patients with atopic dermatitis. J Am Acad Dermatol 2006;55(1):168–70.
116. Lane JE, Cheyney JM, Lane TN, et al. Treatment of recalcitrant atopic dermatitis with omalizumab. J Am Acad Dermatol 2006;54(1):68–72.
117. Ramirez del Pozo ME, Contreras Contreras E, Lopez Tiro J, et al. Omalizumab (an anti-IgE antibody) in the treatment of severe atopic eczema. J Investig Allergol Clin Immunol 2011;21(5):416–7.
118. Sheinkopf LE, Rafi AW, Do LT, et al. Efficacy of omalizumab in the treatment of atopic dermatitis: a pilot study. Allergy Asthma Proc 2008;29(5):530–7.
119. Incorvaia C, Pravettoni C, Mauro M, et al. Effectiveness of omalizumab in a patient with severe asthma and atopic dermatitis. Monaldi Arch Chest Dis 2008;69(2):78–80.
120. Velling P, Skowasch D, Pabst S, et al. Improvement of quality of life in patients with concomitant allergic asthma and atopic dermatitis: one year follow-up of omalizumab therapy. Eur J Med Res 2011;16(9):407–10.
121. Belloni B, Ziai M, Lim A, et al. Low-dose anti-IgE therapy in patients with atopic eczema with high serum IgE levels. J Allergy Clin Immunol 2007;120(5):1223–5.
122. Andres C, Belloni B, Mempel M, et al. Omalizumab for patients with severe and therapy-refractory atopic eczema? Curr Allergy Asthma Rep 2008;8(3):179–80.
123. Krathen RA, Hsu S. Failure of omalizumab for treatment of severe adult atopic dermatitis. J Am Acad Dermatol 2005;53(2):338–40.
124. Heil PM, Maurer D, Klein B, et al. Omalizumab therapy in atopic dermatitis: depletion of IgE does not improve the clinical course—a randomized, placebo-controlled and double blind pilot study. J Dtsch Dermatol Ges 2010;8(12):990–8.
125. Spector SL, Tan RA. Omalizumab also successful in chronic urticaria. J Allergy Clin Immunol 2008;121(3):784 [author reply: 784–5].
126. Romano C, Sellitto A, De Fanis U, et al. Maintenance of remission with low-dose omalizumab in long-lasting, refractory chronic urticaria. Ann Allergy Asthma Immunol 2010;104(1):95–7.
127. Sheikh J. Effect of omalizumab on patients with chronic urticaria: issues with the determination of autoimmune urticaria. Ann Allergy Asthma Immunol 2008;100(1):88 [author reply: 88–9].
128. Saini S, Rosen KE, Hsieh HJ, et al. A randomized, placebo-controlled, dose-ranging study of single-dose omalizumab in patients with H1-antihistamine-refractory chronic idiopathic urticaria. J Allergy Clin Immunol 2011;128(3):567–73, e561.
129. Sabroe RA. Failure of omalizumab in cholinergic urticaria. Clin Exp Dermatol 2010;35(4):e127–9.
130. Metz M, Bergmann P, Zuberbier T, et al. Successful treatment of cholinergic urticaria with anti-immunoglobulin E therapy. Allergy 2008;63(2):L247–9.
131. Siebenhaar F, Kuhn W, Zuberbier T, et al. Successful treatment of cutaneous mastocytosis and Meniere disease with anti-IgE therapy. J Allergy Clin Immunol 2007;120(1):213–5.

132. Johnson P, Glennie M. The mechanisms of action of rituximab in the elimination of tumor cells. Semin Oncol 2003;30(1 Suppl 2):3–8.
133. Kimby E. Tolerability and safety of rituximab (MabThera). Cancer Treat Rev 2005;31(6):456–73.
134. Martin LK, Werth V, Villanueva E, et al. Interventions for pemphigus vulgaris and pemphigus foliaceus. Cochrane Database Syst Rev 2009;1:CD006263.
135. Esposito M, Capriotti E, Giunta A, et al. Long-lasting remission of pemphigus vulgaris treated with rituximab. Acta Derm Venereol 2006;86(1):87–9.
136. Faurschou A, Gniadecki R. Two courses of rituximab (anti CD20 monoclonal antibody) for recalcitrant pemphigus vulgaris. Int J Dermatol 2008;47(3):292–4.
137. Kasperkiewicz M, Shimanovich I, Ludwig RJ, et al. Rituximab for treatment-refractory pemphigus and pemphigoid: a case series of 17 patients. J Am Acad Dermatol 2011;65(3):552–8.
138. Fernando SL, Broadfoot AJ. Treatment options for pemphigus foliaceus. G Ital Dermatol Venereol 2009;144(4):363–77.
139. Anan T, Shimizu F, Hatano Y, et al. Paraneoplastic pemphigus associated with corneal perforation and cutaneous alternariosis: a case report and review of cases treated with rituximab. J Dermatol 2011;38(11):1084–9.
140. Vezzoli P, Berti E, Marzano AV. Rationale and efficacy for the use of rituximab in paraneoplastic pemphigus. Expert Rev Clin Immunol 2008;4(3):351–63.
141. Schierl M, Foedinger D, Geissler K, et al. Paraneoplastic pemphigus despite treatment with rituximab, fludarabine and cyclophosphamide in chronic lymphocytic leukemia. Eur J Dermatol 2008;18(6):717–8.
142. Meurer M. Immunosuppressive therapy for autoimmune bullous disease. Clin Dermatol 2012;30(1):78–83.
143. Schmidt E, Zillikens D. Diagnosis and treatment of patients with autoimmune bullous disorders in Germany. Dermatol Clin 2011;29(4):663–71.
144. Schmidt E, Hunzelmann N, Zillikens D, et al. Rituximab in refractory autoimmune bullous diseases. Clin Exp Dermatol 2006;31(4):503–8.
145. Li Y, Foshee JB, Sontheimer RD. Sustained clinical response to rituximab in a case of life-threatening overlap subepidermal autoimmune blistering disease. J Am Acad Dermatol 2011;64(4):773–8.
146. Kasperkiewicz M, Schmidt E. Current treatment of autoimmune blistering diseases. Curr Drug Discov Technol 2009;6(4):270–80.
147. Niedermeier A, Eming R, Pfutze M, et al. Clinical response of severe mechano-bullous epidermolysis bullosa acquisita to combined treatment with immunoadsorption and rituximab (anti-CD20 monoclonal antibodies). Arch Dermatol 2007;143(2):L192–8.
148. Chiu YE, Co DO. Juvenile dermatomyositis: immunopathogenesis, role of myositis-specific autoantibodies, and review of rituximab use. Pediatr Dermatol 2011;28(4):357–67.
149. Troiano M, Lotti T. Rituximab in dermatological diseases. G Ital Dermatol Venereol 2009;144(4):495–9.
150. Huber AM. Juvenile dermatomyositis: advances in pathogenesis, evaluation, and treatment. Paediatr Drugs 2009;11(6):361–74.
151. Schmidt E, Brocker EB, Goebeler M. Rituximab in treatment-resistant autoimmune blistering skin disorders. Clin Rev Allergy Immunol 2008;34(1):56–64.
152. Nickoloff BJ, Schroder JM, von den Driesch P, et al. Is psoriasis a T-cell disease? Exp Dermatol 2000;9(5):359–75.
153. Okamura H, Tsutsi H, Komatsu T, et al. Cloning of a new cytokine that induces IFN-gamma production by T-cells. Nature 1995;378(6552):88–91.

154. Hong K, Berg EL, Ehrhardt RO. Persistence of pathogenic CD4+ Th1-like cells in vivo in the absence of IL-12 but in the presence of autoantigen. J Immunol 2001;166(7):4765–72.
155. Watanabe H, Kawaguchi M, Fujishima S, et al. Functional characterization of IL-17F as a selective neutrophil attractant is psoriasis. J Invest Dermatol 2009; 129(3):650–6.
156. Aggarwal S, Ghilardi N, Xie MH, et al. Interleukin-23 promotes a distinct CD4 T cell activation state characterized by the production of interleukin-17. J Biol Chem 2003;278(3):1910–4.
157. Leonardi CL, Kimball AB, Papp KA, et al. Efficacy and safety of ustekinumab, a human interleukin-12/23 monoclonal antibody, in patients with psoriasis: 76-week results from a randomized, double-blind, placebo-controlled trial (PHOENIX 1). Lancet 2008;371(9625):1665–74.
158. Gospodarevskaya E, Picot J, Cooper K, et al. Ustekinumab for the treatment of moderate to severe psoriasis. Health Technol Assess (Winchester, England) 2009;13(Suppl 3):61–6.
159. Lebwohl M, Yeilding N, Szapary P, et al. Impact of weight on the efficacy and safety of ustekinumab in patients with moderate to severe psoriasis: rationale for dosing recommendations. J Am Acad Dermatol 2010;63(4):L571–9.
160. Ferrandiz C, Garcia A, Blasco AJ, et al. Cost-efficiency of adalimumab, etanercept, infliximab and ustekinumab for moderate-to-severe plaque psoriasis. J Eur Acad Dermatol Venereol 2012;26(6):768–77.
161. Tsai TF, Ho JC, Song M, et al. Efficacy and safety of ustekinumab for the treatment of moderate-to-severe psoriasis: a phase III, randomized, placebo-controlled trial in Taiwanese and Korean patients. (PEARL). J Dermatol Sci 2011;63(3):154–63.
162. Laws PM, Warren RB. Ustekinumab for the treatment of psoriasis. Expert Rev Clin Immunol 2011;7(2):155–64.
163. Pidala J, Perez L, Beato F, et al. Ustekinumab demonstrates activity in glucocorticoid-refractory acute GVHD. Bone Marrow Transplant 2012;47(5): 747–8.
164. Gulliver WP, Jemec GB, Baker KA. Experience with ustekinumab for the treatment of moderate to severe hidradenitis suppurativa. J Eur Acad Dermatol Venereol 2011. [Epub ahead of print].
165. De Douza A, Ali-Shaw T, Strober BE, et al. Successful treatment of subacute lupus erythematosus with ustekinumab. Arch Dermatol 2011;147(8):896–8.
166. Balestri R, Bardazzi F, Antonucci A. Should ustekinumab really be used as first-line biological therapy in pityriasis rubra pilaris? Br J Dermatol 2010;163(4): 896–7 [author reply: 897–8].
167. Guenova E, Teskek A, Fehrenbacher B, et al. Interleukin 23 expression in pyoderma gangrenosum and targeted therapy with ustekinumab. Arch Dermatol 2011;147(10):1203–5.

The Use of Monoclonal Antibodies in Immune-Mediated Hematologic Disorders

Daan Dierickx, MD[a],*, Emilie Beke, MD[b], Timothy Devos, MD, PhD[a], André Delannoy, MD, PhD[c]

KEYWORDS

- Monoclonal antibodies • Immune-mediated
- Hematologic disorders • Costimulation signals

Key Points

- Monoclonal antibodies have emerged as a promising therapeutic tool in immune-mediated hematologic disorders.
- Monoclonal antibody therapy targets different parts of the immune system, including B cells, T cells, proinflammatory cytokines, and the complement system.
- Despite initially promising results with monoclonal antibody therapy in immune-mediated hematologic disorders, controlled trials have often shown more conflicting results, necessitating further research regarding pathogenesis, mechanism of action, and resistance.
- Although considered a safe therapy compared with chemotherapy and classic immunosuppressive therapy, serious adverse events have been described and the therapy warrants ongoing caution.

BASIC IMMUNOLOGIC CONCEPTS IN AUTOIMMUNE DISORDERS

Over the last decades, the interactions between innate and adaptive immunologic subsystems have been emphasized, in contrast to considering them as 2 separate mechanisms. The innate immune system includes several host defense pathways that range from the nonspecific barrier function of epithelia to the highly selective recognition of pathogens through the use of invariant germline-encoded receptors.[1] Innate immune

[a] Department of Hematology, University Hospitals Leuven, Herestraat 49, 3000 Leuven, Belgium
[b] Department of Internal Medicine, University Hospitals Leuven, Herestraat 49, 3000 Leuven, Belgium
[c] Hôpital de Jolimont, Haine-Saint-Paul and Cliniques Universitaires St Luc, Rue Ferrer 159, 1700 Haine-Saint-Paul, Brussels, Belgium
* Corresponding author.
E-mail address: Daan.dierickx@uzleuven.be

Med Clin N Am 96 (2012) 583–619
doi:10.1016/j.mcna.2012.04.006   **medical.theclinics.com**
0025-7125/12/$ – see front matter © 2012 Elsevier Inc. All rights reserved.

responses are not leading to immunologic memory. For example, toll-like receptors (TLRs) are expressed on innate immune cells, and binding of TLRs to microbial ligands leads to a rapid activation of multiple inflammatory pathways and systemic defense against pathogens. Natural killer (NK) cells, neutrophils, macrophages and dendritic cells (in their role as antigen-presenting cells [APCs]) are part of the innate immune system. On the other hand, B and T lymphocytes are effector cells of the adaptive immune response. Through recombination of their antigen receptor genes, B and T cells can recognize antigens in a flexible way and this antigen-specific response persists in the long-term (immunologic memory). Moreover, cellular cross-talk is important in adaptive immunity because 2 signals are required for lymphocyte activation. For T cells, the activating signal is delivered by a professional APC (**Fig. 1**), and for B lymphocytes the second signal is usually delivered by an activated T cell.

Both innate and adaptive responses play a role in the occurrence of autoimmunity. Autoimmune disorders occur when an adaptive immune response is directed against self-antigens. A priming of autoantigen-specific immune cells, without relevant clinical damage, comes first. This process is controlled by the activation of the nonspecific innate immune system.[2] TLRs play a crucial role in this process, and their inappropriate activation by endogenous or exogenous ligands may lead to the initiation of autoimmunity.[3] NK cells can drive the adaptive responses toward autoimmunity through the secretion of cytokines.[4] Dendritic cells are particularly effective in stimulating T cells. Contrasting roles for macrophage subsets in autoimmunity have been described (protective vs activating), as reviewed recently.[5]

Autoimmunity can occur as a breakdown in immunologic tolerance, leading to the activation of self-reactive T and B cells. Mechanisms of T-cell tolerance are clonal deletion, clonal anergy, ignorance, and active suppression. T cells are educated in the thymus. High-avidity interactions between immature thymocytes caused by a relatively high-affinity contact between a rearranged T-cell receptor (TCR) and a peptide/major histocompatibility complex on APCs in the thymus, result in clonal deletion of these autoreactive thymocytes (**Fig. 2**). When a self-reactive T cell escapes this

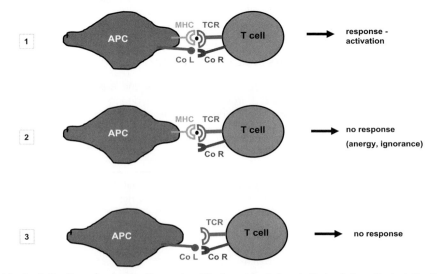

Fig. 1. Activation of naive T cells requires 2 independent signals. To be fully activated, T cells need both the T-cell receptor signal, after encounter with the peptide/major histocompatibility complex, and stimulation through the costimulatory pathway.

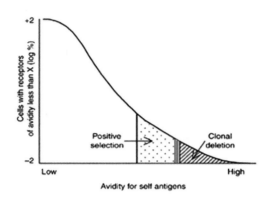

Fig. 2. Selection of the T-cell repertoire as a consequence of TCR avidity for self-antigens expressed in the thymus. Cells of which the receptors have the highest avidities (*stripped area, far right*) undergo negative selection by clonal deletion. Intermediate avidities undergo positive selection. (*From* Schwartz RH. Natural regulatory T cells and self-tolerance. Nat Immunol 2005;6(4):328; with permission.)

mechanism, tolerance induction in the periphery can be obtained through anergy, active suppression (regulatory T cells), ignorance, or deletion (**Fig. 3**). These mechanisms are defective in autoimmune diseases.[6]

B-cell tolerance is also disturbed in autoimmune conditions. B cells are increasingly considered as effectors cells as well as cells with immunoregulatory potential. The improvement seen in autoimmune disease, such as immune thrombocytopenia and

central tolerance

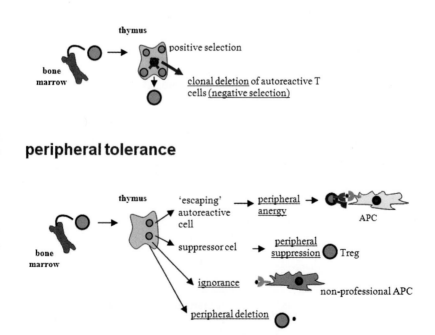

peripheral tolerance

Fig. 3. Mechanisms of central and peripheral tolerance induction.

autoimmune hemolytic anemia (AIHA), after B-cell depleting therapy, documents the important role of B lymphocytes. Interactions between B and T cells are important. After rituximab therapy in patients with lupus nephritis, a reduction of expression of the costimulatory molecule CD40L on CD4$^+$ T cells was seen, leading to the conclusion that B cells can promote autoimmunity in humans by directly influencing T cells.[7]

The increasing knowledge on the pathogenesis of autoimmune disorders has led to an expanding interest in the use of monoclonal antibodies (MAbs) targeting different cells, cytokines, and immunologic interactions. In this review, the currently available evidence on the use of MAb therapy in immune-mediated hematologic disorders is described (**Table 1**).

IMMUNE THROMBOCYTOPENIA

Immune thrombocytopenia (ITP) includes a group of autoimmune disorders characterized by platelet destruction caused by autoantibodies and impaired thrombopoiesis, explaining the high response rate to thrombopoietin receptor agonists. These autoantibodies cause thrombocytopenia and hence related symptoms such as bleeding and purpura.[8] ITP can be classified into primary and secondary ITP. Diagnosis of primary ITP can be made by the finding of an isolated thrombocytopenia ($<100,000/mm^3$) without any obvious initiating or underlying cause. Secondary causes include autoimmune disorders (eg, antiphospholipid syndrome, systemic lupus erythematosus),

Table 1
Available evidence on the use of MAb therapy in immune-mediated hematologic disorders

Target	MAb	Type	Randomized Clinical Trial	Prospective Trial	Retrospective Case Series
CD20	Rituximab	Chimeric	ITP	ITP, AIHA, TTP, cGVHD	ITP, AIHA, ES, TTP, cGVHD, acquired hemophilia, acquired von Willebrand syndrome, APS
CD20	Veltuzumab	Humanized	—	ITP	—
CD52	Alemtuzumab	Humanized	—	aGVHD, AA	ITP, AIHA, ES, aGVHD, AA
CD154	IDEC-131/ E6040	Humanized	—	ITP	—
C5	Eculizumab	Humanized	PNH	PNH	AIHA, PNH
CD25	Inolimomab	Murine	—	—	aGVHD
CD25	Daclizumab	Humanized	aGVHD	aGVHD,AA	aGVHD, cGVHD, AA
CD25	Basiliximab	Chimeric	—	aGVHD	aGVHD,AA
CD147	CBL-1	Murine	—	aGVHD	—
CD147	ABX-CBL	Murine	aGVHD	aGVHD	—
CD3	Muromonab CD3	Murine	aGVHD	aGVHD	aGVHD
CD3	Visilizumab	Humanized		aGVHD	aGVHD
TNF-α	Infliximab	Chimeric	aGVHD	aGVHD	aGVHD, cGVHD

Abbreviations: AA, aplastic anemia; aGVHD, acute graft-versus-host disease; APS, antiphospholipid syndrome; cGVHD, chronic graft-versus-host disease; ES, Evans syndrome; ITP, immune thrombocytopenia; PNH, paroxysmal nocturnal hemoglobinuria; TNF-α, tumor necrosis factor α; TTP, thrombotic thrombocytopenic purpura.

infections (eg, hepatitis C virus, human immunodeficiency virus [HIV], *Helicobacter pylori*), lymphoproliferative disorders, and drugs.[9] During the disease course, 3 different phases can be recognized. In the first 3 months, ITP is named newly diagnosed ITP. If there is no spontaneous or medication-induced remission, this phase is followed by persistent ITP, a term limited to the period between 3 and 12 months after diagnosis. If the disease lasts for more than 12 months, the term chronic ITP is preferred.[9]

In the management of ITP, the cornerstones are evaluation of the risk of severe bleeding and obtaining safe levels of platelet counts, although the use of a predetermined platelet count level necessitating treatment initiation is controversial.[9,10] First-line treatment of ITP is corticosteroids, mainly methylprednisone at a dose of 1 to 2 mg/kg per day. Two-thirds of the patients respond to this therapy and 10% to 15% remain in complete remission after 6 months. Alternatively, high-dose dexamethasone can be used, leading to sustained responses in 70% of patients.[11] If there is no response or relapse after treatment with corticosteroids, other therapeutic strategies need to be considered. The success rate of splenectomy has been studied in a systematic review by Kojouri and colleagues.[12] They found a sustained response in 64% (456 of 707 patients), with a median follow-up of 7.25 years (range, 5–12.75). Although splenectomy has an excellent response rate, many physicians and patients are reluctant to prescribe/undergo this procedure because of its possible complications, such as perioperative thrombosis, bleeding, and infection.[13] Depending on reimbursement differences between countries, new medical treatments including thrombopoietin receptor agonists (romiplostim, eltrombopag) and MAbs (rituximab) can be used in both splenectomized and nonsplenectomized patients.

The use of MAbs in the treatment of ITP has been limited to a few antibodies. Most experience has been obtained with the MAb rituximab, which targets CD20 on B cells. The use of other MAbs is limited to a few patients. Because rituximab is the most used MAb in ITP and most other autoimmune hematologic disorders, its mechanism of action, pharmacodynamics, and resistance issues are briefly described in this article.

Anti-CD20 Therapy

The human CD20 molecule is a transmembrane glycoprotein, expressed on both malignant and normal B cells. In malignant cells, expression is restricted to most mature B-cell non-Hodgkin lymphomas, whereas in normal cells CD20 is expressed on precursor and mature B lymphocytes, but not on pro-B cells and plasma cells.[14] The function and mechanism of action of CD20 are not known, partly because no natural ligand has been identified. Probably CD20 regulates, by participating as a calcium ion channel in B-cell receptor signaling, 1 or more early steps in B-cell proliferation and differentiation.[15]

Rituximab is a chimeric human/murine IgG1 MAb, initially designed for the treatment of B-cell non-Hodgkin lymphomas. Because it binds only CD20 expressing cells, hematopoietic stem cells, myeloid cells, and plasma cells are spared, explaining the low toxicity profile of the antibody.[14]

By binding to CD20, rituximab enhances a cascade of immune reactions, resulting in apoptosis of premature and mature B lymphocytes (**Fig. 4**). Several mechanisms of action have been studied and described. The best-known mechanisms include antibody-dependent cell-mediated cytotoxicity (ADCC), complement-dependent cytotoxicity (CDC), direct apoptosis, disturbed T-cell reactions, and possible vaccinal effects.[16]

ADCC

After binding of hundreds of rituximab molecules with their Fab region to the CD20 receptor on B cells, macrophages and NK cells recognize the Fc portion of the

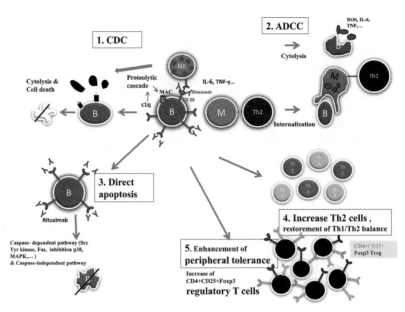

Fig. 4. Mechanisms of action of rituximab (see text).

antibody, leading to binding with their Fcγ receptor (FcγR). This interaction causes activation of the effector cells, leading to phagocytosis, release of cytokines and cytotoxic molecules, and attraction of T$_{H2}$ cells.

CDC
Rituximab can activate complement by the classic pathway. C1q binds to the Fc portion and activates a proteolytic cascade, resulting in the formation of a membrane attack complex, causing lysis of the B cells. Variable degrees of efficacy of CDC action have been described in several lymphoma subtypes treated with rituximab. This finding is possibly related to the expression of different membrane complement regulatory proteins on B cells, including CD55 and CD59 expression, leading to impaired CDC.

Direct apoptosis
Rituximab may promote direct apoptosis, mainly by caspase-dependent but also caspase-independent pathways.

Disturbances of T-cell reactions
Although several T-cell subtypes have been identified, CD4+CD25+FOXP3 regulatory T cells (Tregs) have emerged as key players in autoimmune disorders. Decreased levels of Tregs have been correlated with autoreactivity and enhancement of autoimmune disorders.[17] Deficiency in generation or defective functions of Tregs may contribute to loss of immunologic self-tolerance in autoimmune disorders by failure to suppress autoreactive T and B cells, which results in continued autoantibody production. Li and colleagues[18] reported on 62 patients with ITP treated with glucocorticoids with or without low-dose rituximab. Before start of therapy, the investigators observed significantly decreased levels of Tregs. After therapy, a significant increase of Tregs was seen in both groups, but this upregulation was more pronounced and lasted longer in patients treated with rituximab. Stasi and colleagues[19] observed

similar findings in 26 patients with chronic ITP. Levels of Tregs before treatment were significantly lower compared with the control group. After therapy, amounts of Treg cells significantly improved and the percentage of Tregs was not significantly different between patients in remission and controls. Rituximab restores the T_{H1}/T_{H2} balance. In patients with autoimmune disorders there is a disturbed balance in favor of T_{H1} lymphocytes. Recently, it has been shown that this pattern is skewed toward an increase in T_{H2} cells during remission of ITP, suggesting that active disease may be predominantly caused by T_{H1} activation.[20,21] Stasi and colleagues[22] observed that after treatment with rituximab, amounts of T_{H2} cells increased in responding patients with restoration of T_{H1}/T_{H2} balance, but not in nonresponding patients.

Vaccinal effects
Rituximab might also possess vaccinal effects, in which killing of the cell by rituximab results in the elicitation of a specific T-cell response, as was recently reported in patients with follicular lymphoma.[23–25]

Rituximab is administered intravenously. Treatment with rituximab rapidly leads to depletion of B lymphocytes in peripheral blood, which mostly persists for approximately 6 months, followed by recovery of lymphopenia within 12 months.[16]

The optimal rituximab dosing schedule for autoimmune disorders has not been established, but is in most cases derived from studies in lymphomas. As a consequence, most clinicians use the classic dose of 375 mg/m² once a week for 4 consecutive weeks.[17,18] In recent studies, lower dosing schedules have been proposed because of smaller amounts of B cells that need to be destructed, leading to similar efficacy and possibly a more favorable toxicity profile.[26]

Treatment with rituximab, both in the oncologic and autoimmune setting, is associated with an increasing number of resistant cases, even if initially complete or partial responses were observed. The basis of this resistance is not completely understood, and better understanding will probably lead to improved outcomes.

In lymphomas, loss of the CD20 antigen as a result of repeated rituximab therapy is a well-known cause of secondary resistance to anti-CD20 therapy, which may be partially explained by epigenetic mechanisms.[27,28] Besides, expression of the complement regulatory proteins CD55 and CD59 may contribute to impaired CDC. Another mechanism of resistance includes deregulation of important intracellular proliferation and antiapoptotic pathways, as reviewed by Stolz and Schuler.[29]

However, the best-studied mechanism for resistance is related to impaired ADCC, in particular Fc/FcγR interactions. Most evidence has derived from studies showing that the activating FcγRIIIa on myeloid effectors is critical for ADCC, exemplified by the finding that the higher-affinity 158V allele in FcγRIIIa of patients with lymphoma shows higher response rates compared with patients with the low-affinity 185F allele.[30] However, recent evidence also points to an important role of the inhibitory FcγRIIb on target B cells. Lim and colleagues[31] showed that patients with lymphoma with high FcγRIIb expression showed less durable responses after treatment with rituximab-containing regimens. In this way, optimizing antibody therapy by enhancing interaction with activating FcγRs or blocking binding to the inhibitory FcγRs might improve responses to rituximab treatment.

As shown in **Table 2**, the use of rituximab in ITP has been reported extensively. However, most available evidence is based on retrospective case reports and case series, with only a few uncontrolled prospective trials and only 2 randomized prospective studies. In the first trial, Zaja and colleagues[32] included 103 patients with primary ITP. After inclusion, patients were randomized to receive dexamethasone 40 mg/d for 4 days with or without rituximab 375 mg/m²/wk for 4 consecutive weeks. Sustained

Table 2
Clinical evidence evaluating the efficacy of rituximab in the treatment of ITP

Authors	Number of Patients	Age (y)	Previous Splenectomy (%)	OR/CR Rates (%)	Response Duration (Mo)	Factors Predictive for Better Outcome
Saleh	13	21–77	56	33/22	13–26+	—
Stasi	25	22–74	32	52/20	0.5–26	Women (NS), younger age (NS)
Giagounidis	12	28–71	92	75/41	1–15+	—
Shanafelt	12	22–79	83	50/42	1–11+	—
Zaja	15	26–76	13	53/40	2–16+	—
Cooper	57	21–79	54	54/32	<3–59+	—
Braendstrup	35 (39R)	17–82	46	44/18	2–29,	—
Zaja	37	NR	14	73/54	3–55	—
Penalver	89	4–98	53	55/46	NR in 12	Achievement of CR, fewer previous treatments, longer-lasting ITP
Schweizer	14	16–84	29	64/50	0.5–36	—
Garcia-Chavez	18	17–70	83	56/28	median 54 (CR), 18 (PR)	—
Godeau	60	18–84	0	40/NR	24+	Female, young age (NS), fewer previous treatments (NS)
Pasa	17	24–66	100	82/14	6+	—
Zaja	48	16–74	6	75/43	24 mo relapse free: 45%	Younger age, lower weight

						Younger age, shorter interval between diagnosis and therapy
Medeot	26	18–76	15	69/54	8–69	
Alasfoor	14	12–72	21	93/79,	2–19	None found
Kelly	11	mean: 50	NR	54/NR	NR	—
Dierickx	40 (43R)	9–86	73	70/63	PFS 1 y: 70%	None found
Hasan	37	NA	23	68/46	NR	Previous treatment with rituximab
Aleem	24 (29R)	14–70	46	67/45	0.5–55	No previous splenectomy
Brah	39 (40R)	20–87	15	71.8/56.4	6-mo PFS <50%	Positive antinuclear antibodies (NS)
Gobert	12 (33R with CVID)	12–65	NR	83/80	30-mo RFS 50%	—
Audia	40	30–76	21	42.1/26.3	11.7	—
Zaja	101 (103R)	49 ± 16	NR	63/53	30-mo probability 69%	—
D'Arena	21	46–75	0	86/57	4–49	—
Gobert	22	12–65	18	86/82	2–26	—
Arnold	33	30–59	0	62/53	6	—

Abbreviations: CR, complete response; CVID, common variable immunodeficiency; NR, no response; NS, not significant; PFS, progression-free survival; PR, partial response; R, rituximab courses; RFS, relapse-free survival.

responses (defined as a platelet count 50 $\times$ 10^9/L or greater at 6 months after initiation of treatment) were significantly greater in patients treated with combination therapy (63% vs 36%, P = .004). Patients treated with rituximab showed a higher rate of grade 3/4 adverse events, although the incidence of serious adverse events was similar in both arms. In contrast to the findings of this trial, Arnold and colleagues[33] recently published the results of another randomized prospective trial comparing nonsplenec-tomized patients with newly diagnosed or relapsed ITP. After inclusion, patients were randomized to receive adjunctive therapy with rituximab (4 weekly administrations of 375 mg/m^2) or placebo. After 6 months, no differences were seen in efficacy or bleeding tendency in both arms. Another major limitation of all these publications on the use of rituximab in ITP is the impressive heterogeneity in criteria used for reporting responses and clinical outcomes, as recently reviewed by Ruggeri and colleagues.[34] Despite these drawbacks, rituximab seems to have efficacy in the treatment of ITP with overall response (OR) and complete response (CR) rates exceeding 60% and 40%, respectively. Median time to response is 4 to 6 weeks after first dose, whereas median duration of response is 10.5 months.[26,35] Patients with previous response to rituximab therapy can be successfully retreated in case of relapse. **Table 2** provides an overview of all publications regarding the use of rituximab in adult ITP. Articles in abstract form, articles not written in English, and publications describing fewer than 10 patients are not included in this table. Efficacy of rituximab in immune cytopenia/thrombocytopenia has also been reviewed elsewhere.[36–38]

Initially considered a relatively safe treatment option, rituximab use has been associ-ated with several toxicities. Although most side effects have been reported in heavily treated patients with lymphoma, patients with immune-mediated disorders experi-encing serious complications have also been described, necessitating ongoing caution as well in autoimmune disorders, especially in patients who have received repeated courses of rituximab or who are treated with other immunosuppressive therapy concur-rently. As recently reviewed,[26,35,39] most complications include infusion-related, infec-tious (mainly progressive multifocal leukoencephalopathy and hepatitis B reactivation), and hematologic complications.

Although new-generation anti-CD20 MAbs have been used extensively in the treat-ment of B-cell neoplasms, their use in ITP is limited. Liebman and colleagues[40] reported on 41 evaluable patients, treated in a phase I/II trial with low-dose intravenous or subcutaneous veltuzumab. OR rate was 68%, including CR in 17%. Responses, which were less pronounced in longstanding disease, occurred at all dose levels (ranging from 2 administrations of 80 mg to 2 doses of 320 mg, which has been esti-mated as the fixed dose for the ongoing phase II part), with both intravenous and subcutaneous administrations, with an acceptable toxicity profile.

Other MAbs

The use of the anti-CD52 MAb alemtuzumab (alone or in combination with rituximab) has also been investigated, but only in a few case reports and small series. Gomez-Almaguer and colleagues[41] studied the use of alemtuzumab in combination with rituxi-mab in 11 patients with ITP. Alemtuzumab was given at a fixed dose of 10 mg/d subcutaneously on days 1 to 3, whereas rituximab was administered at a dose of 100 mg/wk intravenously on days 4, 11, 18, and 25. OR rate was 100%, with 58% of the patients showing a CR. All patients showed a response at 1 week. Median dura-tion of response was 46 weeks.

The humanized anti-CD154 MAb is another potentially interesting molecule in the treatment of ITP. By blocking the interaction between CD40 on APCs and CD154 (= CD40 ligand) on activated CD4+ T cells, the autoimmune response is selectively suppressed. Although a phase I trial showed encouraging results, no further trials were set up because of the occurrence of unacceptable, thromboembolic adverse events.[42]

Najaoui and colleagues[43] recently described the finding of autoantibody-mediated complement activation in many patients with chronic ITP, even when no autoantibodies were detectable. Further studies on complement participation in ITP might lead to new therapeutic options targeting complement activation, for example by using the anti-C5 MAb eculizumab.

AIHA

AIHA is an autoimmune disorder caused by formation of antibodies against self red blood cells (RBCs) that can be primary or secondary. The disorder is defined as a hemoglobin level less than 11 mg/L, with signs of hemolysis (increased indirect bilirubin, low haptoglobin, and increased lactate dehydrogenase levels), together with a positive direct antiglobulin test (DAT).

AIHA can be divided into 2 groups based on the characteristics of the antibody causing hemolytic anemia: warm-type antibodies and cold-type antibodies.[44,45]

Eighty percent of cases of AIHA are caused by warm-type autoimmune antibodies. These antibodies are in most cases IgG-type antibodies forming dimers. IgG opsonized RBCs are recognized by macrophages in the spleen, leading to phagocytosis of the RBC. Warm-type antibodies thus cause extravascular hemolysis. Twenty percent to 30% of cases are primary (idiopathic). Secondary causes include viral infections, systemic autoimmune diseases, hematologic malignancies, medication, and immune deficiencies. First-line treatment of warm antibody AIHA are corticosteroids. They are associated with high initial response rates, although they lead to long-term CR in only 20% of patients. Second-line treatment is splenectomy, leading to success rates of 67%. Other second-line options are immunosuppressive therapies, immunomodulators, or MAbs like rituximab.[46]

A second group (20%) of autoimmune antibodies causing AIHA are cold-type antibodies, which are active at a temperature less than 37°C. They are mostly IgM-type antibodies forming pentamers and are powerful complement activators, leading to cytolysis and thus intravascular hemolysis. They can be primary (CAD) or secondary to infections (mostly Epstein-Barr virus [EBV]and *Mycoplasma pneumoniae*), systemic diseases, and lymphoproliferative disorders. Treatment with corticosteroids or splenectomy is generally less effective or even not effective compared with warm-type AIHA. Instead, there is a better response to immunosuppressive therapy and MAbs.[47]

Experience with the use of MAbs in AIHA is even more limited compared with ITP. Most studies have been carried out with rituximab, a few with alemtuzumab.

Anti-CD20 Therapy

Use of rituximab in AIHA is associated with OR rates of about 60%, although relapses are frequent.[26] In this way, together with the fact that response rates and duration of response are also comparable, warm-type AIHA shows a marked similarity with ITP. However, in cold-type AIHA, the situation is different. As mentioned earlier, corticosteroids and splenectomy offer no real benefit for the treatment of these patients. On the other hand, the use of rituximab, especially in primary CAD, is promising, despite the fact that CR rates are low. Prospective evidence is almost exclusively derived from the Scandinavian experience. Berentsen and colleagues[48] studied the use of rituximab in CAD in a prospective trial including 27 patients. OR rate was 54%, although CR was achieved in only 3%. In a second, retrospective follow-up study of 52 patients treated with rituximab, similar results were observed, with OR and CR rates of 50% and 8%, respectively.[49] In another prospective study, Schollkopf and colleagues[50] found similar results. To improve response rates and duration of response, Berentsen and colleagues[51] recently performed an uncontrolled prospective trial combining rituximab and fludarabine, a purine analogue used in several lymphoproliferative disorders, in patients with primary CAD. OR rate was 76%, with 21% of the patients achieving a CR. Response duration was estimated to be more than 66 months, and responses were also observed in patients who had not responded to rituximab monotherapy previously. In contrast to the favorable toxicity profile of rituximab, combination therapy was associated with a higher frequency (41%) of grade III to IV hematologic toxicity.

Autoimmune cytopenia, especially AIHA, is observed in 5% to 10% of patients with chronic lymphocytic leukemia (CLL).[52] In most cases, the autoimmune process can be successfully suppressed with corticosteroids. However, in steroid-refractory patients, the complication seems to respond well to rituximab-containing immunochemotherapy. Most regimens include R-CD (rituximab, cyclophosphamide, and dexamethasone) and R-CVP (rituximab, cyclophosphamide, vincristine, prednisone), leading to an OR rate of 90% to100% and CR rate of up to 60%, with durable responses in many of the patients.[53–56]

Table 3 again shows an overview of all publications regarding the use of rituximab in adult AIHA, according to the same inclusion criteria as described in the section on ITP.[26,36]

Other MAbs

In their prospective study examining the use of combined alemtuzumab and rituximab therapy for patients with steroid-refractory autoimmune cytopenias, Gomez-Almaguer and colleagues[41] also included 8 patients with warm-type AIHA. Promising results were observed with OR and CR rates of 100% and 75%, respectively, with a median duration of CR of 46 weeks. Because all patients were rituximab-naive, it is not clear whether upfront combination therapy offers an advantage to rituximab monotherapy, followed by combination. In another study, Willis and colleagues[57] used alemtuzumab in 21 patients with severe autoimmune cytopenias, including 4 patients with AIHA, 1 with ITP, and 3 with Evans syndrome (ES). Alemtuzumab was given at a dose of 10 mg intravenously daily for 10 days. Although initial response rates for the whole group were promising, relapses and infectious complications were a major concern.

The essential role of the complement system in CAD may have therapeutic implications through introduction of pharmacologic complement inhibition. At least from a theoretic point of view, the anti-C5 MAb eculizumab may be promising.[47] However, only 1 case report has been published, resulting in stable improvement.[58]

ES

ES is defined by the presence of both AIHA and ITP, either sequential or simultaneous. Like other immune-mediated cytopenias, it can be primary or secondary to lymphoproliferative disorders, systemic autoimmune disorders, and primary immune deficiencies. The treatment of ES is not different from that of AIHA and ITP.[59]

Anti-CD20 Therapy

Treatment with rituximab has similar efficacies in patients with ES compared with AIHA and ITP. Michel and colleagues[60] recently published a retrospective cohort study of 68 patients. Rituximab was administered in 11 patients, of whom 5 had

Table 3
Clinical evidence evaluating the efficacy of rituximab in the treatment of AIHA

Authors	Number of Patients (n)	Age (y)	Previous Splenectomy	Warm-type/ Cold-type Antibody	OR/CR Rates	Response Duration (Mo)	Factors Predictive for Better Outcome
Zecca	15	0, 3–14	13	14 warm, 1 cold	87/NR	7–27+	—
Berentsen	27(37R)	51–91	NR	Cold	54/3	2–42	—
Narat	11	18–81	45	Warm	64/27	2.5–20	—
Schollkopf	20	54–86	0	Cold	45/4	2–18+	—
D'Arena	14	48–87	0	Warm	72/22	17	—
Berentsen	52	30–92	NR	Cold	50/8	NR	—
D'Arena	11	23–81	9	Warm	100/73	1–96+	—
Bussone	27	15–81	22	Warm	93/30	NR	—
Kaufmann	20	48–78	5	—	100/NR	5–53+	—
Dierickx	53(68R)	1–87	19	36 warm, 14 cold	79/47	1 y PFS:72%	—
Bowen	17	40–80	NR	—	95/70	22	—
Penalver	36	20–86	36	—	77/61	>6 (if CR)	Previous splenectomy
Berentsen	29	39–87	NR	—	76/21	>33	—
Rossignol	26	36–79	19	—	89,5/83	24	Achievement of CR

Abbreviations: CR, complete response; NR, no response; PFS, progression-free survival; R, rituximab courses.

a previous splenectomy. OR and CR rates were 82% and 45%, respectively, with 64% of the patients showing a long sustained response (more than 42 months).

Rossignol and colleagues[56] studied the combination of rituximab, cyclophosphamide, and dexamethasone in patients with secondary immune deficiencies caused by CLL. Eight of the 48 patients had ES. These investigators found an OR rate of 89.5% and a CR rate in 83%. The outcome was independent of the underlying immunologic disorder.

Other studies have not been carried out yet, and only a few case studies are available. Rituximab thus has a similar efficacy in treatment of Evans syndrome compared with AIHA and ITP and can be administered in primary or secondary (in CLL combined with cyclophosphamide and dexamethasone) ES.

THROMBOTIC MICROANGIOPATHY

Thrombotic microangiopathy (TMA) encompasses a group of life-threatening disorders characterized by the presence of microangiopathic vessel destruction with formation of thrombi, thrombocytopenia, and mechanical (DAT-negative) hemolysis.[61,62] TMA can be divided into 3 main categories: ADAMTS13-deficient thrombotic thrombocytopenic purpura (TTP), hemolytic uremic syndrome (HUS), and secondary TMA (**Table 4**).[63]

ADAMTS13-deficient TTP is a disorder caused by deficiency of ADAMTS13, a desintegrinlike metalloproteinase produced by the liver in response to increased vascular shear stress. In these circumstances, ADAMTS13 cleaves von Willebrand factor (vWF) multimers (which are partially produced in vascular endothelial cells) in inactive cleavage products, thus inhibiting thrombus formation. In the absence of ADAMTS13, unusually large amounts of vWF multimers can be found in the circulation, with a high capacity of thrombus formation, vessel-wall damage, thrombocytopenia, and Coombs-negative hemolytic anemia (**Fig. 5**). A deficiency of ADAMTS13 can be congenital (caused by gene mutations) or acquired, caused by autoantibody formation against ADAMTS13.[64] HUS is defined by the occurrence of mechanical hemolytic microangiopathy, thrombocytopenia, and renal function impairment. HUS can be divided into typical and atypical HUS. In typical HUS, which is mainly observed in childhood, the disorder is caused by Shiga toxin-producing *Escherichia coli*, especially *E coli* 0157:H7. In contrast, atypical HUS is caused by a disorder in the complement alternative pathway, typically caused by mutations in genes encoding for complement regulatory factors and activators. These factors include factor H, factor I, membrane

Table 4	
Classification of TMA	
TMA Subtype	**Cause**
ADAMTS13-deficient TTP	Congenital (mutations in ADAMTS13 gene) Acquired (antibodies against ADAMTS13)
HUS	Typical HUS (Shiga toxin-producing bacteria) Atypical HUS (mutations in complement-regulating factors)
Secondary TMA	Medication (eg, clopidogrel, ticlopidin, mitomycin C, gemcitabin, calcineurin inhibitors) Autoimmune disorders Solid organ transplantation Hematopoietic stem cell transplantation Pregnancy Infections (eg, HIV)

ADAMTS13 released (by endothelium
and liver) in case of increased vascular
shear stress.
Its function is cleavage of ultra-long
very active vWF in cleavage products.

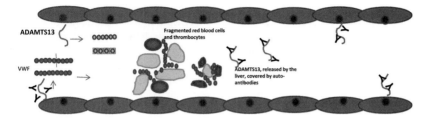

ADAMTS13 loaded with autoantibodies and inactivated.
Large vWF multimers, clotting with
thrombocytes, cause intravascular
hemolysis and thrombocytopenia.

Fig. 5. Pathogenesis of ADAMTS13-deficient TTP.

cofactor protein, thrombomodulin, factor B, and factor C3.[65,66] The disorder can also be caused by formation of autoantibodies against factor H.[67] TMA can be secondary to underlying conditions or disorders, for example medication. In most of these cases ADAMTS13 levels are normal without demonstrable autoantibodies.

Because only acquired ADAMTS13-deficient TTP and a few atypical HUS cases can be considered autoimmune disorders, most evidence of MAbs in these disorders again derives from experience with rituximab. Standard of care treatment of these immune-mediated disorders is based on prompt initiation of daily therapeutic plasma exchange (TPE, with plasma-based substitution fluids), mostly in association with corticosteroids.[61–63]

Anti-CD20 Therapy

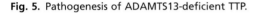

Based on recent literature reviews, almost 150 patients with TTP who received rituximab during their disease course haven been identified.[26,68] In most cases, rituximab was administered because of refractory disease or at relapse, together with reinitiation of TPE, leading to remission rates of more than 85%. The largest detailed case series to date was published by Scully and colleagues,[69] who administered rituximab to 25 patients with relapsing or refractory acquired ADAMTS13-deficiency TTP. All patients showed a complete remission, which occurred within 11 days after rituximab adminis-tration. This study confirmed the inverse relationship between successful rituximab therapy and decreased antibody levels and increased ADAMTS13 activity. The increasing use of rituximab therapy in patients with TTP was recently underscored by a report of the regional United Kingdom TTP Registry, showing that the number of patients having received adjuvant rituximab therapy in period 2004 to 2006 was signifi-cantly increased compared with other adjuvant therapies.[70] Although in most reported cases no relapses were observed, length of follow-up was limited. Chemnitz and colleagues[71] published long-term follow-up data for 12 patients, all achieving an initial remission after application of rituximab. However, after a mean follow-up of 49.6 months, 3 patients relapsed. The investigators conclude that extended follow-up remains neces-sary. Besides its use in relapsing or refractory TTP, rituximab has also been used prophy-lactically in patients with relapsing TTP, with promising responses.[72,73]

These promising results have raised the question whether rituximab can be used upfront together with TPE as standard treatment of newly diagnosed or relapsed TTP. To answer this question, an American multicenter, randomized phase III trial (the STAR study) was initiated in 2009. In this trial, which intended to recruit 220 patients, patients were randomized to receive TPE and corticosteroids with or without rituximab. However, this trial was terminated because of a low enrollment rate (http:// clinicaltrials.gov/ct2/show/NCT00799773). In an open-label prospective study from the French Thrombotic Microangiopathies Reference Center, 22 adult patients with TTP with no response or a disease exacerbation after treatment with TPE were given rituximab therapy. Rituximab 375 mg/m^2 was given on day 0, 3, 7, and 14, with day 0 being the day of diagnosis of suboptimal response to TPE. Compared with historical controls who received TPE with or without vincristine, rituximab therapy was associated with a shorter overall treatment duration and reduced relapse rate at 1 year. No serious side effects were recorded in this trial.[74] In another UK multicenter, nonrandomized phase II trial examining the use of rituximab in newly diagnosed or relapsed patients with TTP, 40 patients were included. In contrast to the French trial, all patients were given rituximab 375 mg/m^2/wk during 4 consecutive weeks, starting within 3 days after diagnosis. Here too the study group was compared with a historical control group who had never received rituximab. Again, rituximab significantly reduced both plasma exchange and hence hospital duration and relapse rate. In 92.5% of the patients ADAMTS13 levels increased, whereas ADAMTS13 antibodies decreased. No excess infections or serious adverse events were observed.[75] Although not confirmed in a randomized setting, these data point to a beneficial role of rituximab in autoimmune subtypes of TMA.

Other MAbs

Based on the major role of complement activation in the pathogenesis of atypical HUS, many case reports have been published showing promising activity of the monoclonal anti-C5 antibody eculizumab in the treatment of relapsed atypical HUS.[66] However, the results of many trials with eculizumab in both typical and atypical HUS need to be awaited to determine its real efficacy and safety profile in this patient population. Whether complement targeting in ADAMTS13-deficient TTP, especially if the kidney is involved, might also offer benefit is not clear.

GRAFT-VERSUS-HOST DISEASE

During the last decades, the use of allogeneic hematopoietic stem cell transplantation for treatment of high-risk hematologic disorders has increased. However, the rate of life-threatening infectious and immunologic complications of this therapy remains high. Graft-versus-host disease (GVHD) arises when donor T lymphocytes recognize major and minor HLA antigens, expressed on different recipient cells. Despite HLA identity between a patient and donor, about 40% of recipients of HLA-identical grafts still develop systemic acute GVHD (aGVHD) requiring treatment.[76]

Initially, GVHD was separated into 2 main subcategories, classified according to its moment of development after transplantation. In this way, the term aGVHD was given if GVHD arose before day 100 after transplant, whereas chronic GVHD (cGVHD) occurred after that time. Because this definition, especially with the introduction of reduced intensity conditioning transplantation, failed to categorize both late-onset aGVHD and overlap syndromes, a new classification was proposed by the US National Institutes of Health.[77]

Although all organs can be targeted in aGVHD, the organ systems most commonly affected are skin (81% of patients), gastrointestinal tract (54%), and liver (50%).[78] The involvement of these 3 organs has led to the aGVHD grading system, in which severity and hence prognosis ranges from grade I (mild) to IV (very severe). In cGVHD, clinical manifestations are different from those seen in aGVHD. cGVHD is characterized by the occurrence of single-organ or multiorgan system involvement similar to those observed in autoimmune disorders.

Based on experimental data derived from mouse models, development and progress of aGVHD can be conceptualized in 3 sequential phases. A first phase involves the activation of APCs by the underlying disorder and the transplantation conditioning regimen (chemotherapy with or without radiotherapy). Tissue damage as a result of these conditions leads to the massive release of proinflammatory cytokines, including tumor necrosis factor α (TNF-α), and to the increased expression of different molecules on APCs, such as costimulatory molecules. In a second phase, donor T cells proliferate and differentiate in response to host APCs and increased costimulatory signals, leading to an increased production of T_{H1} cytokines such as interferon γ (IFN-γ), interleukin 2 (IL-2), and TNF-α. In the last phase of the process, local tissue damage and inflammation are amplified because of synergism between activated cytotoxic cells (T_C and NK) and soluble inflammatory agents, including TNF-α, IFN-γ, and IL-1.[76]

Because of the dramatic impact of GVHD on both survival and quality of life, prophylactic strategies have been incorporated in current transplant protocols. These strategies include negative selection of T cells or positive selection of CD34+ cells ex vivo on one hand and pharmacologic anti–T-cell therapy on the other. However, in this article, only the use of MAbs in the treatment of GVHD are discussed. The use of corticosteroids, which possess both antilymphocytic and anti-inflammatory properties, is considered the cornerstone in the treatment of aGVHD, leading to durable CR in about 35% of patients.[79] However, in steroid resistance, no established salvage therapy exists. Although use of steroids is the standard of care, the treatment of cGVHD is even more difficult, requiring careful balancing of advantages and disadvantages of treatment initiation.

Acute GVHD

The complex immunopathogenesis of aGVHD, including many cell types and cytokines, has made the disorder an attractive target for the use of MAb-based therapy. Theoretically, each step in the pathogenesis may be targeted by different antibodies, although significant overlap exists. For example, TNF-α is critically involved in all phases of aGVHD pathogenesis by activating APCs, recruiting effector cells to different organs, and directly participating in tissue damage.[76]

In this review, we categorize the MAbs into those directed against cell surface antigens on effector cells and those directed against soluble inflammatory mediators, as proposed by Schroeder and colleagues.[80]

MAbs directed against cell surface antigens on effector cells

Because T cells are the most important initiators of GVHD, most antieffector MAbs target T-cell surface antigens. Here we discuss anti-CD25, anti-CD52, anti-CD3, and anti-CD147 MAbs.

Anti-CD25 MAbs IL-2 plays an important role in the effector phase of the GVHD process and binds to the high-affinity IL-2 receptor (IL-2R) (CD25) expressed on activated T cells. Based on decreased acute rejection rates anti-IL-2Rα MAbs have emerged as an important part of immunosuppressive regimens in kidney transplant recipients because of selective depletion of activated T cells. Three MAbs have been used in the treatment of aGVHD. Inolimomab is a murine MAb and basiliximab is chimeric, whereas daclizumab is humanized.[81]

Beside many retrospective series, 4 prospective trials have been published. Prze-piaha and colleagues[82] treated 43 patients with advanced or steroid-refractory aGVHD with daclizumab. About 50% had overall grade II aGVHD at the start of anti-CD25 treatment, of which 2 different dose regiments were evaluated. In the first cohort, daclizumab 1 mg/k was given on days 1, 8, 15, 22, and 29, whereas the second cohort received daclizumab 1 mg/kg on days 1, 4, 8, 15, and 22. CR rates were 29% and 47%, respectively, whereas survival on day 120 was superior in the second cohort (29% vs 53%). This study showed that better responses are obtained if the second dose was administered earlier during the treatment period. No serious adverse effect directly related to daclizumab was observed, although 60% of the patients had died by study day 120, mostly because of ongoing GVHD or infection. In another prospective phase II trial, Willenbacher and colleagues[83] treated 12 patients with steroid-refractory grade III to IV aGVHD with daclizumab, showing an OR rate of 67%, with only 1 patient showing a CR. In contrast to other studies, daclizumab therapy was associated with a high incidence of serious infectious complications. Daclizumab was also tested as first-line therapy in combination with steroids in a multicenter, double-blind, random-ized study. A total of 102 patients presenting with a GVHD skin stage II or overall grade II to IV were randomized to receive steroids + placebo versus steroids + daclizumab. Response rates at study day 42 were similar in both groups (51% vs 53%, $P = .85$). However, after an interim analysis, the study was stopped because of a significant decreased survival at day 100 in the combination group. This worse survival was also observed at 1 year (29% vs 60%; 9 = 0.001).[84] Schmidt-Hieber and colleagues[85] treated 23 patients with steroid-refractory aGVHD II to IV with basiliximab. OR rate was 82.5%, with 4 patients (17.5%) showing a CR. Remissions were observed between 2 and 10 days after first basiliximab dose. Six relapsed patients reached a second remission after treatment with an IL-2Rα antagonist (daclizumab or basilix-imab). Administration of basiliximab was associated with a favorable toxicity profile. Compared with daclizumab and basiliximab, the murine MAb inolimomab may offer the advantage of possessing a lower affinity for soluble IL-2R, which is increased during aGVHD. This finding may explain the high OR and CR rates in a large retrospec-tive analysis of 85 patients with steroid-refractory aGVHD.[86] Further studies are needed to investigate whether the potential theoretic advantage translates into a clinical one. A particular concern in patients treated with anti-CD25 therapy is the observation of a substantial proportion of aGVHD showing flares and progression to cGVHD.[80] This situation could be because these antibodies also target CD4+CD25+FOXP3+ Tregs. Decrease in this subtype of CD4+ T cells is associated with occurrence of cGVHD.[87] The critical role of IL-2 in growth, survival, and activity was recently confirmed in an observational cohort study, showing that daily adminis-tration of low-dose IL-2 was associated with sustained Treg cell expansion and amelioration of cGVHD manifestations in many patients with cGVHD.[88]

Anti-CD147 MAbs CD147 is another cell surface antigen, upregulated in activated lymphocytes, and hence is an attractive target for the use of immunotherapy. In a pilot trial with CBL-1, a murine MAb, 10 pediatric patients with steroid-resistant II to IV aGVHD were included. Five CRs and 4 partial responses were observed. Responses were independent of the organs involved. Immunophenotypic analyses of a subset of patients indicated no further impaired immune reconstitution in patients treated with CBL-1.[89]

In a subsequent phase 1/2 trial, 59 patients with steroid-resistant aGVHD were treated with the murine MAb ABX-CBL. Among 51 evaluable patients, 51% res-ponded, including 25% CRs. Dose-limiting toxicity consisted of myalgias at doses of 0.2 mg/kg/d (given for 7 consecutive days followed by 2 infusions/wk for 2 more weeks). No antibody-related deaths were reported, with 6-month survival of 44%.[90] Because of these promising results, a phase 2/3 multicenter, randomized, clinical trial of 95 patients with steroid-resistant aGVHD was initiated, comparing ABX-CBL with antithymocyte globulin (ATG). ABX-CBL 0.1 mg/kg was given daily for 14 consecutive days followed by up to 6 weeks twice weekly and was compared with equine ATG at a dose of 30 mg/kg every other day for a total of 6 administrations. Response rates were similar in both arms (56% vs 57%). However, probability of survival at day 180 was lower, with ABX-CBL1 (35.4% vs 44.7%), leading to the conclusion that ABX-CBL offers no advantage compared with ATG in the treatment of steroid-refractory acute GVHD.[91]

Anti-CD52 MAbs CD52 is expressed on the surface of normal B and T lymphocytes, NK cells, monocytes, macrophages, and some dendritic cells. Despite its well-established role in the prevention of GVHD,[92] experience with alemtuzumab, a humanized anti-CD52 MAb, in the treatment of aGVHD is limited. Beside some smaller case series and case reports, only 3 studies have been published that include 10 or more patients, of which 2 were prospective.[93–95] Taken together, these studies included 38 patients with steroid-refractory grade II to IV aGVHD. OR rates ranged from 50% to 83%, with 20% to 35% CRs. Alemtuzumab treatment was associated with a high infectious complication rate, necessitating careful monitoring and antibacterial, antiviral, and antifungal prophylaxis. All 3 studies used different dosage regimens (10 mg daily vs 10 mg weekly), duration of treatment (fixed number vs until resolution of symptoms or until unacceptable complications), and administration route (subcutaneous vs intravenous).

Anti-CD3 MAbs CD3 is a cell surface marker expressed on mature T cells. Muromonab CD3 (= OKT3) is a murine MAb targeting CD3. Although OKT3 showed a marked efficacy in the prevention of solid organ transplant recipients, its use has largely been abandoned mainly because of xenosensitization, pulmonary toxicity, and its relationship with malignancies.[96] In hematopoietic stem cell transplantation, early studies in the 1990s in small numbers of patients showed promising results. Based on these results, Knop and colleagues[97] retrospectively evaluated 43 patients with steroid-resistant grade II to IV aGVHD treated with OKT3. Despite an initially high OR rate of 69%, only 12% of the patients showed a CR, especially in skin involvement, whereas durable remission ($\geq$30 days) was observed in only 12% of the patients. Despite these controversial results, a prospective, randomized, multicenter trial was conducted by the European Bone Marrow Transplantation Chronic Leukemia Working Party. In this trial of 80 patients with aGVHD, patients were randomized to receive OKT3 + high-dose steroids or high-dose steroids alone. Combination therapy was associated with a trend toward improved day 100 OR rate and overall survival. The use of OKT3 allowed the steroids to be taped more rapidly, leading to a significant decrease in viral infections. Infusion-related symptoms were seen in 60% of the patients, although none of them was considered grade 3 or 4.[98] Whether OKT3 added to standard dose steroids may offer advantage in the treatment of aGVHD has not been studied.

Visilizumab is a humanized anti-CD3 MAb. After an initial phase 1 trial, showing encouraging results,[99] a phase 2 trial was conducted in 44 patients with grade II to IV steroid-refractory aGVHD. However, this study showed disappointing results, with overall and complete remission rates of only 32% and 14%, respectively.[100] Treatment with visilizumab was associated with a high rate of EBV reactivation, with

2 of 7 patients developing posttransplant lymphoproliferative disorder (PTLD) in the phase I trial. Because of these findings, 17 of 44 (39%) received preemptive treatment with rituximab in the phase 2 trial, with only 1 patient showing biopsy-confirmed PTLD.

MAbs directed against soluble inflammatory cytokine mediators

With increasing knowledge on the pathogenesis of aGVHD, TNF-α is now considered one of the most important players in both initiation and propagation of aGVHD.[1] Pharmacologic blocking of TNF-α has been studied extensively in the treatment of aGVHD. Most of the clinical trials using anti-TNF-α have been developed using either infliximab, a chimeric MAb, or the fusion protein etanercept, which binds soluble TNF-α.

Infliximab has been used in several retrospective trials, of which the 2 largest include 21 and 32 patients. Couriel and colleagues[101] described 21 patients with steroid-refractory aGVHD, of whom only 4 (19%) had grade III to IV aGVHD. OR rate was 67%, including 62% CRs. On the other hand, Patriarca and colleagues[102] reported on 32 patients, of whom most (88%) experienced grade III to IV aGVHD, resulting in fewer CRs (19%) and an OR rate of 59%. The best responses were seen in gastrointestinal GVHD. In both studies, infliximab therapy was associated with a higher-than-expected incidence of fungal and other infections. Because of the high response rates observed in the different retrospective series, Couriel and colleagues[103] conducted a prospective phase 3 trial in 63 patients with newly diagnosed grade II to IV aGVHD. Again, most presented with grade II disease at the start of the trial. After inclusion, patients were randomized to either methylprednisolone 2 mg/kg/d or infliximab 10 mg/kg/wk for 4 consecutive weeks combined with methylprednisolone 2 mg/kg/d. At days 7 and 28, response rates were not significantly different in both arms (52% vs 78% at day 7; 62% vs 58% at day 28), with no differences in nonrelapse mortality (52% vs 36%) and overall survival (17% vs 28%), with a median follow-up of 68 and 59 months, retrospectively. Infection rates were also comparable between both groups. After a futility analysis, it was decided to close this study prematurely.

Because etanercept is not an MAb, its use in the treatment of aGVHD is not reviewed here.

Chronic GVHD

Increasing evidence points to a major role of B cells in the pathogenesis of cGVHD, not only by acting as APCs for T-cell activation but also as antibody-producing cells. Several case reports, retrospective case series, and a few prospective studies have evaluated the role of rituximab in the treatment of cGVHD. The largest retrospective study, from Gruppo Italiano Trapianto di Midollo Osseo (the Italian transplantation group), was an analysis of 38 patients with cGVHD. Most of the patients had received at least steroids (100%) and calcineurin inhibitors (89%), although most had received other therapies as well. Patients were treated with rituximab 375 mg/m^2/wk during 4 consecutive weeks, although 21% received more infusions. OR rate was 65%, with a particularly high response rate for skin involvement.[104] In a small, noncontrolled, prospective trial, 6 patients with therapy-refractory extensive cGVHD were treated with the classic rituximab schedule. If there was a partial response, an additional course for 4 weeks was given, leading to marked clinical improvement in 5 patients.[105] The largest prospective trial was reported by Cutler and colleagues,[106] who reported on 21 patients. Again, patients were able to receive an additional rituximab course if there was an incomplete response. OR rate was 70%, although only 2 patients had a CR. Responses were limited to cutaneous and musculoskeletal manifestations, but were durable for 1 year after therapy, with all responding patients experiencing a significant steroid dose reduction at that time compared with pretreatment doses.

Tolerance was good, with only a few infectious complications. All 4 male patients with transplants from female donors showed significant decrease of alloantibody titers against Y-chromosome-encoded minor HLA antigens. In a third prospective trial in 7 patients with steroid-refractory cGVHD, a durable response was seen in 6 patients (3 partial responses and 3 stable disease at 1 year). However, responses were mostly observed in moderate skin and oral involvement, not in severe manifestations.[107] Similar to the observations in other immune-mediated disorders, von Bonin and colleagues[108] reported on their experience in 13 patients with low-dose rituximab (mostly 4 weekly administrations of 50 mg/m^2/wk), showing comparable OR rates of 69%. Consistent with the other studies, cutaneous, oral, and musculoskeletal symptoms responded most. In a recent meta-analysis on the efficacy of rituximab in steroid-refractory cGVHD, 3 prospective and 4 retrospective studies were included. The investigators confirmed the high response rates (60%) in cutaneous symptoms, compared with other sites of involvement.[109]

MAb therapy shows encouraging results in the treatment of both acute and chronic GVHD. However, the few prospective, multicenter, randomized, controlled trials failed to confirm the promising results observed in the different smaller retrospective and prospective trials. Further understanding of the pathogenesis of human GVHD and the optimal schedules and doses of the different antibodies is needed, taking into account the (mainly infectious) toxicity profile.

ACQUIRED INHIBITORS OF COAGULATION
Acquired Hemophilia

Acquired inhibitors of coagulation leading to bleeding should be distinguished from antiphospholipid antibodies, which result in thrombosis and rarely in bleeding. (Alloantibodies to transfused clotting factors developing in patients with congenital disorders of hemostasis are not discussed here.)

Acquired factor VIII autoantibodies, also named acquired hemophilia A, the most frequent presentation of acquired coagulation inhibitor, are an uncommon disorder, with a yearly incidence between 1.3 and 1.5 cases per million population.[110] No underlying disorder can be identified in half of the patients, whereas pregnancy, postpartum period, systemic lupus erythematosus, rheumatoid arthritis, drug reactions, or malignancies are factors present in the other half.[110]

Bleeding, often severe, is the presenting symptom in most cases. Hematomas, ecchymoses, and epistaxis are common, whereas, in contrast with congenital hemophilia, hemarthrosis is uncommon. The diagnosis relies on the discovery of a prolonged activated partial thromboplastin time left uncorrected after addition of normal plasma. The antibody titer can be quantified by the Bethesda assay based on factor VIII activity assessment after serial dilutions of the patient's plasma incubated with normal plasma. The greater the dilution needed to detect factor VIII activity, the stronger the inhibitor.[111]

Treatment of active bleeding is based on the use of desmopressin and high doses of factor VIII concentrates, if the inhibitor concentration is moderate (<5 Bethesda units), whereas activated prothrombin complex concentrate or recombinant factor VIIa is preferred when the inhibitor titer is higher.[112]

Some inhibitors disappear spontaneously, especially after delivery in pregnancy-associated autoantibodies. In the other cases, immunosuppressive drugs like prednisone and cyclophosphamide can eliminate the inhibitor in most patients.[113] Transfusion of IgG is not effective. Of 19 prospectively assessed patients, 2 responded with a prompt decrease of the inhibitor titer, whereas the antibody titer declined weeks or months later in 4 additional patients.[114]

Anti-CD20 therapy

The experience gained with the use of MAbs relies almost exclusively on treatment with rituximab. Available data from a literature search on Medline, in abstract books from the American Society of Hematology and in the references of recent major reviews on this topic, are presented here.[115–117] For the sake of brevity, the references quoted in full in Garvey's[116] recent and most comprehensive review are not reproduced here.

We identified 46 full papers and abstracts presenting 98 patients given rituximab for acquired hemophilia.[116,118–145] The data presented in such a heterogeneous literature are often incomplete. In addition, the benefits from the use of rituximab are often obscured by the concomitant use of other immunosuppressive agents: of 85 patients with informative data, 53 were given additional immunosuppressive agents during treatment with rituximab or shortly before. The population distribution was as follows: median age, 64 years (range: 18–94 years); male/female ratio: 38:59; inhibitor secondary to an underlying condition, 33 (13 with autoimmune disorders, 12 post-partum, 5 malignancies, 4 drug-induced, 2 pregnancy-associated) versus 47 cases with no underlying condition. Rituximab was started upfront (within 7 days after diagnosis) in 30 cases, after failing to respond to other immunosuppressive agents in 50 cases, and at relapse in 9 patients. Most patients (n = 60) were given 4 infusions of rituximab at the classic dose of 375 mg/m^2/wk, but some were given up to 13 infusions of rituximab, whereas others were given very low doses (as little as 1 single 100-mg infusion). A CR was achieved in 87 patients, whereas 7 obtained a partial response and 2 failed to respond. The distribution of CRs over time is shown in **Fig. 6**. Practically all the CRs were observed during the first year of treatment, whereas approximately one-third of CRs were obtained during the first 3 months. Starting rituximab upfront, in refractory patients or at relapse had no impact on the median time needed to obtain a response (respectively 8, 9, and 10 months in patients given rituximab upfront, after failing on other immunosuppressive drugs, and at relapse, respectively; P = .9, Kruskal-Wallis statistic).

Most CRs proved stable, as shown in **Fig. 7**, with only 14% of patients experiencing a relapse. All relapses occurred during the first year after achieving a CR. However, some patients died while in CR, which points to the severity of the underlying condition and of the infectious complications related to the immunosuppressive treatments (ISTs). Overall median relapse-free survival was 58 months, despite a low relapse rate (see **Fig. 7**).

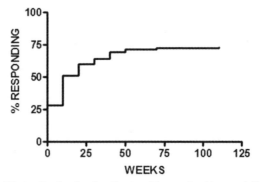

Fig. 6. Cumulative CRs to rituximab of patients with acquired hemophilia over time. Practically all the responses occur during the first year after treatment with rituximab.

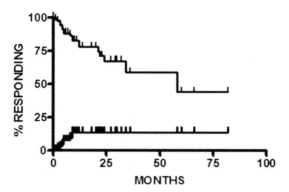

Fig. 7. Relapse-free survival (*upper curve*) and cumulative relapse rate (*lower curve*) of patients with acquired hemophilia. Responses are stable after the first year. However, the relapse-free survival curve keeps going down, as patients continue to die from their underlying disease or from other complications.

The inhibitor titer varied to a large extent (median 33.5 Bethesda units; range, 1–3075). A high inhibitor titer has been associated with resistance to rituximab.[146] We could not confirm this finding from our review. Patients with an inhibitor titer inferior to the median failed to respond to rituximab in 2 cases, whereas 6 patients with an inhibitor titer superior to the median failed to respond ($P = .3$, Fisher exact test). As shown in **Fig. 8**, relapse-free survival resulted unaffected by the strength of the inhibitor ($P = .16$, log rank test).

Interpreting the available data on the use of rituximab in patients with acquired hemophilia is limited by many factors, including bias toward reporting case reports with a favorable outcome, poor follow-up in most cases, and use of rituximab together with other immunosuppressive agents in a disorder with frequent spontaneous remissions. However, it seems that in most cases, the coagulation inhibitor was no longer detected weeks to months after using rituximab. Although most patients experienced a stable response, long-term overall survival was disappointing, because many patients died while in CR.

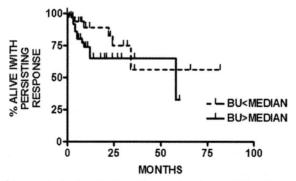

Fig. 8. Relapse-free survival of patients with acquired hemophilia. Comparison between patients with an inhibitor titer superior or inferior to the median titer. Inhibitor titer did not affect relapse-free survival.

Acquired von Willebrand Syndrome

Acquired von Willebrand syndrome is an uncommon condition. In contrast with acquired hemophilia, which practically always results from the presence of neutralizing autoantibodies, acquired von Willebrand syndrome can result from more complex mechanisms, including autoantibodies interfering with collagen or platelet binding or increased clearance of vWF from the plasma.[147] An underlying disorder can be identified in most cases, including monoclonal gammopathy of unknown significance (MGUS), myeloma and other lymphoproliferative conditions, and cardiovascular, myeloproliferative, and autoimmune disorders. The diagnosis is not straightforward and often depends on an array of converging data, including a history of late-onset bleeding, lack of familial history of bleeding, presence of an underlying condition, presence of inhibitors of vWF binding, response to therapy for the underlying disorder or to intravenous polyclonal immune globulins (intravenous IgG [IVIG]) and short-lived response to vWF transfusion and to desmopressin.

Treatment of acute bleeds relies on the use of desmopressin or transfusion of vWF, recombinant factor VIIa, infusion of polyclonal Ig, plasmapheresis, and use of antifibrinolytics. Whenever possible, the underlying disorder should be treated.[147]

Anti-CD20 therapy

Treatment with rituximab was reported, to the best of our knowledge, in 9 patients, 7 with an underlying MGUS, 1 with malignant lymphoma and Sjögren disease, and 1 with no underlying disorder.[148-152] Only the patient with malignant lymphoma achieved a CR, whereas a partial response was obtained in 2 additional patients, both with MGUS.[41] Although data are few, they suggest that, in contrast with acquired hemophilia, acquired von Willebrand disease is relatively insensitive to rituximab, except, possibly, when the underlying disorder is improved by rituximab.

The Antiphospholipid Syndrome

The antiphospholipid syndrome is best defined by a combination of clinical and biologic abnormalities (**Table 5**).

Table 5
The updated International Preliminary Classification Criteria for APS (1 clinical and 1 serologic criterion needed to make the diagnosis)

Clinical Criteria	Laboratory Criteria
Vascular thrombosis	Lupus anticoagulant present in plasma on 2 or more occasions at least 12 wk apart
Pregnancy morbidity	
One or more unexplained death of a normal fetus at or beyond 10 wk of gestation	Anticardiolipin antibodies of IgG or IgM isotype in serum or plasma present in medium or high titers on 2 or more occasions at least 12 wk apart
One or more premature birth of normal neonate before 34 wk of gestation	Anti-β_2 glycoprotein I antibody of IgG or IgM isotype in serum or plasma present on 2 occasions at least 12 wk apart
Three or more unexplained consecutive spontaneous abortions before 10 wk of gestation	—

Data from Miyakis S, Lockshin MD, Atsumi T, et al. International consensus statement on an update of the classification criteria for definite antiphospholipid syndrome (APS). J Thromb Haemost 2006;4(2):295–306.

The catastrophic antiphospholipid syndrome occurs in approximately 0.8% of patients with antiphospholipid syndrome and is characterized by widespread thrombotic disease with multiorgan failure.[153] The basis for the diagnosis of this severe condition is a history of antiphospholipid syndrome, 3 or more new organ thromboses within a week, biopsy confirmation of microthrombosis, exclusion of other causes of multiple organ thrombosis. Despite treatment, the mortality of catastrophic antiphospholipid syndrome is approximately 50%.[154]

Because morbidity and mortality from venous and arterial thrombosis remain the main threat to patients with the antiphospholipid syndrome, long-term anticoagulation with warfarin and aspirin is the basis of treatment in patients with established thrombosis, whereas heparin combined with aspirin is the preferred treatment of pregnant patients with previous obstetric morbidity.

In addition, many anti-inflammatory and immunomodulatory agents are being investigated to alter the course of antiphospholipid syndrome, including statins, hydroxychloroquine, GPIIbIIIa inhibitors, tumor necrosis factor blockade, inhibitors of tissue factor release by endothelial cells, of complement activation, and of nuclear factor κB.[155]

Anti-CD20 therapy
The role of B cells in the pathogenesis of the antiphospholipid syndrome has been proposed and was shown in some experimental models, which prompted the use of rituximab in patients with antiphospholipid syndrome.[156,157]

Again, the few data available on the outcome of patients with the antiphospholipid syndrome treated with rituximab rely on case reports and suffer from the many shortcomings mentioned in the previous sections. In addition to the 12 patients reported in a previous systematic review of off-label use of biologic therapies in autoimmune diseases, we identified 19 patients with the antiphospholipid syndrome given rituximab.[158–178] The major characteristics of the 31 cases were as follows: 11 males/20 females; median age 34 years (range: 2 months to 69 years); rituximab given for resistant disease, relapse, or upfront in 13, 4, and 6 cases, respectively. Concomitant treatments, including steroids, plasmapheresis, cyclophosphamide, IVIG, azathioprine, bendamustine, and polychemotherapy were explicitly mentioned in 20 cases, whereas monotherapy with rituximab was clearly mentioned in 1 single case report.[69] A CR was obtained in 17 cases, whereas response was partial in 12 patients, and 2 additional patients failed to respond. No underlying condition was mentioned in 11 cases, whereas the antiphospholipid was associated with systemic lupus in 7 cases, with catastrophic antiphospholipid syndrome in 5 cases, with malignant lymphoma in 3 patients, with Sjögren syndrome, Evans syndrome, hypoprothrombinemia, transverse myelitis, and cutaneous necrosis in 1 case each.

In most patients, the response proved stable with a median follow-up of 11 months (2–41 months) (**Fig. 9**), with no relapses being mentioned after 10 months.

Conclusions from such heterogeneous data should be regarded as provisional. The available information suggest that in many difficult cases with refractory, severe, or relapsing antiphospholipid syndrome, the use of rituximab, generally combined with anticoagulants, other immunosuppressive agents, and often plasmapheresis can lead to prolonged good-quality responses at the price of manageable toxicity. No additional recommendation can be made from the present evidence.

APLASTIC ANEMIA AND PAROXYSMAL NOCTURNAL HEMOGLOBINURIA

Aplastic anemia (AA) is a bone marrow failure syndrome defined by the combination of pancytopenia, decreased bone marrow cellularity (empty marrow), and a quasiabsence of hematopoietic progenitor cells (HPC). Based on the neutrophil (polymorphonuclear

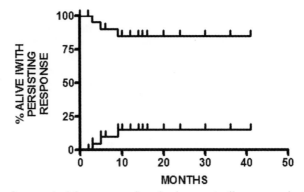

Fig. 9. Relapse-free survival (*upper curve*) and relapse rate (*lower curve*) of patients with antiphospholipid syndrome after treatment with rituximab. Responses remain stable after the first year.

[PMN]) count, the disease is classified as nonsevere (PMN $>0.5 \times 10^9$/L), severe (PMN $0.2–0.5 \times 10^9$/L), or very severe AA (PMN $<0.2 \times 10^9$/L). Seventy percent to 80% of cases of acquired AA are idiopathic. The pathogenesis of AA is explained by the immunologic (classic) hypothesis as an immune attack of autoreactive cytotoxic T cells against the HPC. Over the last decades, awareness has grown that abnormalities in the hematopoietic microenvironment of the bone marrow and autoantibodies contribute to AA development.[179] In addition, toxic and genetic factors may play a role in the occurrence of acquired AA, which makes it a complex and heterogenic disease. For nonsevere forms of AA not requiring transfusions, cyclosporine A treatment is prescribed. For severe cytopenias requiring transfusions, IST or bone marrow transplantation is proposed. IST consists of ATG, which are polyclonal purified IgG fractions of sera of rabbits (rATG) or horses (hATG), immunized with human thymocytes. ATG therapy in combination with cyclosporine A results in response rates of 65% to 75%, and in 20% to 25% of the cases a relapse is seen.[180] Most studies show a better response and survival in first-line treatment with hATG compared with rATG.[181] Bone marrow transplantation is the first-line treatment in young patients with severe AA having an HLA-matched sibling or in patients between 40 and 65 years old after failure of IST. Patients with refractory/relapsed AA, not having a suitable donor, can be offered an alternative treatment with alemtuzumab, a humanized monoclonal anti-CD52 antibody. An OR rate of 54% was obtained in patients with refractory AA, being treated with 75 to 103 mg subcutaneous alemtuzumab in escalating doses over 5 days, followed by cyclosporine A treatment.[182] Studies are now running to compare alemtuzumab and ATG, but the overall expectation is that hATG has a superior outcome in first-line treatment of AA.

Paroxysmal nocturnal hemoglobinuria (PNH) is characterized by the clonal expansion of blood cells, which lack glycosylphosphatidylinositol (GPI) anchored proteins. A mutation in the PIG-A gene, necessary for the synthesis of GPI, causes this clonal stem cell disorder. The clinical picture of PNH consists of intravascular hemolysis and fatigue, hemoglobinuria, smooth muscle dystonia, abdominal pain, and thrombophilia. Forty percent of patients with PNH develop thrombosis and it remains the major cause of death from the disease. Because PNH red cells lack 2 GPI-anchored, complement regulatory proteins (CD55 and CD59), they are more susceptible to complement-mediated lysis. Eculizumab, a humanized MAb, targets the complement protein C5 and inhibits terminal compliment activation and hemolysis in PNH. A placebo-controlled, randomized phase III trial showed that 51% of the patients with PNH achieved transfusion independence in the eculizumab arm compared with 0% in the placebo group.[183] Significant reduction in fatigue and improvement of the quality-of-life scores in the eculizumab arm was also observed. Long-term treatment with eculizumab seems to reduce the risk of thrombosis.[184] The effect of eculizumab in patients with PNH is persistent after 8 years of continuous treatment and improves survival.[185]

More than 10% of patients with AA develop clinically evident PNH, and most AA has a subclinical percentage of granulocytes with PNH phenotype, as shown by flow cytometry. An AA/PNH overlap disease exists. It is crucial to distinguish patients with classic PNH from those with AA/PNH, because the former are excellent candidates for eculizumab therapy. In the latter group, IST and bone marrow transplantation should be considered if there is severe pancytopenia.

SUMMARY

Immune-mediated hematologic disorders include a heterogeneous group of disorders characterized by the loss of self-tolerance to a variety of antigens. One of their most characteristic features is a high relapse rate after initial responses to classic first-line IST. This finding has led to interest in the use of MAbs in these disorders, particularly in relapsed or refractory cases. However, the initially promising results have become more doubtful for different reasons. First, exact responses are unknown because patients not responding are unlikely to be reported and only a few prospective trials have been performed. Second, different reports have been published describing serious (mainly infection-related) complications requiring careful balancing of advantages and disadvantages when treating immune-mediated disorders with MAbs. However, only 7 randomized, controlled trials have been published (2 in ITP, 4 in aGVHD, and 1 in PNH), as shown in **Table 1**.[32,33,84,91,98,103,183] Despite promising results in different retrospective case series and uncontrolled prospective trials, only 2 of these trials showed a significant advantage for the experimental arm.[32,183] Disrupting the immune system by MAb therapy itself may lead to autoimmune adverse events, as recently shown by the high rate of autoimmune complications after ipilimumab (a fully human anti-CTLA4 MAb) treatment in patients with advanced melanoma. These complications were associated with objective and durable clinical responses.[186] Whether these complications (replacing 1 autoimmune manifestation with another) can be tolerated in benign hematologic disorders is questionable. However, it can be expected that by using more potent immunotherapy this ethical discussion might become more relevant.

REFERENCES

1. Clark R, Kupper T. Old meets new: the interaction between innate and adaptive immunity. J Invest Dermatol 2005;125(4):629–37.
2. Recher M, Lang KS. Innate (over) immunity and adaptive autoimmune disease. Curr Top Microbiol Immunol 2006;305:89–104.
3. Papadimitraki ED, Bertsias GK, Boumpas DT. Toll like receptors and autoimmunity: a critical appraisal. J Autoimmun 2007;29(4):310–8.
4. Shi FD, Zhou Q. Natural killer cells as indispensable players and therapeutic targets in autoimmunity. Autoimmunity 2011;44(1):3–10.
5. Murray PJ, Wynn TA. Protective and pathogenic functions of macrophage subsets. Nat Rev Immunol 2011;11(11):723–37.
6. Schwartz RH. Natural regulatory T cells and self-tolerance. Nat Immunol 2005; 6(4):327–30.

7. Sfifakis PP, Boletis JN, Lionaki S, et al. Remission of proliferative lupus nephritis following B cell depletion therapy is preceded by down-regulation of the T cell costimulatory molecule CD40 ligand. Arthritis Rheum 2005;52(2):501–13.

8. Cines DB, Blanchette VS. Immune thrombocytopenic purpura. N Engl J Med 2002;346(13):995–1008.

9. Provan D, Stasi R, Newland AC, et al. International consensus report on the investigation and management of primary immune thrombocytopenia. Blood 2010;115(2):168–86.

10. Neunert C, Lim W, Crowther M, et al. The American Society of Hematology 2011 evidence-based practice guidelines for immune thrombocytopenia. Blood 2011; 117(16):4190–207.

11. Mazzucconi MG, Fazi P, Bernasconi S, et al. Therapy with high-dose dexamethasone (HD-DXM) in previously untreated patients affected by idiopathic thrombocytopenic purpura: a GIMEMA experience. Blood 2007;109(4):1401–7.

12. Kojouri K, Vesely SK, Terrell DR, et al. Splenectomy for adult patients with idiopathic thrombocytopenic purpura: a systematic review to assess long-term platelet count responses, prediction of response, and surgical complications. Blood 2004;104(9):2623–34.

13. Stasi R, Newland A, Thornton P, et al. Should medical treatment options be exhausted before splenectomy is performed in adult ITP patients? A debate. Ann Hematol 2010;89(12):1185–95.

14. Maloney DG, Liles TM, Czerwinski DK, et al. Phase I clinical trial using escalating single-dose infusion of chimeric anti-CD20 monoclonal antibody (IDEC-C2B8) in patients with recurrent B-cell lymphoma. Blood 1994;84(8):2457–66.

15. Van Meerten T, Hagenbeek A. CD20-targeted therapy: the next generation of antibodies. Semin Hematol 2010;47(2):199–210.

16. Smith MR. Rituximab (monoclonal anti-CD20 antibody): mechanisms of action and resistance. Oncogene 2003;22(47):7359–68.

17. Tang Q, Bluestone JA. The Foxp3+ regulatory T cell: a jack of all trades, master of regulation. Nat Immunol 2008;9(3):239–44.

18. Li Z, Mou W, Lu G, et al. Low-dose rituximab combined with short-term glucocorticoids up-regulates Treg cell levels in patients with immune thrombocytopenia. Int J Hematol 2011;93(1):91–8.

19. Stasi R, Cooper N, Del Poeta G, et al. Analysis of regulatory T-cell changes in patients with idiopathic thrombocytopenic purpura receiving B cell-depleting therapy with rituximab. Blood 2008;112(4):1147–50.

20. Semple JW. T cell cytokine abnormalities in patients with autoimmune thrombocytopenic purpura. Transfus Apher Sci 2003;28(3):237–42.

21. Panitsas FP, Theodoropoulou M, Kouraklis A, et al. Adult chronic idiopathic thrombocytopenic purpura (ITP) is the manifestation of a type-1 polarized immune response. Blood 2004;103(7):2645–7.

22. Stasi R, Del Poeta G, Stipa E, et al. Response to B-cell depleting therapy with rituximab reverts the abnormalities of T-cell subsets in patients with idiopathic thrombocytopenic purpura. Blood 2007;110(8):2924–30.

23. Hilchey SP, Hyrien O, Mosmann TR, et al. Rituximab immunotherapy results in the induction of a lymphoma idiotype-specific T-cell response in patients with follicular lymphoma: support for a "vaccinal effect" of rituximab. Blood 2009; 113(16):3809–12.

24. Maloney DG, Grillo-Lopez AJ, White CA, et al. IDEC-C2B8 (Rituximab) anti-CD20 monoclonal antibody therapy in patients with relapsed low-grade non-Hodgkin's lymphoma. Blood 1997;90(6):2188–95.

25. McLaughlin P, Grillo-Lopez AJ, Link BK, et al. Rituximab chimeric anti-CD20 monoclonal antibody therapy for relapsed indolent lymphoma: half of patients respond to a four-dose treatment program. J Clin Oncol 1998;16(8):2825–33.
26. Dierickx D, Delannoy A, Saja K, et al. Anti-CD20 monoclonal antibodies and their use in adult autoimmune hematological disorders. Am J Hematol 2011; 86(3):278–91.
27. Kennedy GA, Tey SK, Cobcroft R, et al. Incidence and nature of CD20-negative relapse following rituximab therapy in aggressive B-cell non-Hodgkin's lymphoma: a retrospective review. Br J Haematol 2002;119(2):412–6.
28. Hiraga J, Tomita A, Sugimoto T, et al. Down-regulation of CD20 expression in B-cell lymphoma cells after treatment with rituximab-containing combination chemotherapies: its prevalence and clinical significance. Blood 2009;113(20): 4885–93.
29. Stolz C, Schuler M. Molecular mechanisms of resistance to rituximab and pharmacological strategies for its circumvention. Leuk Lymphoma 2009;50(6): 873–85.
30. Weng WK, Levy R. Two immunoglobulin G fragment C receptor polymorphisms independently predict response to rituximab in patients with follicular lymphoma. J Clin Oncol 2003;21(21):3940–7.
31. Lim SH, Vaughan AT, Ashton-Key M, et al. Fc gamma receptor IIb on target B cells promotes rituximab internalization and reduces clinical efficacy. Blood 2011;118(9):2530–40.
32. Zaja F, Baccarani M, Mazza P, et al. Dexamethasone plus rituximab yields higher sustained response rates than dexamethasone monotherapy in adults with primary immune thrombocytopenia. Blood 2010;115(14):2755–62.
33. Arnold DM, Heddle NM, Carruthers J, et al. A pilot randomized trial of adjuvant rituximab or placebo for non-splenectomized patients with immune thrombocytopenia. Blood 2012;119(6):1356–62.
34. Ruggeri M, Fortuna S, Rodeghiero F. Heterogeneity of terminology and clinical definitions in adult idiopathic thrombocytopenic purpura: a critical appraisal from a systematic review of the literature. Haematologica 2008;93(1):98–103.
35. Arnold DM, Dentali F, Crowther MA, et al. Systematic review: efficacy and safety of rituximab for adults with idiopathic thrombocytopenic purpura. Ann Intern Med 2007;146(1):25–33.
36. Gobert D, Bussel JB, Cunningham-Rundles C, et al. Efficacy and safety of rituximab in common variable immunodeficiency-associated immune cytopenias: a retrospective multicentre study on 33 patients. Br J Haematol 2011;155(4): 498–508.
37. Brah S, Chiche L, Fanciullino R, et al. Efficacy of rituximab in immune thrombocytopenic purpura: a retrospective survey. Ann Hematol 2012;91(2):279–85.
38. D'Arena G, Capalbo S, Laurenti L, et al. Chronic lymphocytic leukemia-associated immune thrombocytopenia treated with rituximab: a retrospective study of 21 patients. Eur J Haematol 2010;85(6):502–7.
39. Kelesidis T, Daikos G, Boumpas D, et al. Does rituximab increase the incidence of infectious complications? A narrative review. Int J Infect Dis 2011;15(1):e2–16.
40. Liebman HA, Saleh MN, Bussel JB, et al. Phase I/II study of subcutaneous injections of low-dose anti-CD20 veltuzumab in relapsed immune thrombocytopenia. Blood 2011;118:[abstract: 3302].
41. Gomez-Almaguer D, Solano-Genesta M, Tarin-Arzaga L, et al. Low-dose rituximab and alemtuzumab combination therapy for patients with steroid-refractory autoimmune cytopenias. Blood 2010;116(23):4783–5.

42. Kuwana M, Nomura S, Fujimura K, et al. Effect of a single injection of humanized anti-CD154 monoclonal antibody on the platelet-specific autoimmune response in patients with immune thrombocytopenic purpura. Blood 2004;103(4):1229–36.

43. Najaoui A, Backchoul T, Stoy J, et al. Autoantibody-mediated complement activation on platelets is a common finding in patients with immune thrombocytopenic purpura (ITP). Eur J Haematol 2012;88(2):167–74.

44. Gehrs BC, Friedberg RC. Autoimmune hemolytic anemia. Am J Hematol 2002; 69(4):258–71.

45. Trivedi DH, Bussel JB. 21. Immunohematologic disorders. J Allergy Clin Immunol 2003;111(Suppl 2):S669–76.

46. Michel M. Classification and therapeutic approaches in autoimmune hemolytic anemia: an update. Expert Rev Hematol 2011;4(6):607–18.

47. Berentsen S. How I manage cold agglutinin disease. Br J Haematol 2011; 153(5):309–17.

48. Berentsen S, Ulvestad E, Gjertsen BT, et al. Rituximab for primary chronic cold agglutinin disease: a prospective study of 37 courses of therapy in 27 patients. Blood 2004;103(8):2925–8.

49. Berentsen S, Ulvestad E, Langholm R, et al. Primary chronic cold agglutinin disease: a population based clinical study of 86 patients. Haematologica 2006;91(4):460–6.

50. Schöllkopf C, Kjeldsen L, Bjerrum OW, et al. Rituximab in chronic cold agglutinin disease: a prospective study of 20 patients. Leuk Lymphoma 2006;47(2):253–60.

51. Berentsen S, Randen U, Vagan AM, et al. High response rate and durable remissions following fludarabine and rituximab combination therapy for chronic cold agglutinin disease. Blood 2010;116(17):3180–4.

52. Hodgson K, Ferrer G, Pereira E, et al. Autoimmune cytopenia in chronic lymphocytic leukaemia: diagnosis and treatment. Br J Haematol 2011;154(1):14–22.

53. Gupta N, Kavuru S, Patel D, et al. Rituximab-based chemotherapy for steroid-refractory autoimmune hemolytic anemia of chronic lymphocytic leukemia. Leukemia 2002;16(10):2092–5.

54. Kaufman M, Limaye SA, Driscoll N, et al. A combination of rituximab, cyclophosphamide and dexamethasone effectively treats immune cytopenias of chronic lymphocytic leukemia. Leuk Lymphoma 2009;50(6):892–9.

55. Bowen DA, Call TG, Shanafelt TD, et al. Treatment of autoimmune cytopenia complicating progressive chronic lymphocytic leukemia/small lymphocytic lymphoma with rituximab, cyclophosphamide, vincristine and prednisone. Leuk Lymphoma 2010;51(4):620–7.

56. Rossignol J, Michallet AS, Oberic L, et al. Rituximab-cyclophosphamide-dexamethasone combination in the management of autoimmune cytopenias associated with chronic lymphocytic leukemia. Leukemia 2011;25(3):473–8.

57. Willis F, Marsh JC, Bevan DH, et al. The effect of treatment with Campath-1H in patients with autoimmune cytopenias. Br J Haematol 2011;114(4):891–8.

58. Röth A, Hüttmann A, Rother RP, et al. Long-term efficacy of the complement inhibitor eculizumab in cold agglutinin disease. Blood 2009;113(16):3885–6.

59. Norton A, Roberts I. Management of Evans syndrome. Br J Haematol 2006; 132(2):125–37.

60. Michel M, Chanet V, Dechartres A, et al. The spectrum of Evans syndrome in adults: new insight into the disease based on the analysis of 68 cases. Blood 2009;114(15):3167–72.

61. Murrin RJ, Murray JA. Thrombotic thrombocytopenic purpura: aetiology, pathophysiology and treatment. Blood Rev 2006;20(1):51–60.

62. George JN. Thrombotic thrombocytopenic purpura. N Engl J Med 2006; 354(18):1927–35.
63. Sadler JE. Thrombotic thrombocytopenic purpura: a moving target. Hematology Am Soc Hematol Educ Program 2006;415–20.
64. Sadler JE. Von Willebrand factor, ADAMTS13, and thrombotic thrombocytopenic purpura. Blood 2008;112(1):11–8.
65. Loirat C, Frémeaux-Bacchi V. Atypical hemolytic uremic syndrome. Orphanet J Rare Dis 2011;6:60–89.
66. Kavanagh D, Goodship TH. Atypical hemolytic uremic syndrome, genetic basis, and clinical manifestations. Hematology Am Soc Hematol Educ Program 2011; 2011:15–20.
67. Moore I, Strain L, Pappworth I, et al. Associations of factor H autoantibodies with deletions of CFHR1, CFHR3, CFHR4, and with mutations in CHF, CFI, CD46, and C3 in patients with atypical hemolytic uremic syndrome. Blood 2010;115(2):379–87.
68. Caramazza D, Quintini G, Abbene I, et al. Relapsing or refractory idiopathic thrombotic thrombocytopenic purpura-hemolytic uremic syndrome: the role of rituximab. Transfusion 2010;50(12):2753–60.
69. Scully M, Cohen M, Cavenagh J, et al. Remission in acute refractory and relapsing thrombotic thrombocytopenic purpura following rituximab is associated with a reduction in IgG antibodies to ADAMTS-13. Br J Haematol 2007; 136(3):451–61.
70. Scully M, Yarranton H, Liesner R, et al. Regional UK TTP registry: correlation with laboratory ADAMTS 13 analysis and clinical features. Br J Haematol 2008; 142(5):819–26.
71. Chemnitz JM, Uener J, Hallek M, et al. Long-term follow-up of idiopathic thrombotic thrombocytopenic purpura treated with rituximab. Ann Hematol 2010; 89(10):1029–33.
72. Fakhouri F, Vernant JP, Veyradier A, et al. Efficiency of curative and prophylactic treatment with rituximab in ADAMTS13-deficient thrombotic thrombocytopenic purpura: a study of 11 cases. Blood 2005;106(6):1932–7.
73. Bresin E, Gastoldi S, Daina E, et al. Rituximab as pre-emptive treatment in patients with thrombotic thrombocytopenic purpura and evidence of anti-ADAMTS13 autoantibodies. Thromb Haemost 2009;101(2):233–8.
74. Froissart A, Buffet M, Veyradier A, et al. Efficacy and safety of first-line rituximab in severe, acquired thrombotic thrombocytopenic purpura with a suboptimal response to plasma exchange. Experience of the French Thrombotic Microangiopathies Reference Center. Crit Care Med 2012;40(1):104–11.
75. Scully M, McDonald V, Cavenagh J, et al. A phase 2 study of the safety and efficacy of rituximab with plasma exchange in acute acquired thrombotic thrombocytopenic purpura. Blood 2011;118(7):1746–53.
76. Ferrara JL, Levine JE, Reddy P, et al. Graft-versus-host disease. Lancet 2009; 373(9674):1550–61.
77. Filipovich AH, Weisdorf D, Pavletic S, et al. National Institutes of Health consensus development project on criteria for clinical trials in chronic graft-versus-host disease: I. Diagnosis and staging working group report. Biol Blood Marrow Transplant 2005;11(12):945–56.
78. Martin PJ, Schoch G, Fisher L, et al. A retrospective analysis of therapy for acute graft-versus-host disease. Blood 1990;76(8):1464–72.
79. MacMillan ML, Weisdorf DJ, Wagner JE, et al. Response of 443 patients to steroids as primary therapy for acute graft-versus-host disease: comparison of grading systems. Biol Blood Marrow Transplant 2002;8(7):387–94.

80. Schroeder T, Haas R, Kobbe G. Treatment of graft-versus-host disease with monoclonal antibodies and related fusion proteins. Expert Rev Hematol 2010; 3(5):633–51.

81. Campara M, Tzvetanov IG, Oberholzer J. Interleukin-2 receptor blockade with humanized monoclonal antibody for solid organ transplantation. Expert Opin Biol Ther 2010;10(6):959–69.

82. Przepiorka D, Kernan NA, Ippoliti C, et al. Daclizumab, a humanized anti-interleukin-2 receptor α chain antibody, for treatment of acute graft-versus-host disease. Blood 2000;95(1):83–9.

83. Willenbacher W, Basara N, Blau IW, et al. Treatment of steroid refractory acute and chronic graft-versus-host disease with daclizumab. Br J Haematol 2001; 112(3):820–3.

84. Lee SJ, Zahrieh D, Agura E, et al. Effect of up-front daclizumab when combined with steroids for the treatment of acute graft-versus-host disease: results of a randomized trial. Blood 2004;104(5):1559–64.

85. Schmidt-Hieber M, Fietz T, Knauf W, et al. Efficacy of the interleukin-2 receptor antagonist basiliximab in steroid-refractory acute graft-versus-host disease. Br J Haematol 2005;130(4):568–74.

86. Bay JO, Dhédin N, Goerner M. Inolimomab in steroid-refractory acute graft-versus-host disease following allogeneic hematopoietic stem cell transplantation: retrospective analysis and comparison with other interleukin-2 receptor antibodies. Transplantation 2005;80(6):782–8.

87. Zorn E, Kim HT, Lee SJ, et al. Reduced frequency of FOXP3+ CD4+CD25+ regulatory T cells in patients with chronic graft-versus-host disease. Blood 2005;106(8):2903–11.

88. Koreth J, Matsuoka K, Kim HT, et al. Interleukin-2 and regulatory T cells in graft-versus-host disease. N Engl J Med 2011;365(22):2055–66.

89. Heslop HE, Benaim E, Brenner MK. Response of steroid-resistant graft-versus-host disease to lymphoblast antibody CBL1. Lancet 1995;346(8978):805–6.

90. Deeg HJ, Blazar BR, Bolwell BJ, et al. Treatment of steroid-refractory graft-versus-host with anti-CD147 monoclonal antibody ABX-CBL. Blood 2001; 98(7):2052–8.

91. MacMillan ML, Couriel D, Weisdorf DJ, et al. A phase 2/3 multicenter randomized clinical trial of ABX-CBL versus ATG as secondary therapy for steroid-resistant acute graft-versus-host disease. Blood 2007;109(6):2657–62.

92. Kanda J, Lopez RD, Rizzieri DA. Alemtuzumab for the prevention and treatment of graft-versus-host disease. Int J Hematol 2011;93(5):586–93.

93. Schnitzler M, Hasskarl J, Egger M, et al. Successful treatment of severe acute intestinal graft-versus-host resistant to systemic and topical steroids with alemtuzumab. Biol Blood Marrow Transplant 2009;15(8):910–8.

94. Gomez-Almaguer D, Ruiz-Arguelles GJ, del Carmen Tarin-Arzaga L, et al. Alemtuzumab for the treatment of steroid-refractory acute graft-versus-host disease. Biol Blood Marrow Transplant 2008;14(1):10–5.

95. Martinez C, Solano C, Ferra C, et al. Alemtuzumab as treatment of steroid-refractory acute graft-versus-host disease: results of a phase II study. Biol Blood Marrow Transplant 2009;15(5):639–42.

96. Burk ML, Matuszewski KA. Muromonab-CD3 and antithymocyte globulin in renal transplantation. Ann Pharmacother 1997;31(11):1370–7.

97. Knop S, Hebart H, Gscheidle H, et al. OKT3 muromonab as second-line and subsequent treatment in recipients of stem cell allografts with steroid-resistant acute graft-versus-host disease. Bone Marrow Transplant 2005;36(9):831–7.

98. Knop S, Hebart H, Gratwohl A, et al. Treatment of steroid-resistant acute GVHD with OKT3 and high-dose steroids results in better disease control and lower incidence of infectious complications when compared to high-dose steroids alone: a randomized multicenter trial by the EBMT Chronic Leukemia Working Party. Leukemia 2007;21(8):1830–3.
99. Carpenter PA, Appelbaum FR, Corey L, et al. A humanized non-FcR-binding anti-CD3 antibody, visilizumab, for treatment of steroid-refractory acute graft-versus-host disease. Blood 2002;99(8):2712–9.
100. Carpenter PA, Lowder J, Johnston L, et al. A phase II multicenter study of visilizumab, humanized anti-CD3 antibody, to treat steroid-refractory acute graft-versus-host disease. Biol Blood Marrow Transplant 2005;11(6):465–71.
101. Couriel D, Saliba R, Hicks K, et al. Tumor necrosis factor-α blockade for the treatment of acute GVHD. Blood 2004;104(3):649–54.
102. Patriarca F, Sperotto A, Damiani D, et al. Infliximab treatment for steroid-refractory acute graft-versus-host disease. Haematologica 2004;89(11):1352–9.
103. Couriel DR, Saliba R, de Lima M, et al. A phase III study of infliximab and corticosteroids for the initial treatment of acute graft-versus-host disease. Biol Blood Marrow Transplant 2009;15(12):1555–62.
104. Zaja F, Bacigalupo A, Patriarca F, et al. Treatment of refractory chronic GVHD with rituximab: a GITMO study. Bone Marrow Transplant 2007;40(3):273–7.
105. Caninga-van Dijk MR, van der Straaten HM, Fijnheer R, et al. Anti-CD20 monoclonal antibody treatment in 6 patients with therapy-refractory chronic graft-versus-host disease. Blood 2004;104(8):2603–6.
106. Cutler C, Miklos D, Kim HT, et al. Rituximab for steroid-refractory chronic graft-versus-host disease. Blood 2006;108(2):756–62.
107. Teshima T, Nagafuji K, Henzan H, et al. Rituximab for the treatment of corticosteroid-refractory chronic graft-versus-host disease. Int J Hematol 2009;90(2):253–60.
108. von Bonin M, Oelschlagel U, Radke J, et al. Treatment of chronic steroid-refractory graft-versus-host disease with low-dose rituximab. Transplantation 2008;86(6):875–9.
109. Kharfan-Dabaja MA, Mhaskar AR, Djulbegovic B, et al. Efficacy of rituximab in the setting of steroid-refractory chronic graft-versus-host disease: a systematic review and meta-analysis. Biol Blood Marrow Transplant 2009;15(9):1005–13.
110. Collins PW, Hirsch S, Baglin TP, et al. Acquired hemophilia A in the United Kingdom: a 2-year national surveillance study by the United Kingdom Haemophilia Centre Doctors' Organisation. Blood 2007;109(5):1870–7.
111. Kasper CK, Aledort L, Aronson D, et al. Proceedings: a more uniform measurement of factor VIII inhibitors. Thromb Diath Haemorrh 1975;34(2):612.
112. Hay CR, Brown S, Collins PW, et al. The diagnosis and management of factor VIII and IX inhibitors: a guideline from the United Kingdom Haemophilia Centre Doctors Organisation. Br J Haematol 2006;133(6):591–605.
113. Green D, Rademaker AW, Briët E. A prospective, randomized trial of prednisone and cyclophosphamide in the treatment of patients with factor VIII autoantibodies. Thromb Haemost 1993;70(5):753–7.
114. Schwartz RS, Gabriel DA, Aledort LM, et al. A prospective study of treatment of acquired (autoimmune) factor VIII inhibitors with high-dose intravenous gammaglobulin. Blood 1995;86(2):797–804.
115. Franchini M. Rituximab in the treatment of adult acquired hemophilia A: a systematic review. Crit Rev Oncol Hematol 2007;63(1):47–52.

116. Garvey B. Rituximab in the treatment of autoimmune haematological disorders. Br J Haematol 2008;141(2):149–69.
117. Barcellini W, Zanella A. Rituximab therapy for autoimmune haematological diseases. Eur J Intern Med 2011;22(3):220–9.
118. Tamponi G, Schinco P, Borchiellini A, et al. Acquired factor VIII deficiency: rapid and complete remission after immunosuppressive therapy with high dose cyclophosphamide and rituximab. Blood 2002;100:101b.
119. Low B, Cohen A. Complete remission in high-titer acquired factor VIII inhibitor after rituximab therapy. Blood 2003;102:101b.
120. Mazj S, Li H, Lichtman S, et al. Successful treatment of acquired factor VIII inhibitor with rituximab in 4 patients. Blood 2003;102:798a.
121. Grimley C, Dolan G. Successful treatment of acquired hemophilia unresponsive to conventional immunosuppression with rituximab (anti-CD20 antibody). Haemophilia 2004;10(Suppl 3):58.
122. Riess H. Successful treatment of refractory acquired hemophilia with the anti-CD20 antibody rituximab. Haemophilia 2004;10(Suppl 3):62.
123. Krause M, Königs C, Kessel C, et al. Epitope mapping of inhibitory antibodies and inhibitor elimination with rituximab in patients with acquired haemophilia. J Thromb Haemost 2005;3(Suppl 1):P0201.
124. Maruscak M, Cohan B, Aghakhanian L, et al. Rituximab in the treatment of factor VIII inhibitor. Blood 2005;106 [abstract: 4064].
125. Hat-Kuhne A, Lages P, Zimmermann R. Successful inhibitor elimination with rituximab in acquired hemophilia A and a patient with a carrier status for hemophilia A–two case reports. J Thromb Haemost 2005;3(Suppl 1):P1830.
126. Malato A, Siragusa S, Anastasio R, et al. Successful treatment of acquired hemophilia with FEIBA and rituximab. J Thromb Haemost 2005;3(Suppl 1):P1398.
127. Teitel J. Acquired hemophilia following treatment with trimethoprim/sulfamethoxazole in a young woman. Haemophilia 2006;12(Suppl 2):PO18.
128. De Souza J, Escobar M. Rituximab as a treatment option for acquired inhibitors. Blood 2006;108 [abstract: 4065].
129. Millet A, Decaux O, Bareau B, et al. Efficiency of rituximab in acquired hemophilia: report of two cases and review of literature. Rev Med Interne 2007; 28(12):862–5.
130. Machado P, Raya JM, Martín T, et al. Successful response to rituximab in two cases of acquired haemophilia refractory to standard-therapy. Int J Hematol 2008;87(5):545–9.
131. Cretel E, Jean R, Chiche L, et al. Successful treatment with rituximab in an elderly patient with acquired factor VIII inhibitor. Geriatr Gerontol Int 2009; 9(2):197–9.
132. Dedeken L, St-Louis J, Demers C, et al. Postpartum acquired haemophilia: a single centre experience with rituximab. Haemophilia 2009;15(5):1166–8.
133. Stockschläder M, Ruf L, Linderer A, et al. Induction of tolerance after combined immunosuppression and -adsorption in two patients with acquired haemophilia after severe haemorrhages controlled by sequential administration of rFVIIa and FEIBA. Thromb Haemost 2009;101(3):586–90.
134. Ichikawa S, Kohata K, Okitsu Y, et al. Acquired hemophilia A with sigmoid colon cancer: successful treatment with rituximab followed by sigmoidectomy. Int J Hematol 2009;90(1):33–6.
135. Kruse-Jarres R, Fang J, Leissinger CA, et al. Rituximab therapy modulates IFN-gamma and IL-4 gene expression in a patient with acquired haemophilia A. Br J Haematol 2010;148(1):176–8.

136. Wermke M, von Bonin M, Gehrisch S, et al. Successful eradication of acquired factor-VIII-inhibitor using single low-dose rituximab. Haematologica 2010;95(3): 521–2.

137. Braunert L, Bruegel M, Pfrepper C, et al. Rituximab in the treatment of acquired haemophilia A in a patient with polymyalgia rheumatica. Hamostaseologie 2010; 30(Suppl 1):S40–3.

138. Singh AG, Hamarneh IS, Karwal MW, et al. Durable responses to rituximab in acquired factor VIII deficiency. Thromb Haemost 2011;106(1):172–4.

139. Castaman G, Tosetto A. Is a reduced intensity treatment with Rituximab effective in acquired haemophilia A? Haemophilia 2011;17(5):817–8.

140. Wilson B, Means RT Jr. Acquired factor VIII inhibitor as initial manifestation of collagen vascular disease: response to combination immunosuppression as first-line therapy. Am J Med Sci 2011;342(1):70–2.

141. García-Chávez J, Vela-Ojeda J, García-Manzano A, et al. Long-term response to rituximab in a patient with acquired hemophilia. Rev Invest Clin 2011;63(2): 210–2.

142. Mei-Dan E, Walfisch A, Martinowitz U, et al. A rapidly progressive, life-threatening postpartum hemorrhage: successful treatment with anti-CD-20 monoclonal antibody. Obstet Gynecol 2009;114(2 Pt 2):417–9.

143. Ayoola A, Mohsini W, Aung S. Acquired factor VIII inhibitor in a patient with dermatomyositis–a case study. Acta Haematol 2008;119(1):8–11.

144. Mota K, Bastos N. Rituximab in the treatment of acquired hemophilia A: a novel eradicating therapy? Blood 2008;112:[abstract: 4533].

145. Theodossiades G, Nomikou E, Tsevrenis V, et al. Acquired hemophilia A with severe hematuria and response to rituximab. Haemophilia 2006;12(Suppl 2):PO19.

146. Boles JC, Key NS, Kasthuri E, et al. Single-center experience with rituximab as first-line immunosuppression for acquired hemophilia. J Thromb Haemost 2011; 9(7):1429–31.

147. Tiede A, Rand JH, Budde U, et al. How I treat the acquired von Willebrand syndrome. Blood 2011;117(25):6777–85.

148. Grimaldi D, Bartolucci P, Gouault-Heilmann M, et al. Rituximab failure in a patient with monoclonal gammopathy of undetermined significance (MGUS)-associated acquired von Willebrand syndrome. Thromb Haemost 2008;99(4):782–3.

149. Singh P, Siegel J, Caro J, et al. Rituximab use in four patients with acquired von Willebrand's syndrome. Blood 2006;108 [abstract: 4045].

150. Iwabuchi T, Kimura Y, Suzuki T, et al. Successful treatment with rituximab in a patient with primary thymic MALT lymphoma complicated with acquired von Willebrand syndrome and Sjögren syndrome. Rinsho Ketsueki 2011;52(4): 210–5.

151. Mazoyer E, Fain O, Dhote R, et al. Is rituximab effective in acquired von Willebrand syndrome? Br J Haematol 2009;144(6):967–8.

152. Moll S, Fuller E, Cassara J, et al. Acquired von Willebrand's disease not responding to rituximab. J Thromb Haemost 2003;1(Suppl 1):CD050.

153. Erkan D, Espinosa G, Cervera R. Catastrophic antiphospholipid syndrome: updated diagnostic algorithms. Autoimmun Rev 2010;10(2):74–9.

154. Espinosa G, Santos E, Cervera R, et al. Adrenal involvement in the antiphospholipid syndrome: clinical and immunologic characteristics of 86 patients. Medicine (Baltimore) 2003;82(2):106–18.

155. Mehdi AA, Uthman I, Khamashta M. Antiphospholipid syndrome: pathogenesis and a window of treatment opportunities in the future. Eur J Clin Invest 2010; 40(5):451–64.

156. Youinou P, Renaudineau Y. The antiphospholipid syndrome as a model for B cell-induced autoimmune diseases. Thromb Res 2004;114(5–6):363–9.
157. Kahn P, Ramanujam M, Bethunaickan R, et al. Prevention of murine antiphospholipid syndrome by BAFF blockade. Arthritis Rheum 2008;58(9): 2824–34.
158. Ramos-Casals M, Brito-Zerón P, Muñoz S, et al; BIOGEAS Study Group. A systematic review of the off-label use of biological therapies in systemic autoimmune diseases. Medicine (Baltimore) 2008;87(6):345–64.
159. Binstadt BA, Caldas AM, Turvey SE, et al. Rituximab therapy for multisystem autoimmune diseases in pediatric patients [erratum in: J Pediatr 2004;144(4):558]. J Pediatr 2003;143(5):598–604.
160. Weide R, Heymanns J, Pandorf A, et al. Successful long-term treatment of systemic lupus erythematosus with rituximab maintenance therapy. Lupus 2003;12(10):779–82.
161. Tomietto P, Gremese E, Tolusso B, et al. B cell depletion may lead to normalization of anti-platelet, anti-erythrocyte and antiphospholipid antibodies in systemic lupus erythematosus. Thromb Haemost 2004;92(5):1150–3.
162. Shurafa M, Babbar N, Khairullah Q. Resolution of catastrophic antiphospholipid syndrome with acute renal failure after treatment with rituximab. Blood 2004;104: [abstract: 4089].
163. Harner KC, Jackson LW, Drabick JJ. Normalization of anticardiolipin antibodies following rituximab therapy for marginal zone lymphoma in a patient with Sjogren's syndrome. Rheumatology (Oxford) 2004;43(10):1309–10.
164. Ahn ER, Lander G, Bidot CJ, et al. Long-term remission from life-threatening hypercoagulable state associated with lupus anticoagulant (LA) following rituximab therapy. Am J Hematol 2005;78(2):127–9.
165. Bern M. Rituximab immunotherapy for the antiphospholipid syndrome. Blood 2005;106:[abstract: 4163].
166. Chavez J, Mendoza-Torres M, Vela-Ojeda J, et al. Rituximab in warfarin resistance treatment in patients with thrombophilia due to primary antiphospholipid syndrome: a pilot study. Blood 2007;110:[abstract: 4001].
167. Rückert A, Glimm H, Lübbert M, et al. Successful treatment of life-threatening Evans syndrome due to antiphospholipid antibody syndrome by rituximab-based regimen: a case with long-term follow-up. Lupus 2008;17(8):757–60.
168. Manner H, Jung B, Tonassi L, et al. Successful treatment of catastrophic antiphospholipid antibody syndrome (CAPS) associated with splenic marginal-zone lymphoma with low-molecular weight heparin, rituximab and bendamustine. Am J Med Sci 2008;335(5):394–7.
169. Erre GL, Pardini S, Faedda R, et al. Effect of rituximab on clinical and laboratory features of antiphospholipid syndrome: a case report and a review of literature. Lupus 2008;17(1):50–5.
170. Espinosa G, Mendizábal A, Mínquez S, et al. Transverse myelitis affecting more than 4 spinal segments associated with systemic lupus erythematosus: clinical, immunological, and radiological characteristics of 22 patients. Semin Arthritis Rheum 2010;39(4):246–56.
171. Nageswara Rao A, Arteaga G, Reed A, et al. Rituximab for successful management of probable pediatric catastrophic antiphospholipid syndrome. Pediatr Blood Cancer 2008;52(4):536–8.
172. Ketari Jamoussi S, Zaghdoudi I, Ben Dhaou B, et al. Catastrophic antiphospholipid syndrome and rituximab: a new report. Tunis Med 2009;87(10): 699–702.

173. Costa R, Fazal S, Kaplan RB, et al. Successful plasma exchange combined with rituximab therapy in aggressive APS-related cutaneous necrosis. Clin Rheumatol 2010. [Epub ahead of print].
174. Iglesias-Jiménez E, Camacho-Lovillo M, Falcón-Neyra D, et al. Infant with probable catastrophic antiphospholipid syndrome successfully managed with rituximab. Pediatrics 2010;125(6):e1523–8.
175. Haque W, Kadikoy H, Pacha O, et al. Osteonecrosis secondary to antiphospholipid syndrome: a case report, review of the literature, and treatment strategy. Rheumatol Int 2010;30(6):719–23.
176. Tsagalis G, Psimenou E, Nakopoulou L, et al. Effective treatment of antiphospholipid syndrome with plasmapheresis and rituximab. Hippokratia 2010;14(3):215–6.
177. Sciascia S, Naretto C, Rossi D, et al. Treatment-induced downregulation of antiphospholipid antibodies: effect of rituximab alone on clinical and laboratory features of antiphospholipid syndrome. Lupus 2011;20(10):1106–8.
178. Elazary AS, Klahr PP, Hershko AY, et al. Rituximab induces resolution of recurrent diffuse alveolar haemorrhage in a patient with primary antiphospholipid antibody syndrome. Lupus 2012;21(4):438–40.
179. Chao YH, Peng CT, Harn HJ, et al. Poor potential of proliferation and differentiation in bone marrow mesenchymal stem cells derived from children with severe aplastic anemia. Ann Hematol 2010;89(7):715–23.
180. Young NS, Calado RT, Scheinberg P. Current concepts in the pathophysiology and treatment of aplastic anemia. Blood 2006;108(8):2509–19.
181. Dufour C, Bacigalupo A, Oneto R, et al. Rabbit ATG for aplastic anemia treatment: a backward step? Lancet 2011;378:1831–3.
182. Risitano AM, Selleri C, Serio B, et al. Alemtuzumab is safe and effective as immunosuppressive treatment for aplastic anemia and single-lineage marrow failure: a pilot study and a survey from the EBMT WPSAA. Br J Haematol 2010;148:791–6.
183. Hillmen P, Young NS, Schubert J, et al. The complement inhibitor eculizumab in paroxysmal nocturnal hemoglobinuria. N Engl J Med 2006;355(12):1233–43.
184. Hillmen P, Muus P, Dührsen U, et al. Effect of the complement inhibitor eculizumab on thromboembolism in patients with paroxysmal nocturnal hemoglobinuria. Blood 2007;110(12):4123–8.
185. Kelly RJ, Hill A, Arnold LM, et al. Long term treatment with eculizumab in paroxysmal nocturnal hemoglobinuria: sustained efficacy and improved survival. Blood 2011;117(25):6786–92.
186. Weber J. Ipilimumab: controversies in its development, utility and autoimmune adverse events. Cancer Immunol Immunother 2009;58(5):823–30.

Immunotherapies in Diabetes Mellitus Type 1

Smita Gupta, MD

KEYWORDS

- Diabetes mellitus type 1 • Immunosuppressants
- Immunomodulators • Immunotherapies • Transplantation

Key Points

- Type 1 diabetes is an autoimmune disease with gradual destruction of insulin-producing beta cells.
- In addition to genetic susceptibility, various environmental agents and autoantigens have been identified over the years that trigger the autoimmune response.
- Immunotherapies, that can change the course of immune-mediated destruction and preserve and possibly regenerate the pancreatic beta cells, seem to be promising in preclinical trials but so far have been unsuccessful in human studies.
- Stem cell transplant and combination therapies using monoclonal antibodies might hold some promise in future.

Type 1 diabetes is characterized by a progressive loss of insulin-producing beta cells as a result of inflammation and autoimmune reactivity caused by a complex interplay of environmental and genetic factors. It involves pathogenic autoreactive CD4 and CD8 T cells and antiinflammatory regulatory T cells, which suppress the activity of pathogenic effector cells. In addition to T cells, B cells, natural killer cells, and dendritic cells cause direct activation of T cells in response to specific antigens.[1]

The presence of HLA DR, HLA DQ, and protein tyrosine phosphatase N22 genotypes confers high risk for diabetes type 1. However, because many children with high-risk genotypes do not develop diabetes and because of a low concordance among identical twins, it is believed that environmental factors also have a role in the development of this disease. It is hypothesized that a lack of early childhood exposure to infectious agents increases susceptibility to autoimmune diseases later in life (hygiene hypothesis).[2]

Various environmental agents and autoantigens have been suggested to trigger the autoimmune response. Insulin, and more specifically the β chain insulin peptide, has been suggested as the primary autoantigen. Other candidate autoantigens include glutamic acid decarboxylase (GAD), the tyrosine phosphatase–related insulinoma-associated protein 2 molecule (IA-2), islet cell–specific glucose 6-phosphatase

---

Diabetes and Endocrinology Consultants, 8435 Clearvista Place, Suite 101 Indianapolis, IN 46256, USA
E-mail address: drsmitagupta@yahoo.com

Med Clin N Am 96 (2012) 621–634
doi:10.1016/j.mcna.2012.04.008
0025-7125/12/$ – see front matter © 2012 Elsevier Inc. All rights reserved.

medical.theclinics.com

catalytic subunit-related protein, heat shock protein peptide 277, zinc transporter 8 (ZnT8), and chromogranin A.

Autoantibodies are excellent markers of beta cell destruction and appear long before the clinical onset of the disease. However, these antibodies themselves are not pathogenic or deleterious. Five disease-related autoantibodies have been described that predict the clinical manifestation of type 1 diabetes. These include islet cell antibodies, insulin autoantibodies (IAAs), and autoantibodies to GAD, IA-2, and ZnT8.[3,4] Positivity for 2 or more antibodies signals a risk of 50% to 100% for the development of type 1 diabetes over the course of 5 to 10 years.[5] Predicting the likelihood of diabetes based on antibody status has more sensitivity in children and young adults than in older individuals and those at low genetic risk.[6]

The genetically susceptible models of type 1 diabetes that have been widely used in preclinical trials are the nonobese diabetic (NOD) mice and diabetes-prone biobreeding (BB) rat. Early experiments in these rodent models were able to demonstrate that the disease could be induced in syngeneic hosts following adoptive transfer of T cells from the diseased animals.[7] Studies in NOD mice models of spontaneous type 1 diabetes provide proof of concept that the disease is preventable. However, there has been a disconnect between the preclinical data in mouse and rat models of type 1 diabetes and the outcomes in human trials, mainly because of issues such as dosing and timing of intervention, shorter life span of rodents, heterogeneity of human disease, and less ability of human beta cells to regenerate and replicate.[8] Animal studies are done in controlled settings, which is difficult to be carried out in human trials.

Despite years of basic and clinical research, no cure for type 1 diabetes has been found yet. There is a growing interest in immunotherapies that are being used in other autoimmune diseases. Theoretically, identifying the high-risk population by genetic study and high autoantibody titers and initiating immunomodulation in such individuals would have high success in mitigating the onset of the disease. In animals, most studies were true prevention studies with intervention initiated even before the onset of disease. However, in a human trial, this would mean intervening in healthy people, which could lead to the obvious dilemma of whether the prevention is worth the risk of adverse effects of immunosuppressants and immunomodulators. Furthermore, the current tests available to detect at-risk patients lack absolute precision and require screening of a large population.

Only few interventions would be successful once autoimmunity sets in, but this still seems to be a more realistic approach. Studies done in individuals with diabetes at the time of clinical onset have the advantage of clear-cut diagnosis, but the beta cell reserve is already low, although still preserved at 20% to 30%, at the time of onset of hyperglycemia. Therefore the treatment needs to be instituted within days of diagnosis. These studies aim to preserve residual beta cell mass for easier glycemic management with less hypoglycemia and ketoacidosis. Preserving even modest beta cell function with a stimulated C-peptide level greater than 0.2 pmol/mL has been shown to reduce long-term complications.[9]

Current approaches of preventive trials for type 1 diabetes are based on avoidance of environmental triggers, inducing autoantigen-specific tolerance by regulatory T-cell induction, immunomodulation that targets effector T cells, immunosuppression, and beta cell regeneration.[10]

These approaches can be categorized into primary, secondary, and tertiary prevention strategies based on the phase of disease they target.

PRIMARY PREVENTION TRIALS

The incidence of type 1 diabetes is rising faster than it had previously among children, particularly among those younger than 5 years.[11] Accumulating evidence suggests that beta cell autoimmunity may be induced early in life, as early as 3 months of age.[12,13] Consensus exists that intervening early in life or primary prevention has the best chance of success in eradicating type 1 diabetes.

Dietary Modifications

Food content in early childhood may modify the risk of type 1 diabetes later in life. This has been reported to be successful in experimental models of autoimmune diabetes, although the data are not consistent.[14,15] A short duration of breastfeeding and early exposure to complex dietary proteins, such as cow milk proteins and cereals, or fruits, berries, and roots have been implicated as risk factors for beta cell autoimmunity and clinical type 1 diabetes.[16,17]

A Finnish study in children genetically at high risk of diabetes showed that weaning to highly hydrolyzed formula during infancy was associated with fewer signs of autoimmunity up to 10 years of age.[18] The Trial to Reduce Insulin-dependent diabetes mellitus in the Genetically at Risk (TRIGR) is an ongoing international, randomized, double-blind, controlled intervention trial designed to find whether weaning to an extensively hydrolyzed formula in infancy in comparison with standard intact foreign cow's milk protein formula will decrease the risk of type 1 diabetes by 10 years of age.[19] Possible mechanisms for the beneficial effect of hydrolyzed formula include reduced gut permeability, modification of gut microflora, and induction of maturation of regulatory T cells in the gut-associated lymphoid tissue.

Inconsistent data are found regarding the risk of diabetes and duration of breastfeeding. The BABYDIAB study followed up newborn children of parents with type 1 diabetes. The study showed that reduced total or exclusive breastfeeding duration did not significantly increase the risk of developing islet autoantibodies,[20] although one single-cohort study showed increased risk of GAD and IAAs with shorter duration of breastfeeding.[21]

Food supplementation with gluten-containing foods before 3 months of age, however, was associated with significantly increased islet autoantibody risk. Children who first received gluten foods after 6 months of age did not have increased risks for islet autoantibodies.[20]

Vitamin D

Studies in vitro have shown that vitamin D3 is immunosuppressive or immunomodulating by arresting the ongoing immune process initiated in susceptible individuals by early environmental exposures. Studies in experimental models of autoimmunity, including one for autoimmune diabetes, have shown vitamin D to be protective. Most of the data regarding vitamin D supplementation and diabetes come from case-control and cohort studies. The EURODIAB study was a large case-control study conducted in 7 European centers. The study suggested the beneficial effect of supplementation of vitamin D in infancy.[22] Similar results were reported in another study, which recommended that supplementation of 2000 IU/d of vitamin D seemed to reduce the risk of diabetes type 1.[23] A dose of 0.25 μg/d of calcitriol did not seem to protect from developing diabetes mellitus type 1.[24]

Omega-3 Polyunsaturated Fatty Acids

The DAISY (Diabetes Autoimmunity Study in the Young) study assessed development of islet autoimmunity in association with reported dietary intake of polyunsaturated fatty acids starting at age 1 year.[25] The study concluded that dietary intake of omega-3 fatty acids is associated with reduced risk of islet autoimmunity in children at increased genetic risk for type 1 diabetes.

SECONDARY PREVENTION TRIALS

A prolonged gradual metabolic deterioration with persistence of substantial beta cell function until at least 6 months is present in several individuals in the preclinical phase after the autoimmunity sets in and before the development of clinical diabetes.[26] This period offers the opportunity for secondary prevention.

Nicotinamide

Nicotinamide prevents autoimmune diabetes in animal models, possibly through inhibition of the DNA repair enzyme poly(adenosine diphosphate–ribose) polymerase and prevention of beta cell nicotinamide adenine dinucleotide depletion, thereby promoting DNA repair and limiting DNA damage. Small trials in humans showed benefit, but a large prevention trial, the ENDIT (European Nicotinamide Diabetes Intervention Trial), that examined the effects of oral modified release nicotinamide, 1.2 gm/m[2], in nondiabetic relatives of patients with type 1 diabetes with positive islet cell antibodies (ICA) over 5 years showed no difference in the development of diabetes between the treated and untreated groups.[27]

Insulin

Development of an autoimmune response to insulin molecule itself is a key event in the pathogenesis of type 1 diabetes, which starts shortly after birth, reflected by the presence of IAAs as early at 6 to 12 months of age. Secondary interventions that can restore immune tolerance to insulin represent a sensible approach to prevent progression of diabetes.

The Diabetes Prevention Trial–Type 1 (DPT-1) with parenteral insulin that included 339 relatives of patients with type 1 diabetes with elevated ICAs and a high 5-year projected risk greater than 50% and low first-phase insulin response. The intervention consisted of low-dose subcutaneous Ultralente insulin and continuous infusion of intravenous insulin for 4 days annually. Intravenous insulin did not delay or prevent diabetes in this trial.[28]

It was hypothesized that oral administration of insulin, which is an autoantigen in diabetes, suppresses autoimmunity by inducing antigen-specific regulatory T cells in the gut, which act by releasing inhibitory cytokines at the target organ. Animal studies showed the preventive effect of oral insulin in young prediabetic mice and in transgenic mouse model of virus-induced diabetes.[29–32] The DPT-1 done with oral insulin at a dose of 7.5 mg/d was conducted in relatives with a moderate risk (projected 5-year risk of 26%–50%) with ICAs and IAAs but normal first-phase insulin response. This trial also failed to show benefit in prevention or delay in the development of diabetes. However, a subgroup analysis showed some beneficial effect of oral insulin in subjects with a confirmed IAA titer greater than 80 neutralizing units (nU)/mL, and a trend suggesting detrimental effect was seen in those with an IAA titer of less than 80 nU/mL.[33] The results were analyzed in a 9-year follow-up study on the same subjects, and it was seen that the effect of oral insulin treatment seemed to be maintained in individuals with a confirmed IAA of 80 nU/mL or more. However, once therapy stopped, the rate of developing diabetes in the oral insulin group increased to a rate similar to that in the placebo group.[34]

Similarly, a Finnish study (the type 1 Diabetes Prediction and Prevention study) performed using intranasal insulin in high-risk newborn babies identified by HLA genotyping, as possessing high-risk HLA-DQB1 genotype and at least 2 types of autoantibodies, failed to show any benefit in prevention of diabetes, even though the treatment began as soon as the antibodies arose.[35]

The Pre-POINT (Primary Oral/INtranasal Insulin Trial), a dose-finding safety and immune efficacy pilot study, is underway for primary mucosal insulin therapy in islet autoantibody–negative children at high genetic risk for type 1 diabetes who naturally first develop autoimmunity to insulin. This study aims to identify an optimal insulin dose and a route of application (orally or intranasally) that are well tolerated and can induce an immune response to insulin for additional use in a phase II/III primary prevention trial in children at risk.[36]

BCG

Initial success in animal studies led to trial in humans, which were ultimately disappointing in preserving beta cell function.

TERTIARY PREVENTION TRIALS

These trials, which have been conducted in subjects with newly diagnosed diabetes, aim to preserve the remaining beta cells to prolong the "honeymoon" phase or induce partial remission. This may translate clinically into lower insulin requirements, simplified dosing regimen with lesser risk of hypoglycemia, and reduced risk of long-term complications.

Immunosuppressants and immunomodulators have been shown to be effective in animal and human studies, but their benefits are overshadowed by the unacceptable side effects and other risks of global immunosuppression.

Cyclosporine

Cyclosporine is a calcineurin inhibitor that blocks the production of cytokines such as interferon (IFN) γ and tumor necrosis factor α (TNF-α) by T cells. These cytokines are important mediators of beta cell destruction. Cyclosporine was one of the first immunosuppressive agents evaluated after successful results in preclinical animal models. The Canadian cyclosporine A pilot study reported remission rates between 30% and 50%. Later studies also reported a remission rate of 39% after 6 months of therapy. The studies showed a greater rate and length of diabetes remission in subjects with recent onset of diabetes (<6 weeks) and with higher cyclosporine trough levels, but the effect of cyclosporine waned after discontinuation of therapy.[37–40] The main limitation of cyclosporine therapy was nephrotoxicity. The cosmetic side effects (hypertrichosis, gingival hyperplasia) were also undesirable. Lifelong administration of this drug is not a feasible option.

Azathioprine

Azathioprine is an immunosuppressive agent that prevents T-cell response to antigen. A trial by Silverstein and colleagues,[41] which investigated the effect of immunosuppression with prednisone and azathioprine, showed that 50% of treated patients achieved an HbA$_{1c}$ level less than 6.8%, a stimulated peak C-peptide response of less than 0.5 nmol/L, and an insulin dose of less than 0.4 U/kg/d in comparison with only 15% of the controls. However, at the end of 1 year, remission was observed in only 3 of 20 immunosuppressed patients. Some other trials were not encouraging and showed absence of maintenance of long-term remission.[42,43]

Anti-CD3 Monoclonal Antibodies

The pathogenesis of type 1 diabetes involves the selective destruction of pancreatic beta cells by autoreactive CD4$^+$ and CD8$^+$ cells. This has sparked interest in immunomodulators that are directed at T cells. Studies have shown that short intervention with Fc receptor (FcR) nonbinding CD3-specific monoclonal antibodies not only arrested ongoing autoimmunity but also had an ongoing long-term effect through induction of immune tolerance. The postulated mode of action involves 2 phases.[44] The initial phase covers the short-term effect during the period of antibody administration in which these antibodies cause antigenic modulation of T-cell receptor–CD3 complex, induction of apoptosis of the activated T cells, and induction of anergy in the T cells. These processes lead to physical and functional debulking of pathogenic T cells, clearance of insulitis, and disease reversal. The second phase seen after the completion of treatment is the immune tolerance mediated by induction of transforming growth factor β–dependent regulatory T cells, which effectively control the pathogenic effector cells.

Studies in NOD mouse, streptozotocin-treated CD1 mice, and rat insulin promoter/lymphocytic choriomeningitis virus models indicated that short-term treatment with monoclonal antibodies against CD3 could prevent and even induce long-term remission of established disease.

Two humanized, nonmitogenic, Fc-mutated CD3 antibodies have been studied in humans: hOKT3γ1(Ala-Ala) and ChAglyCD3.

In a small trial with hOKT3γ1(Ala-Ala)/teplizumab, after a single course of treatment, the C-peptide response was significantly preserved for at least 2 years in patients with recent onset of type 1 diabetes.[45,46] In the 2-year Protégé study performed in patients with diabetes for less than 12 weeks, after 1 year the primary end point of HbA_{1c} less than 6.5% and insulin dose less than 0.5 units/kg/day was not reached in the teplizumab-treated and placebo groups, but there was preservation of C-peptide secretion, allowing glycemic control to be achieved at a lower insulin dose in the teplizumab groups. A greater proportion of patients in the teplizumab groups were able to discontinue or use very low doses of insulin in comparison with that in the placebo group.[47]

Another phase II multicenter European trial done with 8 mg of ChAglyCD3 (otelixizumab) performed in 80 patients showed better C-peptide response and decreased the insulin requirements for 18 months following treatment in newly diagnosed diabetes.[48] The effect was sustained for 48 months in patients with higher baseline residual beta cell function and a younger age.[49]

Side effects include those related to cytokine release such as rash, fever, headache, and mild self-limiting gastrointestinal manifestations. Another important adverse effect is reactivation of Epstein-Barr virus, but this was found to be transient in duration, and did not involve reactivation of other viruses. There is no sustained lymphocyte depletion, and subjects are usually fully immunocompetent by a month after the short-term treatment ends. Forty percent of patients also develop anti-idiotypic antibodies, which can potentially neutralize the effect of CD3-specific antibody, but they appear 2 to 3 weeks after the last treatment dose and do not represent a problem unless repeated treatments are anticipated.

Abatacept

Abatacept, a cytotoxic T lymphocyte antigen 4 immunoglobulin, is a monoclonal antibody that binds to the costimulatory molecules CD80 and CD86, blocking the costimulation that is required for full T-cell activation. In a multicenter randomized placebo-controlled trial that included 112 subjects, it was observed that costimulation modulation with abatacept slowed reduction in beta cell function over 2 years. However, after 6 months, the slope of decrease in beta cell function in the treatment group was parallel to that the placebo group.[50] This finding indicated that T-cell activation occurs early at the time of diagnosis when the abatacept is effective, but later the T-cell activation diminishes and the drug is no longer effective.

Etanercept

TNF-α and other cytokines have an important role in the pathogenesis of diabetes mellitus type 1. These cytokines are produced by CD4$^+$ T cells within inflamed islets during the development of diabetes, and they potentiate the destruction of beta cells by other cytokines such as interleukin (IL)-1β and IFN-γ. Etanercept, which has been used in other autoimmune diseases, is a recombinant soluble TNF-α receptor fusion protein that binds to TNF-α and acts by clearing TNF-α from circulation, thereby blocking the biological activity of this inflammatory cytokine and improving insulin signaling. A small pilot study in a pediatric population with newly diagnosed diabetes type 1 showed that a 24-week course of etanercept resulted in lower HbA$_{1c}$ levels (5.9% vs 7%) and increased endogenous insulin production (area under the curve for C-peptide, 39% increase vs 20% decrease), suggesting preservation of beta cell function. Larger trials with this agent are still needed to assess its efficacy.[51]

Rituximab

Rituximab is a humanized anti-CD20 monoclonal antibody. CD20 antigen is expressed on B lymphocytes, and this antibody causes rapid and prolonged depletion of B cells, reducing not only autoantibody production but also antigen presentation to T cells.[52,53]

Rituximab has shown beneficial effects in autoantibody-mediated autoimmune diseases such as rheumatoid arthritis, lupus, antineutrophil cytoplasmic autoantibody–positive Wegener granulomatosis, vasculitis, idiopathic thrombocytopenic purpura, and autoimmune hemolytic anemia as well as in lymphoma and transplant recipients. Encouraging data in preclinical studies led to trials with rituximab in T-cell–mediated autoimmune diseases, such as multiple sclerosis and diabetes mellitus type 1.[54] In the Trial Net study, use of 4 weekly infusions of rituximab showed a 20% higher mean area under the curve for C-peptide in the rituximab group, indicating reduced loss of C-peptide with improved HbA$_{1c}$ and lower insulin dose at 1 year.[55] The most common adverse reaction is infusion reaction due to cytokine release, although occurrence of neutropenia and rare infections are still potential risks of this therapy.

Basiliximab and Daclizumab

IL-2 plays an important role in the autoimmune process of diabetes, and monoclonal antibodies that bind to CD25, the alpha subunit of IL-2 receptor expressed on activated lymphocytes, have shown promise in transplant cases. Humanized anti-CD25 monoclonal antibodies, basiliximab, and daclizumab do not cause cytokine release syndrome but are used only in combination therapies for type 1 diabetes.

Mycophenolate mofetil (MMF), which has a cytostatic effect on lymphocytes, and daclizumab have shown promising results in other autoimmune diseases and in animal models of type 1 diabetes. However, in human studies, neither MMF alone nor MMF in combination with daclizumab had an effect on the loss of C-peptide in subjects with new-onset type 1 diabetes after 2 years.[56] Adverse events were more frequent in the active therapy groups, and the trial was halted earlier.

Interferon-α

Recombinant IFN-α administration potently prevents diabetes in the NOD mouse by inhibiting the developing of insulitis. This inhibition of the islet inflammatory process seems to be because of an indirect decrease in anti-islet effector cell activity by recombinant IFN-α.[57] Ingested human recombinant IFN-α was safe at the doses used in the trials. In a trial on 128 patients, subjects in the 5000 units daily human recombinant IFN-α treatment group maintained more beta cell function by showing a smaller percentage loss of mixed meal–stimulated C-peptide 1 year after study enrollment than individuals in the placebo group. This effect was not observed in patients who received 30,000 units daily of human recombinant IFN-α.[58]

Anakinra

Anakinra is an IL-1 receptor antagonist. Recent studies from animals, in vitro cultures, and clinical trials provide evidence that IL-1β has a causative role in the autoinflammatory process that results in beta cell death. Inhibition of the action of these cytokines reduce diabetes incidence in animal models of type 1 diabetes and islet graft destruction. However, in human studies, the gene expression, HbA$_{1c}$ levels, and mixed meal tolerance test response did not change significantly after anakinra therapy in patients with diabetes, but these patients had lower insulin requirements 1 and 4 months after diagnosis than that in controls.[59]

Antithymocyte Globulin (Thymoglobulin)

Treatment of overtly diabetic NOD mice with antilymphocyte serum, a polyclonal anti–T-cell antibody, leads to cure of diabetes.[60,61] In NOD mice with recent-onset diabetes, antithymocyte globulin (ATG) can induce remission of diabetes. In human trials, equine ATG was shown to prolong the honeymoon phase of the disease. Side effects are related to cytokine release and serum sickness.

Autoantigen-Based Therapy/Antigen-Based Vaccines

By interfering with the interaction between pathogenic T cells and their target antigens, the autoantigen therapy tends to promote a regulatory immune response, resulting in downregulation of autoimmunity or deletion of autoaggressive antigen-specific T cells.

GAD65, the 65-kD isoform of GAD, is an important autoantigen targeted by autoreactive T cells in patients with diabetes type 1. GAD-alum (Diamyd; Diamyd Medical, Stockholm, Sweden) is an adjuvant-formulated vaccine incorporating recombinant human GAD65, the specific isoform of GAD expressed in human pancreatic beta cells. Intermittent vaccination with this protein is theorized to induce immune tolerance to GAD65, thereby potentially interrupting further beta cell destruction. Injection of this antigen in NOD mice showed slowing of disease progression.[62,63] A dose-finding study in patients with latent autoimmune diabetes showed that a primary injection and a booster injection of 20 μg each of recombinant human GAD in a standard vaccine formulation with alum (GAD-alum/Diamyd) might preserve residual insulin secretion.[64] Antibody levels against GAD were not increased except at a dose of 500 μg.[65] In a randomized placebo-controlled trial with GAD-alum, the vaccine did not show any change in fasting C-peptide level at 15 months, which was the primary end point of the study. However, a subgroup analysis showed that in patients treated within 6 months of diagnosis, the stimulated C-peptide level at 15 and 30 months were significantly higher in the GAD-alum group, although HbA$_{1c}$ and insulin requirements did not differ between the groups.[66] Conversely, 2 subsequent studies did not show any significant reduction in the loss of stimulated C-peptide, HbA$_{1c}$ level reduction, and decrease in insulin requirements over a period of 12 to 15 months.[67,68]

DiaPep277 is a peptide found to be an immunodominant epitope of heat shock protein 60 and is found in insulin secretory granules of beta cell. It is postulated to be an autoantigen and induces T regulatory cells via toll-like receptors. This immunomodulatory peptide arrested beta cell destruction and maintained insulin production in newly diagnosed diabetic NOD mice. In phase II clinical trials, DiaPep277 has shown suggestive evidence of preservation of beta cell function; the intervention group preserved mean C-peptide levels and required less exogenous insulin, indicating preservation of beta cell mass.[69–71] However, no beneficial effect on metabolic parameters and beta cell function was noted in another study in children.[72] A recent exploratory study suggested that adults with type 1 diabetes with low- and moderate-risk HLA genotypes benefit the most from intervention with DiaPep277. In this study, the subgroup with an increase in C-peptide levels at 12 months after diagnosis was the low-risk DiaPep277-treated subgroup.[73]

Incretin-Based Therapies

The effects of incretin-based agents have also been tested in animal models. In the NOD mouse model of autoimmune diabetes, exendin-4 showed a beneficial effect on beta cell mass by enhancing beta cell replication and neogenesis, protecting against IFN-γ–mediated cell death, and increased T regulator frequency when administered together with anti-CD3 antibodies or alone without any concomitant immune intervention.[74,75] Similarly, sitagliptin showed an improvement of islet graft survival and can partially reverse diabetes in NOD mice through T-cell modulation and by the incretin effect.[76] Incretin-based agents may protect beta cells from proinflammatory cytokines locally released during the autoimmune process.[77] A pilot trial of exenatide and anti-CD25 monoclonal antibodies in patients with long-standing type 1 diabetes showed no effects on residual beta cell function, suggesting that the ideal time for using incretin-based agents is likely before or immediately after diagnosis, when a significant beta cell mass is still viable.[78,79]

Gastrin, epidermal growth factor, and islet neogenesis–associated protein have also shown promising results in animals in promoting beta cell neogenesis and preserving beta cell mass.

Further well-designed and adequately powered trials are needed with these groups of agents.

Transplantation

Islet transplantation generated a lot of excitement, but long-term results were less encouraging because only less than 10% of the recipients remained insulin free by 5 years, indicating the decrease in the transplanted islet cell function over time.

Stem cell transplantation provides an exciting approach for curing type 1 diabetes. Human embryonic stem cells and induced pluripotent stem cells can be directed to become fully developed beta cells. Autologous nonmyeloablative hematopoietic stem cell transplantation yielded beneficial results in those with newly diagnosed type 1 diabetes.[80–82] Studies on stem cell transplant are still in their nascent stage and have a long way to go.

FUTURE DIRECTION

It seems that the research is now heading toward combination therapy. These combination therapies target different components in the immunopathogenesis of diabetes type 1. Several trials are underway with varying combinations of agents consisting of beta cell–derived antigen vaccine that can induce and expand T regulator cells, immunomodulators that can reduce T effector cell function, antiinflammatory agents that can neutralize the inflammatory cytokines, and agents that can protect and support regeneration of beta cells. Combination trials using mycophenolate mofetil with daclizumab and exenatide with daclizumab have been disappointing, but several other combination trials are underway, such as ATG-granulocyte colony-stimulating factor, GAD-alum/ sitagliptin/lansoprazole, epidermal growth factor/gastrin, IL-2/gastrin. Monoclonal-based therapies also maintain a crucial place in these combination therapies.

SUMMARY

Despite the continued increase in the knowledge of different aspects of type 1 diabetes and multiple clinical trials over the last 30 years to prevent or reverse this disease, the efforts have not been successful in providing long-term benefits to the patient. Therefore, there is a need to devise a form of immunotherapy that can create long-term tolerance to beta cells while circumventing unacceptable side effects from chronic immunosuppression. It seems that a one-time resetting intervention and monotherapy cannot eliminate, control, or decimate the autoreactive memory pool sufficiently, so interest in combination therapies is growing. Islet cell regeneration strategies and stem cell transplantation also hold a promise in the future.

REFERENCES

1. Phillips B, Trucco M, Giannoukakis N. Current state of type 1 diabetes immunotherapy: incremental advances, huge leaps, or more of the same? Clin Dev Immunol 2011;2011:432016.
2. Bach JF. Infections and autoimmune diseases. J Autoimmun 2005;25(Suppl): 74–80.
3. Knip M. Can we predict type 1 diabetes in the general population? Diabetes Care 2002;25:623–5.
4. Wenzlau JM, Juhl K, Yu L, et al. The cation transporter ZnT8 (Slc30A8) is a major antigen in human type 1 diabetes. Proc Natl Acad Sci U S A 2007;104:17040–5.
5. Knip M. Should we screen for risk of type 1 diabetes? Diabetes Care 2008;31: 622–3.
6. Bingley PJ, Gale EA. Progression to type 1 diabetes in islet cell antibody-positive relatives in the European Nicotinamide Diabetes Intervention trial: the role of additional immune, genetic and metabolic markers of risk. Diabetologia 2006;49: 881–90.
7. Like AA, Weringer EJ, Holdash A, et al. Adoptive transfer of autoimmune diabetes in biobreeding/Worcester (BB/W) inbred and hybrid rats. J Immunol 1985;134: 1583–7.
8. Bresson D, von Herrath M. Immunotherapy for the prevention and treatment of type 1 diabetes: optimizing the path from bench to bedside. Diabetes Care 2009;32(10):1753–68.
9. Steffes MW, Sibley S, Jackson M, et al. Beta cell function and the development of diabetes related complications in the Diabetes Control and Complications Trial. Diabetes Care 2003;26(3):832–6.
10: Rewers M, Gottlieb P. Immunotherapy for the prevention and treatment of type 1 diabetes: human trials and a look into the future. Diabetes Care 2009;32(10): 1769–82.
11. Patterson CC, Dahlquist GG, Gyurus E, et al. Incidence trends in for childhood type 1 diabetes in Europe during 1989-2003 and predicted new cases 2005-20; multicentre prospective registration study. Lancet 2009;373:2027–33.
12. Ziegler A-G, Hummel M, Schenker M, et al. Autoantibody appearance and risk for development of childhood diabetes in offspring of parents with type 1 diabetes: the 2-year analysis of the German BABYDIAB Study. Diabetes 1999;48:460–8.
13. Kimpimaki T, Kupila A, Hamalainen AM, et al. The first signs of β-cell autoimmunity appear in infancy in genetically susceptible children from the general population: the Finnish type 1 diabetes prediction and prevention Study. J Clin Endocrinol Metab 2001;86:4782–8.

14. Karges W, Hammond-McKibben D, Cheung RK, et al. Immunological aspects of nutritional diabetes prevention in NOD mice: a pilot study for the cow's milk based IDDM prevention trial. Diabetes 1997;46:557–64.
15. Malkani S, Nompleggi D, Hansen JW, et al. Dietary cow's milk protein does not alter the frequency of diabetes in the BB rat. Diabetes 1997;46:1133–40.
16. Virtanen SM, Knip M. Nutritional risk predictors of β cell autoimmunity and type 1 diabetes at a young age. Am J Clin Nutr 2003;78:1053–67.
17. Knip M, Virtanen SM, Akerblom HK. Infant feeding and risk of type 1 diabetes. Am J Clin Nutr 2010;91(Suppl):1506S–13S.
18. Knip M, Virtanen SM, Becker D, et al, TRIGR Study Group. Early feeding and risk of type 1 diabetes: experiences from the Trial to Reduce Insulin-dependent diabetes mellitus in the Genetically at Risk (TRIGR). Am J Clin Nutr 2011; 94(Suppl 6):1814S–20S.
19. TRIGR Study Group, Akerblom HK, Krischer J, et al. The Trial to Reduce IDDM in the Genetically at Risk (TRIGR) study: recruitment, intervention and follow-up. Diabetologia 2011;54(3):627–33.
20. Ziegler AG, Schmid S, Huber D, et al. Early infant feeding and risk of developing type 1 diabetes-associated autoantibodies. JAMA 2003;290(13):1721–8.
21. Holmberg H, Wahlberg J, Vaarala O, et al. Short duration of breast feeding as a risk factor for beta cell auto-antibodies in 5 year old children from the general population. Br J Nutr 2007;97:111–6.
22. The EURODIAB Substudy 2 Study Group. Vitamin D supplement in early childhood and risk for Type I (insulin-dependent) diabetes mellitus. Diabetologia 1999;42(1):51–4.
23. Hyppönen E, Läärä E, Reunanen A, et al. Intake of vitamin D and risk of type 1 diabetes: a birth-cohort study. Lancet 2001;358(9292):1500–3.
24. Bizzarri C, Pitocco D, Napoli N, et al, IMDIAB Group. No protective effect of calcitriol on beta-cell function in recent-onset type 1 diabetes: the IMDIAB XIII trial. Diabetes Care 2010;33(9):1962–3.
25. Norris JM, Yin X, Lamb MM, et al. Omega-3 polyunsaturated fatty acid intake and islet autoimmunity in children at increased risk for type 1 diabetes. JAMA 2007; 298(12):1420–8.
26. Sosenko JM, Palmer JP, Greenbaum CJ, et al. Patterns of metabolic progression to type 1 diabetes in the Diabetes Prevention Trial-Type 1. Diabetes Care 2006; 29(3):643–9.
27. Gale EA, Bingley PJ, Emmett CL, et al, European Nicotinamide Diabetes Intervention Trial (ENDIT) Group. European Nicotinamide Diabetes Intervention Trial (ENDIT): a randomised controlled trial of intervention before the onset of type 1 diabetes. Lancet 2004;363(9413):925–31.
28. Diabetes Prevention Trial–Type 1 Diabetes Study Group. Effects of insulin in relatives of patients with type 1 diabetes mellitus. N Engl J Med 2002;346:1685–91.
29. Bergerot I, Fabien N, Maguer V, et al. Oral administration of human insulin to NOD mice generates CD4+ T cells that suppress adoptive transfer of diabetes. J Autoimmun 1994;7:655–63.
30. Polanski M, Melican NS, Zhang J, et al. Oral administration of the immunodominant B-chain of insulin reduces diabetes in a co-transfer model of diabetes in the NOD mouse and is associated with a switch from Th1 to Th2 cytokines. J Autoimmun 1997;10:339–46.
31. Ploix C, Bergerot I, Fabien N, et al. Protection against autoimmune diabetes with oral insulin is associated with the presence of IL-4 type 2 T-cells in the pancreas and pancreatic lymph nodes. Diabetes 1998;47:39–44.

32. von Herrath MG, Dyrberg T, Oldstone MB. Oral insulin treatment suppresses virus-induced antigen-specific destruction of beta cells and prevents autoimmune diabetes in transgenic mice. J Clin Invest 1996;98:1324–31.
33. Skyler JS, Krischer JP, Wolfsdorf J, et al. Effects of oral insulin in relatives of patients with type 1 diabetes: the Diabetes Prevention Trial—Type 1. Diabetes Care 2005;28(5):1068–76.
34. Vehik K, Cuthbertson D, Ruhlig H, et al, DPT-1, TrialNet Study Groups. Long-term outcome of individuals treated with oral insulin: diabetes prevention trial-type 1 (DPT-1) oral insulin trial. Diabetes Care 2011;34(7):1585–90.
35. Näntö-Salonen K, Kupila A, Simell S, et al. Nasal insulin to prevent type 1 diabetes in children with HLA genotypes and autoantibodies conferring increased risk of disease: a double-blind, randomised controlled trial. Lancet 2008; 372(9651):1746–55.
36. Achenbach P, Barker J, Bonifacio E, Pre-POINT Study Group. Modulating the natural history of type 1 diabetes in children at high genetic risk by mucosal insulin immunization. Curr Diab Rep 2008;8(2):87–93.
37. Stiller CR, Dupré J, Gent M, et al. Effects of cyclosporine immunosuppression in insulin-dependent diabetes mellitus of recent onset. Science 1984;223(4643): 1362–7.
38. Dupré J, Stiller CR, Gent M, et al. Effects of immunosuppression with cyclosporine in insulin-dependent diabetes mellitus of recent onset: the Canadian open study at 44 months. Transplant Proc 1988;20(3 Suppl 4):184–92.
39. Chase HP, Butler-Simon N, Garg SK, et al. Cyclosporine A for the treatment of new-onset insulin-dependent diabetes mellitus. Pediatrics 1990;85(3):241–5.
40. Stiller CR, Dupre J, Gent M, et al. Effects of cyclosporine in recent-onset juvenile type 1 diabetes: impact of age and duration of disease. J Pediatr 1987;111(6 Pt 2):1069–72.
41. Silverstein J, Maclaren N, Riley W, et al. Immunosuppression with azathioprine and prednisone in recent-onset insulin-dependent diabetes mellitus. N Engl J Med 1988;319(10):599–604.
42. Cook JJ, Hudson I, Harrison LC, et al. Double-blind controlled trial of azathioprine in children with newly diagnosed type I diabetes. Diabetes 1989;38(6):779–83.
43. Harrison LC, Colman PG, Dean B, et al. Increase in remission rate in newly diagnosed type I diabetic subjects treated with azathioprine. Diabetes 1985;34(12): 1306–8.
44. Chatenoud L, Bluestone JA. CD3-specific antibodies: a portal to the treatment of autoimmunity. Nat Rev Immunol 2007;7(8):622–32.
45. Herold KC, Gitelman SE, Masharani U, et al. A single course of anti-CD3 monoclonal antibody hOKT3g1 (Ala-Ala) results in improvement in C peptide responses and clinical parameters for at least 2 years after onset of type 1 diabetes. Diabetes 2005;54(6):1763–9.
46. Herold KC, Hagopian W, Auger JA, et al. Anti CD3 monoclonal antibody in new onset type 1 diabetes mellitus. N Engl J Med 2002;346(22):1692–8.
47. Sherry N, Hagopian W, Ludvigsson J, et al. Teplizumab for treatment of type 1 diabetes (Protégé study):1-year results from a randomised placebo-controlled trial. Lancet 2011;378:487.
48. Keymeulen B, Vandemeulebroucke E, Ziegler AG, et al. Insulin needs after CD3 antibody therapy in new onset type 1 diabetes. N Engl J Med 2005;352(25): 2598–608.
49. Keymeulen B, Walter M, Mathieu C, et al. Four-year metabolic outcome of a randomised controlled CD3-antibody trial in recent-onset type 1 diabetic patients

depends on their age and baseline residual beta cell mass. Diabetologia 2010; 53(4):614–23.

50. Orban T, Bundy B, Becker DJ, et al, Type 1 Diabetes TrialNet Abatacept Study Group. Co-stimulation modulation with abatacept in patients with recent-onset type 1 diabetes: a randomised, double-blind, placebo-controlled trial. Lancet 2011;378(9789):412–9.

51. Mastrandrea L, Yu J, Behrens T, et al. Etanercept treatment in children with new-onset type 1 diabetes: pilot randomized, placebo-controlled, double-blind study. Diabetes Care 2009;32(7):1244–9.

52. Falcone M, Lee J, Patstone G, et al. B lymphocytes are crucial antigen-presenting cells in the pathogenic autoimmune response to GAD65 antigen in non obese diabetic mice. J Immunol 1998;179:1004–12.

53. Bour-Jordan H, Bluestone JA. B cell depletion: a novel therapy for autoimmune diabetes? J Clin Invest 2007;117(12):3642–5.

54. Serreze DV, Chapman HD, Varnum DS, et al. B lymphocytes are essential for the initiation of T-cell mediated autoimmune diabetes: analysis of a new "speed congenic" stock of NOD.Ig mu null mice. J Exp Med 1996;184:2049–53.

55. Pescovitz MD, Greenbaum CJ, Krause-Steinrauf H, et al. Rituximab, B-lymphocyte depletion, and preservation of beta cell function. N Engl J Med 2009; 361(22):2143–52.

56. Gottlieb PA, Quinlan S, Krause-Steinrauf H, et al; Type 1 Diabetes TrialNet MMF/DZB Study Group. Failure to preserve beta-cell function with mycophenolate mofetil and daclizumab combined therapy in patients with new-onset type 1 diabetes. Diabetes Care 2010;33(4):826–32.

57. Sobel DO, Ahvazi B. Alpha-interferon inhibits the development of diabetes in NOD mice. Diabetes 1998;47(12):1867–72.

58. Rother KI, Brown RJ, Morales MM, et al. Effect of ingested interferon-alpha on beta-cell function in children with new-onset type 1 diabetes. Diabetes Care 2009;32(7):1250–5.

59. Sumpter KM, Adhikari S, Grishman EK, et al. Preliminary studies related to anti-interleukin-1β therapy in children with newly diagnosed type 1 diabetes. Pediatr Diabetes 2011;12(7):656–67.

60. Ogawa N, Minamimura K, Kodaka T, et al. Short administration of polyclonal anti-T cell antibody (ALS) in NOD mice with extensive insulitis prevents subsequent development of autoimmune diabetes. J Autoimmun 2006;26(4): 225–31.

61. Simon G, Parker M, Ramiya V, et al. Murine antithymocyte globulin therapy alters disease progression in NOD mice by a time-dependent induction of immunoregulation. Diabetes 2008;57(2):405–14.

62. Tian J, Clare-Salzler M, Herschenfeld A, et al. Modulating autoimmune responses to GAD inhibits disease progression and prolongs islet graft survival in diabetes-prone mice. Nat Med 1996;2(12):1348–53.

63. Tisch R, Liblau RS, Yang XD, et al. Induction of GAD65-specific regulatory T-cells inhibits ongoing autoimmune diabetes in nonobese diabetic mice. Diabetes 1998;47(6):894–9.

64. Agardh CD, Cilio CM, Lethagen A, et al. Clinical evidence for the safety of GAD65 immunomodulation in adult-onset autoimmune diabetes. J Diabetes Complications 2005;19(4):238–46.

65. Bekris LM, Jensen RA, Lagerquist E, et al. GAD65 autoantibody epitopes in adult patients with latent autoimmune diabetes following GAD65 vaccination. Diabet Med 2007;24(5):521–6.

66. Ludvigsson J, Faresjö M, Hjorth M, et al. GAD treatment and insulin secretion in recent onset type 1 diabetes. N Engl J Med 2008;359(18):1909–20.
67. Wherrett DK, Bundy B, Becker DJ, et al, Type 1 Diabetes TrialNet GAD Study Group. Antigen-based therapy with glutamic acid decarboxylase (GAD) vaccine in patients with recent-onset type 1 diabetes: a randomised double-blind trial. Lancet 2011;378(9788):319–27.
68. Ludvigsson J, Krisky D, Casas R, et al. GAD65 antigen therapy in recently diagnosed type 1 diabetes mellitus. N Engl J Med 2012;366(5):433–42.
69. Raz I, Avron A, Tamir M, et al. Treatment of new-onset type 1 diabetes with peptide DiaPep277 is safe and associated with preserved beta-cell function: extension of a randomized, double-blind, phase II trial. Diabetes Metab Res Rev 2007;23(4):292–8.
70. Raz I, Elias D, Avron A, et al. Beta-cell function in new-onset type 1 diabetes and immunomodulation with a heat-shock protein peptide (DiaPep277): a randomised, double-blind, phase II trial. Lancet 2001;358(9295):1749–53.
71. Huurman VA, Decochez K, Mathieu C, et al. Therapy with the hsp60 peptide DiaPep277 in C-peptide positive type 1 diabetes patients. Diabetes Metab Res Rev 2007;23(4):269–75.
72. Lazar L, Ofan R, Weintrob N, et al. Heat-shock protein peptide DiaPep277 treatment in children with newly diagnosed type 1 diabetes: a randomised, double-blind phase II study. Diabetes Metab Res Rev 2007;23(4):286–91.
73. Buzzetti R, Cernea S, Petrone A, et al, DiaPep Trialists Group. C-peptide response and HLA genotypes in subjects with recent-onset type 1 diabetes after immunotherapy with DiaPep277: an exploratory study. Diabetes 2011;60(11): 3067–72.
74. Sherry NA, Chen W, Kushner JA, et al. Exendin-4 improves reversal of diabetes in NOD mice treated with anti-CD3 monoclonal antibodies by enhancing recovery of β-cells. Endocrinology 2007;148:5136–44.
75. Hadjiyanni I, Baggio LL, Poussier P, et al. Exendin-4 modulates diabetes onset in nonobese diabetic mice. Endocrinology 2008;149:1338–49.
76. Kim SJ, Nian C, Doudet DJ, et al. Dipeptidyl peptidase IV inhibition with MK0431 improves islet graft survival in diabetic NOD mice partially via T-cell modulation. Diabetes 2009;58:641–51.
77. Blandino-Rosano M, Perez-Arana G, Mellado-Gil JM, et al. Anti-proliferative effect of pro-inflammatory cytokines in cultured β-cells is associated with extracellular signal-regulated kinase 1/2 pathway inhibition: protective role of glucagon-like peptide-1. J Mol Endocrinol 2008;41:35–44.
78. Rother KI, Spain LM, Wesley RA, et al. Effects of exenatide alone and in combination with daclizumab on β-cell function in long-standing type 1 diabetes. Diabetes Care 2009;32:2251–7.
79. Bosi E. Time for testing incretin therapies in early type 1 diabetes? J Clin Endocrinol Metab 2010;95(6):2607–9.
80. Voltarelli JC, Couri CE, Stracieri AB, et al. Autologous nonmyeloablative hematopoietic stem cell transplantation in newly diagnosed type 1 diabetes mellitus. JAMA 2007;297(14):1568–76.
81. Couri CE, Oliveira MC, Stracieri AB, et al. C-peptide levels and insulin independence following autologous nonmyeloablative hematopoietic stem cell transplantation in newly diagnosed type 1 diabetes mellitus. JAMA 2009;301(15):1573–9.
82. Gitelman SE, Haller MJ, Schatz D. Autologous nonmyeloablative hematopoietic stem cell transplantation in newly diagnosed type 1 diabetes mellitus. JAMA 2009;302(6):624 [author reply: 624–5].

Immunotherapy in Miscellaneous Medical Disorders Graves Ophthalmopathy, Asthma, and Regional Painful Syndrome

Michael Gonzales, MD[a], Carmel Fratianni, MD[b],
Chaitanya Mamillapali, MBBS, MRCP[b], Romesh Khardori, MD, PhD[a],*

KEYWORDS

- Graves' • Ophthalmopathy • Asthma • Allergy
- Painful neuropathy

Key Points

- Immunotherapy is favorably affecting outcome in Graves ophthalmopathy.
- Immunotherapy in patients with asthma is significantly and favorably helping patients with allergic asthma and its role is expanding.
- Painful neuropathy is associated with immune activation, and suppression of immune activation helps alleviate chronic pain.

GRAVES OPHTHALMOPATHY
Background and Epidemiology

Graves disease (GD) is the most common cause of hyperthyroidism and is well recognized to have extrathyroidal manifestations, affecting both the eyes and skin. It is the result of stimulatory autoantibodies that bind to the thyrotropin receptor (TSH-R) and activate thyroid gland with resultant diffuse toxic goiter and clinical hyperthyroidism.

---

[a] Division of Endocrinology and Metabolism, Department of Internal Medicine, Strelitz Center for Diabetes and Endocrine Disorders, Eastern Virginia Medical School, 855 West Brambleton Avenue, Norfolk, VA 23510, USA
[b] Division of Endocrinology and Metabolism, Department of Internal Medicine, Southern Illinois University School of Medicine, 801 North Rutledge, Springfield, IL 62794-9636, USA
* Corresponding author.
E-mail address: khardoRK@evms.edu

Med Clin N Am 96 (2012) 635–654
doi:10.1016/j.mcna.2012.04.013
0025-7125/12/$ – see front matter © 2012 Elsevier Inc. All rights reserved.
medical.theclinics.com

Those with severe disease and high circulating titers of TSH-R antibody develop more extrathyroidal manifestations.[1] Overall it affects approximately 2% of the adult population,[2] and between 20% and 50% of those affected will evolve demonstrable ocular involvement known variably as Graves ophthalmopathy (GO). The underlying autoimmunity in GD sets up an inflammatory process that leads to remodeling of orbital tissues resulting in GO. Severe, potentially blinding orbital inflammation develops in about 5% to 6% of these patients.[3] The inflammation causes muscle and soft tissue swelling, which when progressive, results in clinical features of proptosis, exposure keratopathy, and compressive optic neuropathy. GD and GO affect more than 20 million adults and the peak incidence is in the fourth and fifth decades.[4] Although both GD and GO are more frequent in women than in men, in severe forms of the eye disease the female-to-male ratio is only 1:4.[4] suggesting that advanced eye disease is more prevalent among men. It has been demonstrated that patients older than 60 with GD, and men in particular, are at risk of developing severe eye disease.[5] GO is relatively uncommon in children, and is usually mild when it occurs, responding to biochemical control of hyperthyroidism and local measures. Graves optic neuropathy has not been reported in the pediatric population.[6]

The immune response in GO is both humoral and cell-mediated with an acute phase driven by mononuclear cells (primarily lymphocytes and mast cells) that infiltrate the extraocular muscles, orbital fat and periorbital tissues. Unique site-specific resident fibroblasts highly responsive to proinflammatory cytokines orchestrate the recruitment of immunocompetent cells and initiate tissue remodeling. These activated fibroblasts drive the disease process through expression of molecular mediators including cytokines and chemoattractants that both promote ongoing inflammation and immune recruitment.[7–9] The hallmark of active GO is inflammation-mediated production and accumulation of orbital glycosaminoglycans.[10–12] The highly charged, hydrophilic, hyaluronan molecules attract water, and thereby contribute to orbital tissue expansion and orbital congestion. The combination of muscle and fat expansion results in proptosis, restricted eye muscle movement, and, in some patients, optic neuropathy. Irreversible changes occur when fibroblast activity induces fibrosis at the level of the fibrovascular matrix of the orbital soft tissue.[13,14]

The eye disease of GO varies from mild, self-limited illness to severe, potentially sight-threatening disease seen in a minority, 3% to 5% of cases.[15] The clinical spectrum of ocular involvement is variable: from minor irritation or discomfort to severe and intense ocular pain with visual loss, which can rarely be permanent. It is notable that GO can manifest either before or after recognition of clinical hyperthyroidism. Although recognition of hyperthyroidism usually precedes or is concomitant with recognition of GO, about 10% of patients with GO will not have clinical or biochemical hyperthyroidism at presentation with their eye disease. The vast majority of patients, approximately 85% will have subsequent evolution of thyroid eye disease within 18 months of the onset of hyperthyroidism.[16]

Clinical Signs and Symptoms; Natural History

Patients with GO may commonly present with symptoms of light sensitivity and increased tearing in addition to a gritty ocular sensation, or retro-orbital pressure sensation or pain.[17] Blurry vision and diminished color perception or visual acuity may be a manifestation of optic neuropathy that requires appropriate emergent clinical evaluation. Other urgent presentations include corneal ulceration, globe subluxation, and severe periorbital edema with chemosis.[18] Double vision may also be noted, which may be a manifestation of extra ocular muscle (EOM) involvement. Proptosis, lid retraction, and edema of lids and/or periorbital tissues may also be seen on physical examination in conjunction with swelling of the conjunctivae. Only a minority of patients demonstrate severe and chronic disease progression.[19] Indeed, the natural history of GO is one of spontaneous remission in most individuals, especially those with milder disease.[4] In one study of patients with GO followed over a median of 12 months, spontaneous improvement in ocular manifestations were noted in approximately two-thirds, stability in 20%, and worsening in 14% to the extent that immunosuppression was required.[20]

Although eye manifestations are usually clinically obvious, more subtle manifestation of ocular involvement can be demonstrated by sophisticated imaging techniques with increased sensitivity for orbital involvement.[21,22] Where imaging is clinically indicated, magnetic resonance imaging is the radiologic procedure of choice on the basis of high image resolution and the absence of ionizing radiation, a risk factor for subsequent cataract formation.[21]

Histology/Immunohistochemistry

An immunohistochemical analysis of orbital tissue in thyroid-associated orbitopathy (TAO) suggests that most of the infiltrating lymphocytic cells in the active stage of GO are clearly T cells, and a significant number of them are CD45RO+ cells. Infiltration of orbital connective tissue by HLA-Dr+, CD25+, and tumor necrosis factor α (TNF-α) cells suggests that Th1-type immune reaction with the interference of proinflammatory cytokine(s) (TNF-α) may be of relevance in the pathogenesis of disease.[23]

Risk Factors Promoting GO

- Smoking
- The therapeutic administration of radioactive iodine for hyperthyroidism
- Posttreatment hypothyroidism
- Additional contributing factors:
    - Prominently elevated pretreatment levels of T3 and TSH-R autoantibody titers
    The severity of hyperthyroidism as manifested by high pretreatment T3 is an additional risk factor for the evolution or deterioration of GO.[24] Furthermore, high serum T3 level in patients treated with radioactive iodine (RAI) was associated with worse clinical outcome.[25] The risk for developing or worsening of GO was 22% for a patient with serum T3 levels above 5 nmol/L compared with only a 2% risk if serum T3 levels were below this threshold. Thyroid-stimulating immunoglobulins, in contrast, have been found in more than 90% of patients with active GD and in 50% to 90% of euthyroid thyroid eye disease (TED) patients. In addition, high TSH-R autoantibody titers and post-RAI–induced hypothyroidism are additional independent risk factors for the evolution of GO following RAI.[26]
    - The role of adipocytes in orbital tissue expansion
    The role of 11 beta hydroxysteroid dehydrogenase-1 (11 beta HSD1) as a determinant of adipocyte differentiation and its role in the inflammatory pathways in the orbital fat from patients with GO has been studied and compared with normal orbital fat (OF).[27] Fat was harvested from the orbits of 46 patients with GO and 44 controls undergoing orbital surgery. Samples were examined by a combination of immunohistochemistry, real-time reverse transcriptase polymerase chain reaction, primary cell culture, specific enzyme assays, colorimetric proliferation assays, and bead-based enzyme-linked immunosorbent assay (ELISA). Primary cultures of GO OF stromal cells demonstrated greater 11-beta HSD1 oxoreductase activity, which was regulated by cytokines, most notably TNF and interleukin (IL)-6,

compared with controls. Activity increased across differentiation, and this was most marked in GO cells. Similarly, stromal cell proliferation was limited by incubation with cortisol in GO cells. This evidence suggests that 11 beta HSD1 may have a role in regulating the inflammatory process in the OF in GO.

○ Role of the orbital fibroblast

The orbital fibroblast is clearly central to the autoimmune attack in the orbit and the pathogenesis of GO.[24] The recruitment of immune cells within the orbit is associated with fibroblast activation, which is a chief determinant of the expansion of orbital tissue responsible for ocular protrusion (proptosis) that is the hallmark of GO.[28] Pritchard and colleagues[29] reported that immunoglobulin G (IgG) isolated from patients with GD (GD-IgG) upregulates T-lymphocyte chemoattractant activity in fibroblasts from orbit, thyroid, and skin in GD . This chemoattraction is specific to donors with GD, and is absent in fibroblasts from donors without thyroid disease. In addition, this chemoattraction can be partially neutralized by antibodies directed against IL-16 and RANTES (Regulated upon Activation, Normal T cell Expressed and Secreted). IL-16 is a CD4(+)-specific chemoattractant, whereas RANTES is a C-C chemokine that targets D4+ memory, activated naive T lymphocytes and monocytes, basophils, and eosinophils.[30] IL-16 is expressed by CD8+ and CD4+ lymphocytes in addition to eosinophils, fibroblasts, and thyrocytes.[31]

Specifically GD-IgG in GD fibroblasts acts to increase protein levels of the CD4+-specific chemoattractant IL-16 and the C-C type chemokine, RANTES. Protein levels of IL-16 and RANTES are substantially elevated by GD-derived IgG acting on fibroblasts in GD. It is notable that the addition of the macrolide, rapamycin, to fibroblast culture medium prevented upregulation by GD-IgG of IL-16, thus implicating the mTOR pathway in the induction of IL-16 expression. These findings suggest a specific mechanism for fibroblast activation in GD, which results in T-cell recruitment.[29]

○ The role of insulinlike growth factor 1 (IGF-1)

Evidence now suggests that IGF-1/IGF-1R pathway is implicated as a mechanism by which GD fibroblasts are activated.[32] When this auto-antigen is activated in GD fibroblasts by IGF-1 or GD-IgG, the production of both IL-16 and RANTES is increased, resulting in both T-lymphocyte chemoattraction and hyaluronan synthesis.[30] IGF-1 and GD-IgG potentially induce both IL-16 and RANTES in human thyrocyte culture. This induction was attenuated by dexamethasone and unaltered by TSH.

Rapamycin, a specific inhibitor of the FKBP12 rapamycin-associated protein (FRAP)/mammalian target of rapamycin/p70s6k pathway, prevented IL-16 synthesis induced by GD-IgG. The use of a monoclonal antibody directed at IGF-IR also blocked the induction of chemoattraction as well as synthesis of RANTES mRNA. The findings of Giannoukakis and Smith[33] suggest that thyrocytes can be activated by GD-IgG and IGF-1 to elaborate powerful T-cell chemoattractants. Because TSH did not alter induction of chemoattractants, these actions of GD-IgG would not appear to be mediated via the TSH receptor. However, in GD, thyrocytes may participate directly in lymphocyte recruitment to the thyroid via IL-16 and RANTES expression.[30]

Management

Appropriate management of GO must address both the thyroid dysfunction and the orbitopathy concomitantly. Euthyroidism should be restored promptly and stably maintained. During the initial phases of treatment when changes of thyroid status are anticipated, monitoring of thyroid status and indices every 4 to 6 weeks is mandatory.[34] A multidisciplinary team of both endocrinologists and ophthalmologists is often required and referral to specialist center, support of smoking cessation including identification of patients who are at risk of second-hand smoke exposures, and prompt treatment to restore and maintain euthyroidism are strongly advocated by present guidelines.[34]

There is retrospective evidence that smoking cessation is associated with better clinical outcomes in GO, and all patients with GO should be encouraged to stop smoking. Current guidelines advocate that all patients with GD should be informed of the risks of smoking and its detrimental effects on the development of GO, the potential deterioration of preexisting GO, the decreased effectiveness of treatments for GO in the presence of ongoing tobacco use, and the potential progression of GO following RAI.[34]

The most widely used disease activity classification system is NOSPECS, which is an acronym that documents the presence of specific symptoms and signs, of which only some are characteristic of active disease.[35] More recently, the modified clinical activity score (CAS) has been used to assess disease activity. The CAS assigns a point to each symptom or sign when it is present (retrobulbar pain or spontaneous ocular pain, and pain with ocular movements, eyelid edema, eyelid erythema, conjunctival injection, chemosis, and swelling of the caruncle) and is a simple summation that does not provide information regarding overall progression or severity. GO is considered active when the sum (CAS) is at least 3/7 and this is predictive of the responsiveness of GO to steroids.[34] Used in conjunction with this is a classification schema stratifying GO into mild, moderate, or severe and sight threatening depending on the degree of lid retraction, soft tissue involvement, proptosis, degree of extraocular muscle involvement (the presence or absence or diplopia), corneal involvement, and the optic nerve status. For example, mild ophthalmopathy is usually defined as proptosis of less than 22 mm, intermittent or diplopia or none, an absence of optic neuropathy, and mild conjunctival and periorbital inflammation. Moderate or severe disease on the other hand is associated with significant proptosis (which can vary by race), increased inflammation of soft tissues, and constant diplopia. In practice, the identification of active GO remains imperfect, relying on the combination of the patient's dynamic clinical picture and the clinician's snapshot interpretation of the corresponding physical signs and symptoms.

In general, the management of thyrotoxicosis is an equally important yet separate goal in patients with GO. RAI therapy without concurrent corticosteroids, antithyroid drugs, such as methimazole (ATD), and thyroidectomy are equally acceptable therapeutic options in patients with Graves hyperthyroidism and inactive ophthalmopathy. Of the 3 established treatments (ATDs, RAI, and thyroidectomy), RAI is the only one possibly associated with a progression of GO; however, this can be prevented by concomitant steroid prophylaxis. In patients with GD and mild active GO, RAI therapy, methimazole, and thyroidectomy are equally acceptable therapeutic options in managing the thyrotoxicosis; however, concurrent treatment with oral corticosteroids should be considered in these patients who have no other risk factors for deterioration of their eye disease and who elect radiation therapy. Mild or inactive disease also may be treated with local measures, such as artificial tears to keep the ocular surface moist and do not require immunosuppressive therapy. Patients with Graves hyperthyroidism and active, moderate-to-severe or sight-threatening ophthalmopathy probably should not be treated with radioactive iodine, but instead treated with either methimazole or surgery and the inflammation controlled with intravenous (IV) glucocorticoids. Patients with inactive, moderate to severe GO should be referred to specialist centers for rehabilitative ocular surgery. It is unclear if radioactive therapy will be beneficial for this group of patients because of the risk of worsening ophthalmopathy. Patients with sight-threatening dysthyroid optic neuropathy should receive intravenous glucocorticoids, and if a poor clinical response is noted after 2 weeks, or there is intolerance to therapy, patients should be referred for prompt orbital decompressive surgery or receive adjunctive orbital radiation.

A significant minority of patients do not respond to strategic immunosuppression for GO, at least in part because it would be expected that only patients in the active stages of disease would respond. Although patients may be selected on the basis of GO severity, only the patients with signs and symptoms of active, inflammatory GO would be anticipated to respond. Patients with severe but fibrotic GO lacking a significant inflammatory component, would not be expected to respond to anti-inflammatory and immunosuppressive strategies.

Anti-inflammatory and Immunomodulatory Therapies

Steroids

Generally, glucocorticoids provide nonspecific immunosuppression in GO, but they have many side effects. Their efficacy is modest, as one-third of the patients do not respond, and the improvement in responders is limited. There is evidence for efficacy with therapy with oral, IV, and peribulbar use corticosteroids.[36] In one multicenter randomized prospective study, patients with GO of less than 6 months' duration, were treated with either 4 doses of 20 mg of triamcinolone acetate 40 mg/mL in a peribulbar injection to the inferolateral orbital quadrant or placebo. Triamcinolone injection was effective in decreasing diplopia and the sizes of extraocular muscles in recent-onset ophthalmopathy without systemic or ocular side effects.[37] Oral prednisone with typical doses of 30 to 40 mg per day has been shown to be effective in the treatment of active, moderate to severe GO. The duration of therapy may extend as far as 3 months but patients should be assessed for response within 4 to 6 weeks, after which other therapies should be considered if no improvement is seen. IV steroids, however, have been shown to have many advantages over oral streroids in terms of greater clinical response and improvement, and fewer adverse events.

According to the European Group on Graves' Orbitopathy recommendations, sight-threatening GO should be treated first with IV glucocorticoids. The clinical goal is to diminish orbital inflammation and congestion, and to prevent advancement of the autoimmune pathology. Response to therapy should be assessed after 1 to 2 weeks, and if poorly responsive, referral for urgent surgical decompression considered.[38]

A 6- to 12-week course of high-dose IV glucocorticoid pulse is first line for active moderate to severe GO. This regimen is preferred over oral treatment regimens with fewer adverse events. Careful patient selection is indicated to avoid exacerbation of preexisting diseases, such as diabetes. Before IV steroid administration, it is recommended that patients should be screened for liver dysfunction, uncontrolled diabetes mellitus, and glaucoma. High doses of IV glucocorticoids have been associated with significant toxicity. Hepatotoxicity with severe liver damage occurred in 7 of approximately 800 patients with GO treated in Italy with IV high-dose steroids, and of those 7, 3 died.[39] However, no cases of liver failure have been reported in patients with GO receiving oral steroids or a cumulative dose of IV methylprednisolone of less than 8 g, although care should be taken and administered only in experienced centers. There is evidence that an early response to IV glucocorticoid for severe GO predicts treatment outcome. In a nonrandomized prospective series of 15 patients treated with high-dose pulse methylprednisolone, 83% of patients with severe GO showed clinically significant response by the end of the first week.[40]

Steroid prophylaxis in patients receiving RAI
Most studies of patients with GD suggest that radioiodine therapy can cause the onset or worsening of ophthalmopathy compared with antithyroid drug therapy or sugery.[26,41,42] It may also be associated with the appearance or exacerbation of infiltrative dermopathy (pretibial myxedema).[43] The reason for this is unknown, but it is speculated that it is related to a rise in serum thyrotropin receptor antibodies, and other thyroid antigens may be a factor.[44] Multiple prospective studies show substantial benefit of steroid prophylaxis for GO in patients with GD without moderate to severe eye disease who elect to receive radioiodine. Randomized trials from Italy evaluated the use of prednisone subsequent to RAI therapy. In the trial by Bartalena and colleagues,[42] the dosage used was 0.4 to 0.5 mg/kg of body weight per day for 1 month starting at 1 to 3 days after radioiodine, and then tapered over 3 months. This study was designed primarily to address in a randomized fashion the effects of treatment of GD with methimazole or radiotherapy alone, as well as the effects of glucocorticoids in patients with mild or moderate GO or none. Patients were evaluated for progression of ophthalmopathy at intervals of 1 to 2 months for 12 months. Another important feature in this study was that hypothyroidism and persistent hyperthyroidism were promptly corrected, which was likely based on a prior Swedish retrospective analysis of 492 patients with GD that suggested early administration of LT4 decreased the occurrence of GO and that both hyperthyroidism and hypothyroidism can exacerbate GO.[45] Ophthalmopathy developed or worsened in 23 (15%) of 150 patients treated with RAI at 2 to 6 months after treatment. None of the 55 other patients in this group who had ophthalmopathy at baseline had improvement in their eye disease. Among the 145 patients treated with both RAI and prednisone, 50 (67%) of the 75 with ophthalmopathy at baseline had improvement, and no patient had progression. It is notable that the prevalence of permanent hypothyroidism after RAI was similar in patients treated with RAI alone (62%) versus RAI followed by steroids (66%). Therefore, it does not appear that post-RAI glucocorticoids affect the biochemical therapeutic outcome of RAI for hyperthyroidism. Therefore, consistent with the European Group of Graves Orbitopathy recommendations, glucocorticoids can be safely given following RAI without concern for decreased treatment efficacy. Among 148 patients treated with methimazole alone, 3 (2%) with ophthalmopathy at baseline improved, whereas 4 (3%) showed worsening of eye disease.

In a subsequent retrospective cohort study, a lower starting dose of steroids (0.2 mg/kg body weight) was compared with previously reported doses (>0.3 mg/kg body weight), with tapering over 6 weeks. The lower dose and shorter treatment period was also shown to be effective in preventing exacerbations of ophthalmopathy in most patients. In addition, there was less body weight increase in the patients who received a lower steroid dose.[46]

The use of RAI in patients with severe GO has not been studied. It is recommended that smokers with preexisting GO and those with severe hyperthyroidism or high thyrotropin receptor antibody titers should be considered for glucocorticoid prophylaxis before RAI, as these are clear risk factors for deterioration of GO after RAI.

Steroids versus surgery
In patients with active GO and optic neuropathy, surgical decompression was compared with IV corticosteroids as first-line treatment with change in visual acuity as the primary outcome.[47] In the surgically treated group, 83% of patients eventually needed additional IV corticosteroid therapy, whereas in the IV corticosteroid group, 56% of patients needed additional therapy (either surgery or orbital radiotherapy).

Orbital irradiation
Radiation therapy is believed to kill retro-orbital T cells and fibroblasts and arrest the immune inflammatory response. There have been 3 controlled trials to date of orbital radiotherapy using sham radiotherapy as control for patients with moderately severe GO.[48–50] The administered retrobulbar radiotherapy totaled 20 Gy in 10 divided fractions of 2 Gy each. Follow-up varied from 6 to 12 months, and overall it was shown that there was no advantage with radiotherapy or x-ray therapy (XRT) over the control group in terms of the CAS score, proptosis, or lid aperture. There was the suggestion that XRT was better than control in terms of diplopia reduction in 2 of the 3 trials on the basis of improvement in extraocular muscle function and motility impairment. Overall adverse events from orbital radiotherapy were generally mild but could include cataracts, radiation retinopathy, and radiation optic neuropathy and without an increased risk of cancer with 30-year follow-up.[51]

Although there have been 2 studies comparing high-dose versus low-dose radiation (16.0 vs 2.4 Gy and 20 Gy vs 10 Gy), in neither trial was there a significant difference between low-dose versus high-dose radiation.[52,53] It is important to note that retrobulbar irradiation is not indicated in children with GO because of the theoretical risk of subsequent tumor induction,[54] although this has not been demonstrated in adults after a 30-year follow-up.[55]

Orbital irradiation alone and in combination versus steroids
In one trial, orbital radiation was felt to be more effective than a 3-month course of oral glucocorticoids for patients with moderately severe GO (using NOSPECS). Both groups showed improvements in total and subjective eye score and a decrease in eye-muscle volume; however, orbital radiation had fewer side effects compared with steroids[56] Combination treatment of systemic corticosteroids and radiotherapy was compared with steroid treatment alone in 2 trials and with radiotherapy alone in 1 trial.[57–59] Treatment with combination of orbital radiotherapy and corticosteroids was significantly better than with either treatment alone. In the subgroup of orbital radiotherapy plus corticosteroids versus corticosteroids alone, the addition of radiotherapy resulted in significantly better results. There was no difference between groups in proptosis and visual acuity at the end of follow-up.

Somatostatin analogs
IGF-1 receptor antibodies have been demonstrated in most patients with GD and may play a role in GO pathogenesis via fibroblast and thyrocyte stimulation and expansion of memory T cells. Somatostatin analogs are thought to inhibit both lymphocyte proliferation and activation, and their accumulation in the orbital tissue of patients with GO. Despite the significant insights into the underlying pathophysiology of GO, which implicate IGF-1 in disease pathogenesis, the clinical outcomes of somatostatin analogs in GO have either been either conflicting or disappointing.

Three double-blind, placebo-controlled trials of octreotide long-acting release (LAR) of 30 mg monthly for 12 to 16 weeks in patients with moderate to severe GO showed no significant therapeutic effect of octreotide LAR. The reduction in soft tissue inflammation and CAS were similar in both groups.[60] A similar study from the Mayo Clinic showed no significant difference between octreotide LAR and the placebo group except for improvement in eyelid fissure in the treatment group.[61]

Cyclosporine
Cyclosporine modulates T-cell function by preventing the dephosphorylation of lymphocyte transcription factors through its binding with cyclophilins. This results in inhibition of lymphokine production and interleukin release and leads to a reduced

function of effector T cells. Two trials have evaluated the effect of immunomodulation with cyclosporine in patients with active GO. The first evaluated cyclosporine in addition to oral corticosteroids versus oral corticosteroids alone. In the combination group, there was a greater reduction in a defined activity score and a lower relapse rate after corticosteroid discontinuation.[62] The second study showed better response rate with oral corticosteroids as a single therapy.[63]

Etanercept

To date, the only clinical data with the anti-TNF agent, etanercept, in GO is a small, noncontrolled pilot study involving 10 patients with recent-onset, active, mildly-to-moderately severe GO treated with subcutaneous injections of 25 mg etanercept (Enbrel) twice weekly over 12 weeks.[64] After therapy, the mean CAS fell by 60%. The main decrease in scores was seen at 6 weeks of treatment. Improvement was particularly evident with respect to soft tissue changes, periocular chemosis, and erythema; however, no change was observed in mean exophthalmometry measurements. GO flared after cessation of etanercept therapy in 3 patients, but no serious adverse events were reported with etanercept over a mean follow-up time of 18 months.

Rituximab

Rituximab (RTX) is an anti-CD20 monoclonal antibody that induces transient B-cell depletion as an anti-inflammatory strategy in the orbit.[65] CD20 is expressed on all immature B cells but not stem cells or most plasma cells. The rationale for this strategy is that B lymphocytes are important antigen-presenting cells and present self-antigens similarly. They are also precursors for antibody-secreting plasma cells. It has been shown that RTX induces not only a fall in peripheral lymphocytes but also it can also inhibit B-cell antigen presentation,[66] and cause depletion of intraorbital CD20+ lymphocytes.[67] RTX has been postulated to cause a fall in TSH receptor antibody levels[68]; however, this has not been demonstrated in other studies.[69,70] A number of studies have indicated that some patients with severe Graves orbitopathy may respond dramatically to B-cell depletion induced by RTX. In a small, open-pilot study comparing RTX to glucocorticoids, peripheral B-cell depletion was achieved in all patients after the first RTX infusion and only minor side effects were reported in 3 patients.[71] CAS values with RTX decreased more significantly compared with IV glucocorticoids. Relapse of active GO was not seen in RTX-treated patients, although relapse was noted in 10% of those treated with IV glucocorticoids. The steroid-treated patients also had more adverse events. There are other few small, uncontrolled studies that have showed some effects of RTX, particularly in glucocorticoid-resistant GO.[69,72,73]

Caution is indicated in consideration of this drug, however, because of reports of significant adverse events and even therapeutic nonresponse.[74] Patients may develop a serum-sicknesslike reaction, iridocyclitis, polyarthralgia, and inflammatory bowel disease after treatment with RTX.[75] Although it might represent a useful treatment for the orbitopathy of GD, randomized clinical trials are needed to establish its ultimate role.

Azathioprine

Azathioprine is not effective in treatment of patients with moderately severe thyroid-associated ophthalmopathy. In a small study involving 20 patients with moderately severe GO, 10 patients received azathioprine, whereas the other 10 matched patients served as controls.[5] Although azathioprine did induce a significant fall in thyroid auto-immunity, with fall in titers of both thyroid microsomal and thyroid-stimulating hormone binding inhibiting immunoglobulin index, no improvement in clinical ocular parameters were seen with azathioprine. With time, however, intraocular pressure fell in both groups, suggesting a spontaneous improvement in moderate-severity GO over time.

Selenium

A recent randomized, double-blind, placebo-controlled trial investigated the effect of the antioxidant selenium in 159 Italian patients with mild Graves orbitopathy.[76] Patients were given selenium (100 μg twice daily), pentoxifylline (600 mg twice daily), or placebo (twice daily) orally for 6 months and were then followed for 6 months after withdrawal of treatment. Primary outcomes at 6 months were evaluated by means of an overall ophthalmic assessment, conducted by an ophthalmologist unaware of the treatment assignments, and a Graves orbitopathy–specific quality-of-life question-naire, completed by the patient. Secondary outcomes were evaluated with the use of a CAS and a diplopia score. At the 6-month evaluation, selenium, but not pentoxifyl-line, was significantly associated with improved quality of life compared with placebo. It also slowed the progression of Graves orbitopathy compared with placebo. The CAS decreased in all groups, but the change was significantly greater in selenium-treated patients. No adverse events were seen with selenium. The investigators concluded that selenium administration significantly improved quality of life, reduced ocular involvement, and slowed disease progression in patients with mild Graves orbitopathy.

Potential future therapeutic agents for GO

Imatinib mesylate Imatinib is a tyrosine kinase inhibitor that blocks the platelet-derived growth factor (PDGF) receptor, and c-Abl and c-Kit activity. In an in vitro tissue culture model, Van Steensel and colleagues[77] recently reported on the potential effi-cacy of imatinib for the treatment of GO. Orbital fat from 10 patients with GO was grown in tissue culture (n = 10) and cultured with or without imatinib mesylate or ada-limumab. PDGF-B and TNF-α mRNA expression levels were determined in the primary orbital tissue, and IL-6 and hyaluronan were measured in tissue-culture supernatants. Imatinib mesylate significantly diminished both IL-6 and hyaluronan production. The inhibition of hyaluronan production correlated with the PDGF-B mRNA level in the primary tissue. Imatinib mesylate can be expected to reduce inflammation and tissue remodeling in GO, whereas adalimumab would be mainly expected to reduce inflam-mation. To date, no clinical trials of imatinib in GO have been published.

Pirfenidone Perfenidone is a preclinical agent that has been shown to have significant effects on animal model of bleomycin induced pulmonary fibrosis where expression of transforming growth factor (TGF)-beta 1 and tissue inhibitors of metalloproteinase (TIMP)-1 in lung tissue was inhibited.[78] Kim and colleagues[79] recently examined the effects of IL-1beta and fibroblast growth factor (FGF), PDGF, and TGF-beta on the induction of TIMP-1 in orbital fibroblasts of patients with TAO. TIMP-1 protein levels were measured by ELISA and Western blot, and TIMP-1 activity assessed by reverse zymography. The actions of pirfenidone on TIMP-1 induction in orbital fibroblasts were compared with dexamethasone as a reference agent. A hydroxyproline assay assessed the effect of pirfenidone and dexamethasone on collagen production in orbital fibroblasts. IL-1beta increased the level of active TIMP-1 protein in a dose-dependent fashion, (whereas FGF, PDGF, and TGF-beta did not induce TIMP-1). Pir-fenidone was more effective than dexamethasone in blocking IL-1beta–induced increases in TIMP-1, reducing TIMP-1 levels to less than those in untreated controls at a minimal concentration (5 mM). Moreover, pirfenidone effectively decreased hydroxyproline levels in orbital fibroblasts, suggesting a decrease in collagen levels, whereas dexamethasone had no such effect. Pirfenidone decreases TIMP-1 and collagen levels in orbital fibroblasts of patients with GO, thereby exerting an antifibrotic effect.

SUMMARY

GO can have frightening consequences for a significant number of patients. Immunotherapy is offering a real opportunity of reducing bad outcomes that lead to disfigurement and impairment of vision. These therapies are not perfect yet; however, we now have a real chance to achieve better outcomes.

IMMUNOTHERAPY OF ASTHMA

Asthma is the most common chronic respiratory disease. It is defined as a chronic inflammatory disease of the airways associated with enhanced airway narrowing response to triggers, such as allergens and exercise. This leads to a multitude of episodic symptoms, such as coughing, chest tightness, dyspnea, and wheezing. It was Salter, a London physician, who in 1860 defined asthma with remarkable precision, "Paroxysonal dyspnea of a peculiar character with intervals of healthy respiration between attacks," and attributed these episodes to contractions of smooth muscles.[80] In the United States, asthma affects 25 million people, resulting in incremental cost to society totaling $18 billion (with direct cost of $10 billion).[81] Given the ever-increasing cost to the society, effective treatment(s) remain top priority. How treatments have evolved and changed over time can be gauged from a 200th anniversary *New England Journal of Medicine* article by Mutius and Drazen[82] using 3 account/views of consultation for a patient with asthma when seen in 1829, 1928, and 2012. Current approach to management is patient centered and targets medication selection, and their dose and delivery systems. There has been significant impact on clinical outcomes, but still more can be done.

Pathophysiology

For a long time asthma was considered as a disease of bronchoconstriction and treated predominantly with bronchodilators; however, presently it is considered as an inflammatory disease of the lungs/airways and corticosteroids are viewed as the mainstay of asthma therapeutics. Because of earlier emphasis on bronchoconstriction, therapies were mostly directed at relieving bronchospasm. This phase was followed by appreciation of asthma as an inflammatory disorder that currently seems to hold sway. Asthma is now recognized as a triad of intermittent airway obstruction, bronchial smooth muscle cell hyperactivity to bronchoconstrictors, and chronic bronchial inflammation. The entire process unfolds in 2 phases: an induction phase and chronic phase. Present accumulated knowledge places IgE at the center of the allergen trigger, helping initiate and maintaining allergic response. Although IgE is an important trigger for inflammation, disease chronicity is a function of recruitment and activation of T_H^2-type T cells that secrete a wide range of cytokines and chemokines that are proallergic. It should be noted that a second-tier control mechanism to regulate T_H^2 responses has been recognized, and this includes regulatory T (Treg) cells that suppress T_H^2 responses partially through generation of cytokine IL-10.[83] Alternatively, therefore, asthma could be considered as a consequence of defective Treg cell inhibitors of T_H^2 responses.

During the induction phase, allergen-specific $CD4^+$ T_H^2 cells secrete a range of cytokines, such as IL-5, IL-9, IL-13, and granulocyte-macrophage colony-stimulating factor. IL-4 and IL-3 promote B-cell class switch, resulting in production of allergen-specific IgE antibody. Allergen-specific IgE antibody binds to mast cells and basophils through high-affinity receptor for IgE, thus resulting in sensitization of the patient to the allergen. This entire process is presaged by activation of dendritic cells and antigen presentation to CD4$^+$ cells. Once IgE is secreted, it binds to the surface of mast cells that release the contents of their granules, which include histamine, prostaglandins, and leukotrienes. Additionally, chemokines released from the mast cells promote eosinophil recruitment.

Better understanding of pathogenesis offers greater potential for targeted therapeutics, starting from allergen avoidance and conventional immunosuppression (using steroids) to suppression/antagonism of cytokines/chemokines involved in the cascading inflammatory response. A comprehensive and elegant review on pathophysiology of asthma has recently been published by Holgate.[84]

Current Treatments

Presently the goal of asthma management revolves around achieving and maintaining control of the disease to prevent exacerbations. In most cases, control can be achieved through the use of avoidance measures coupled with the pharmacologic interventions. The principles of the treatment can be classified as controllers (taken daily, on a long-term basis to achieve control mainly through anti-inflammatory effects) and relievers (used on an as-needed basis for quick relief of bronchospasm) (**Table 1**).

A simple and concise review on asthma and its therapeutics may be found in a recent article by Kim and Mazza.[85] Long-acting beta$_2$-agonist (LABA) monotherapy is not recommended because it does not affect inflammation and is associated with increased risk of morbidity/mortality. These are recommended only in combination with inhaled corticosteroids. Given that asthma is an inflammatory disorder with strong underpinning of immune dysfunction, immunotherapy has been the focus of attention starting with corticosteroids used as the mainstay of effective therapeutic regimens. With better appreciation of pathways involved, newer vistas are being explored.

IMMUNOTHERAPEUTICS IN ASTHMA
Subcutaneously Injected Allergen Immunotherapy

Subcutaneously injected allergen immunotherapy was first developed in 1911 at St. Mary's Hospital in London.[86] It was designed to treat seasonal allergic rhinoconjunctivitis. Only during the second half of the 20th century was allergen-specific immunotherapy attempted in patients with asthma. It involved subcutaneous injections of gradually increasing quantities of relevant allergens until an effective dose is reached, which induces immunologic tolerance to the antigen. A Cochrane review

Table 1
Therapeutic classes

Controllers	Relievers
• Inhaled corticosteroids (ICS)[a]	• Rapid-acting inhaled B$_2$-agonists[b]
• Leukotriene receptor antagonists (LTRAs)	• Inhaled anticholinergic bronchodilators
• Long-acting beta$_2$-agonists (LABAs) in combination with an ICS	
• Anti-IgE therapy	

[a] Systemic corticosteroids may be needed for acute asthma or severe exacerbations.
[b] Formoterol, a LABA, has a rapid onset of action and may be used as a reliever.

of 75 randomized controlled trials examining allergen-specific immunotherapy in asthma management confirmed efficacy, as reflected in symptom score improvements and reduction in dosage of medication requirements.[87] Similar benefits have been observed with sublingual immunotherapy (SLIT).[88] The current international recommendations for subcutaneous immunotherapy and SLIT were recently reviewed in 2011 by Calderon and colleagues.[89] At present, allergen-specific immunotherapy is not universally accepted in all clinical practice guidelines and it should be considered on a case-by-case basis. SLIT is an approved treatment for allergic rhinitis in many countries. In January 2011, the Joint Task Force on Practice Parameters, representing the American Academy of Allergy, Asthma and Immunology and the American College of Allergy, Asthma and Immunology, updated its practice guidelines.[90] A recent review of current understanding of the mechanisms of allergen-specific immunotherapy suggests that Treg lymphocytes are the key orchestrators of immunotherapy-induced allergen tolerance.[91] Allergen-specific immunotherapy is better avoided in children younger than 6 years; in women who are pregnant; in elderly individuals; and in patients with malignancy, immunodeficiency, or autoimmune diseases. It should also be avoided in those with cardiovascular disability, uncontrolled and severe asthma, and those receiving beta blockers. The World Allergy Organization has developed an elaborate grading system (Grades I to V) for systemic reactions to subcutaneous immunotherapy.[92] This should guide future standardization of adverse reactions.

Monoclonal Antibodies in Treatment of Asthma

Use of monoclonal antibodies represents a form of immunotherapy using passive immunity. In 1986, OKT^3 anti-CD_3 (muromonab-CD_3) used for prevention of acute renal transplant rejection became the first murine monoclonal antibody approved for human use by the Food and Drug Administration.[93] Since then a variety of monoclonal antibodies have been approved for clinical use in a variety of disorders.

Asthma, in most patients, can be controlled by regular use of inhaled corticosteroids combined with short-acting $beta_2$ agonists. In some patients, however, exacerbations continue to remain frequent, necessitating higher doses of steroids and adding other available medications. This often leads to noncompliance and/or adverse side effects from chronic high-dose steroid exposure. Alternative therapies are being explored basing rationale on complex cellular and inflammatory/immune phenotypes encountered in patients with asthma. This has broadened the targets of therapeutic intervention(s) bringing within its ambit mast cells, eosinophils, macrophages, dendritic cells, epithelial cells, activated T-cells ($T_H{}^1$, $T_H{}^2$, Tregs), and related cytokines/chemokines. A variety of antibodies have undergone trials to determine efficacy and safety for possible human use. Currently omalizumab is the only monoclonal antibody approved as add-on therapy for use in severe, persistent allergic asthma.

Omalizumab (Xolair) is a recombinant DNA-derived humanized, IgG_1k monoclonal antibody. It selectively binds to circulating human IgE. Once antibody engages circulating IgE, it becomes biologically inactive because binding of IgE to receptor sites is prevented. The level of circulating IgE progressively decreases as it is removed via the reticuloendothelial system. Subcutaneous administration of omalizumab has been known to decrease asthma exacerbations, improve symptom score, and reduce frequency of asthma attacks.

Omalizumab use requires documentation of serum total IgE levels between 30 and 700 IU/mL, evidence of specific allergen sensitivity, and presence of frequent exacerbations. At this time, the steroid-sparing effect remains to be established. In patients not well controlled with high-dose corticosteroids and LABA, use of omalizumab reduced exacerbations by 25%.[94] Monoclonal antibodies against other targets[95] that are currently unapproved for clinical use include the following:

a. Monoclonal antibodies against TNF-α
b. Monoclonal antibodies against IL-5
c. Anti-CD4 monoclonal antibody
d. Monoclonal antibodies targeting IL-4/IL-13 pathways
e. (c-kit)/PDGF receptor-tyrosine kinase inhibitor.

None of these has reached a stage of proven efficacy to start large-scale trials.

SUMMARY

Asthma is a disorder of airways inflammation manifesting as a syndrome of episodic bronchoconstriction attended by shortness of breath and wheezing. Although a variety of new treatments are available, a major reliance is placed on corticosteroid therapy, which exposes the patient to adverse side effects from steroid use. Immune therapy using passive immunity targeting key proinflammatory cytokine/chemokines and medications of their effects has opened a new avenue of research into a safe and durable therapy. Currently one such agent, omalizumab, appears to be safe and effective in clinical use.

IMMUNOTHERAPY IN REGIONAL PAINFUL SYNDROME

The complex regional painful syndrome has an incidence of 2.6 per 10,000 person years.[96] Depending on absence or presence of injury to major nerves, it may be classified as type 1 or type 2. Previously, it was known as Causalgia Sudeck Atrophy, reflex sympathetic dystrophy, and algodystrophy.

Patients have a difficult time with recovery, and the experience can be frustrating. Treatments are often ineffective and frustrating. There is growing evidence of immune activation.[97,98] This has brought to realization the possibility of immunomodulation for alleviating the pain.

In a recent trial of 13 eligible patients who had pain intensity greater than 4 on an 11-point scale and complex regional pain syndrome for 6 to 30 months refractory to standard treatment, intravenous immunoglobulin (IVIG) treatment was compared against normal saliva treatment. Twelve patients completed the trial.[99]

In this study, IVIG 0.5 g/kg administration reduced pain intensity by 1.55 units more than after saliva treatment. In 3 patients, pain intensity was reduced 501% more than after saliva (each patient received 2 treatments of IVIG or saliva). It is than possible that immune mechanisms may be involved in sustaining long-standing pain, and that IVIG may moderate pain sensitivity by reducing immune activation.

REFERENCES

1. Lazarus JH. Acute pretibial myxedema, Graves' disease and radioiodine therapy. Clin Endocrinol 1995;42:661.
2. Weetman AP. Graves' disease. N Engl J Med 2000;343:1236–48.
3. Ludgate M, Baker G. Unlocking the immunological mechanisms of orbital inflammation in thyroid eye disease. Clin Exp Immunol 2002;127:193–8.
4. Wiersinga WM, Bartalena L. Epidemiology and prevention of Graves' ophthalmopathy. Thyroid 2002;12(10):855–60.
5. Perros P, Weightman DR, Crombie AL, et al. Azathioprine in the treatment of thyroid-associated ophthalmopathy. Acta Endocrinol (Copenh) 1990;122(1):8–12.

6. Goldstein SM, Katowitz WR, Moshang T, et al. Pediatric thyroid-associated orbit-opathy: the Children's Hospital of Philadelphia experience and literature review. Thyroid 2008;18(9):997–9.

7. Smith TJ, Koumas L, Gagnon A, et al. Orbital fibroblast heterogeneity may determine the clinical presentation of thyroid-associated ophthalmopathy. J Clin Endocrinol Metab 2002;87:385–92.

8. Smith TJ. Orbital fibroblasts exhibit a novel pattern of responses to proinflammatory cytokines: potential basis for the pathogenesis of thyroid-associated ophthalmopathy. Thyroid 2002;12:197–203.

9. Bahn RS, Gorman CA, Woloschak GE, et al. Human retroocular fibroblasts in vitro: a model for the study of Graves' ophthalmopathy. J Clin Endocrinol Metab 1987;65:665–70.

10. Wang HS, Cao HJ, Winn VD, et al. Leukoregulin induction of prostaglandin-endoperoxide H synthase-2 in human orbital fibroblasts. J Biol Chem 1996;271: 22718–28.

11. Cao HJ, Wang HS, Zhang Y, et al. Activation of human orbital fibroblasts through CD40 engagement results in a dramatic induction of hyaluronan synthesis and prostaglandin endoperoxide H synthase-2 expression. Insights into potential pathogenic mechanisms of thyroid-associated ophthalmopathy. J Biol Chem 1998;273:29615–25.

12. Smith TJ, Bahn RS, Gorman CA, et al. Stimulation of glycosaminoglycan accumulation by interferon gamma in cultured human retroocular fibroblasts. J Clin Endocrinol Metab 1991;72:1169–71.

13. Yang D, Hiromatsu Y, Hoshino T, et al. Dominant infiltration of T (H) 1-type CD4+ T cells at the retrobulbar space of patients with thyroid-associated ophthalmopathy. Thyroid 1999;9:305–10.

14. Aniszewski JP, Valyasevi RW, Bahn RS. Relationship between disease duration and predominant orbital T cell subset in Graves' ophthalmopathy. J Clin Endocrinol Metab 2000;85:776–80.

15. Bartalena L, Pinchera A, Marcocci C. Management of Graves' ophthalmopathy: reality and perspectives. Endocr Rev 2000;21:168–99.

16. Marcocci C, Bartalena L, Bogozzi F, et al. Studies on the occurrence of ophthalmopathy in Graves' disease. Acta Endocrinol (Copenh) 1989;120:473–8.

17. Bahn RS. Assessment and management of the patient with Graves' opthalmopathy. Endocr Pract 1995;1:172–8.

18. Bahn RS, Bartley GB, Gorman CA. Emergency treatment of Graves' ophthalmopathy. Baillieres Clin Endocrinol Metab 1992;6(1):95–105.

19. Prabhakar BS, Bahn RS, Smith TJ. Current perspective on the pathogenesis of Graves' disease and ophthalmopathy. Endocr Rev 2003;24(6):802–35.

20. Perros P, Crombie AL, Kendall-Taylor P. Natural history of thyroid associated ophthalmopathy. Clin Endocrinol (Oxf) 1995;42(1):45.

21. Pichler R, Sonnberger M, Dorninger C, et al. Ga-68-DOTA-NOC PET/CT reveals active Graves' orbitopathy in a single extraorbital muscle. Clin Nucl Med 2011; 36(10):910–1.

22. Kahaly GJ. Recent developments in Graves' ophthalmopathy imaging. J Endocrinol Invest 2004;27(3):254–8.

23. Avunduk AM, Avunduk MC, Pazarli H, et al. Immunohistochemical analysis of orbital connective tissue specimens of patients with active Graves ophthalmopathy. Curr Eye Res 2005;30:631–8.

24. Wiersinga WM, Prummel MF. Pathogenesis of Graves' ophthalmopathy—current understanding. J Clin Endocrinol Metab 2001;86(2):501–3.

25. Törring O, Tallstedt L, Wallin G, et al. Graves' hyperthyroidism: treatment with anti-thyroid drugs, surgery, or radioiodine—a prospective, randomized study. Thyroid Study Group. J Clin Endocrinol Metab 1996;81(8):2986–93.
26. Träisk F, Tallstedt L, Abraham-Nordling M, et al, Thyroid Study Group of TT 96. Thyroid-associated ophthalmopathy after treatment for Graves' hyperthyroidism with antithyroid drugs or iodine-131. J Clin Endocrinol Metab 2009;94(10):3700–7.
27. Tomlinson JW, Durrani OM, Bujalska IJ, et al. The role of 11beta-hydroxysteroid dehydrogenase 1 in adipogenesis in thyroid-associated ophthalmopathy. J Clin Endocrinol Metab 2010;95(1):398–406.
28. van Steensel L, Dik WA. The orbital fibroblast: a key player and target for therapy in Graves' ophthalmopathy. Orbit 2010;29(4):202–6.
29. Pritchard J, Horst N, Cruikshank W, et al. Igs from patients with Graves' disease induce the expression of T cell chemoattractants in their fibroblasts. J Immunol 2002;168(2):942–50.
30. Schall TJ, Bacon K, Toy KJ, et al. Selective attraction of monocytes and T lymphocytes of the memory phenotype by cytokine RANTES. Nature 1990; 347:669–71.
31. Douglas RS, Gianoukakis AG, Kamat S, et al. Aberrant expression of the insulin-like growth factor-1 receptor by T cells from patients with Graves' disease may carry functional consequences for disease pathogenesis. J Immunol 2007; 178(5):3281–7.
32. Douglas RS, Naik V, Hwang CJ, et al. B cells from patients with Graves' disease aberrantly express the IGF-1 receptor: implications for disease pathogenesis. J Immunol 2008;181(8):5768–74.
33. Gianoukakis AG, Smith TJ. Recent insights into the pathogenesis and management of thyroid-associated ophthalmopathy. Curr Opin Endocrinol Diabetes Obes 2008;15(5):446–52.
34. Bartalena L, Baldeschi L, Dickinson A, et al. Consensus statement of the European Group on Graves' Orbitopathy (EUGOGO) on management of GO. Eur J Endocrinol 2008;158:273–85.
35. Werner SC. Modification of the classification of the eye changes of Graves' disease: recommendations of the Ad Hoc Committee of the American Thyroid Association. J Clin Endocrinol Metab 1977;44:203–4.
36. Wiersinga WM. Immunosuppressive treatment of Graves' ophthalmopathy. Thyroid 1992;2(3):229.
37. Ebner R, Devoto MH, Weil D, et al. Treatment of thyroid associated ophthalmopathy with periocular injections of triamcinolone. Br J Ophthalmol 2004;88(11):1380–6.
38. Zang S, Ponto KA, Kahaly GJ. Clinical review: intravenous glucocorticoids for Graves' orbitopathy: efficacy and morbidity. J Clin Endocrinol Metab 2011; 96(2):320–32.
39. Marino M, Morabito E, Brunette MR, et al. Acute and severe liver damage associated with intravenous glucocorticoid pulse therapy in patients with Graves' ophthalmopathy. Thyroid 2004;14:403–6.
40. van Geest RJ, Sasim IV, Koppeschaar HP, et al. Methylprednisolone pulse therapy for patients with moderately severe Graves' orbitopathy: a prospective, randomized, placebo-controlled study. Eur J Endocrinol 2008;158(2): 229–37.
41. Tallstedt L, Lundell G, Tørring O, et al. Occurrence of ophthalmopathy after treatment for Graves' hyperthyroidism. The Thyroid Study Group. N Engl J Med 1992; 326(26):1733.

42. Bartalena L, Marcocci C, Bogazzi F, et al. A relation between therapy for hyper-thyroidism and the course of Graves' ophthalmopathy. N Engl J Med 1998; 338(2):73.

43. Harvey RD, Metcalfe RA, Morteo C, et al. Acute pre-tibial myxoedema following radioiodine therapy for thyrotoxic Graves' disease. Clin Endocrinol (Oxf) 1995; 42(6):657.

44. McGregor AM, Petersen MM, Capiferri R, et al. Effects of radioiodine on thyrotro-phin binding inhibiting immunoglobulins in Graves' disease. Clin Endocrinol (Oxf) 1979;11(4):437.

45. Tallstedt L, Lundell G, Blomgren H, et al. Does early administration of thyroxine reduce the development of Graves' ophthalmopathy after radioiodine treatment? Eur J Endocrinol 1994;130(5):494–7.

46. Lai A, Sassi L, Compri E, et al. Lower dose prednisone prevents radioiodine-associated exacerbation of initially mild or absent Graves' orbitopathy: a retrospec-tive cohort study. J Clin Endocrinol Metab 2010;95(3):1333–7.

47. Wakelkamp IM, Baldeschi L, Saeed P, et al. Surgical or medical decompression as a first-line treatment of optic neuropathy in Graves' ophthalmopathy? A randomized controlled trial. Clin Endocrinol (Oxf) 2005;63:323–8.

48. Prummel MF, Terwee CB, Gerding MN, et al. A randomized controlled trial of orbital radiotherapy versus sham irradiation in patients with mild Graves' oph-thalmopathy. J Clin Endocrinol Metab 2004;89:15–20.

49. Gorman CA, Garrity JA, Fatourechi V, et al. A prospective, randomized, double-blind, placebo-controlled study of orbital radiotherapy for Graves' ophthalmop-athy. Ophthalmology 2001;108:1523–34.

50. Mourits MP, van Kempen-Harteveld ML, Garcia MB, et al. Radiotherapy for Graves' orbitopathy: randomised placebo-controlled study. Lancet 2000;355: 1505–9.

51. Marquez SD, Lum BL, McDougall IR, et al. Long-term results of irradiation for patients with progressive Graves' ophthalmopathy. Int J Radiat Oncol Biol Phys 2001;51(3):766–74.

52. Gerling J, Kommerell G, Henne K, et al. Retrobulbar irradiation for thyroid-associated orbitopathy: double-blind comparison between 2.4 and 16 Gy. Int J Radiat Oncol Biol Phys 2003;55:182–9.

53. Kahaly GJ, Rosler HP, Pitz S, et al. Low- versus high-dose radiotherapy for Graves' ophthalmopathy: a randomized, single blind trial. J Clin Endocrinol Metab 2000;85:102–8.

54. Krassas GE, Gogakos A. Thyroid-associated ophthalmopathy in juvenile Graves' disease—clinical, endocrine and therapeutic aspects. J Pediatr Endocrinol Metab 2006;19(10):1193–206.

55. Schaefer U, Hesselmann S, Micke O, et al. A long-term follow-up study after retro-orbital irradiation for Graves' ophthalmopathy. Int J Radiat Oncol Biol Phys 2002; 52(1):192–7.

56. Prummel MF, Mourits MP, Blank L, et al. Randomized double-blind trial of predni-sone versus radiotherapy in Graves' ophthalmopathy. Lancet 1993;342(8877):949.

57. Ng CM, Yuen HK, Choi KL, et al. Combined orbital irradiation and systemic steroids compared with systemic steroids alone in the management of moderate-to-severe Graves' ophthalmopathy: a preliminary study. Hong Kong Med J 2005;11:322–30.

58. Bartalena L, Marcocci C, Chiovato L, et al. Orbital cobalt irradiation combined with systemic corticosteroids for Graves' ophthalmopathy: comparison with systemic corticosteroids alone. J Clin Endocrinol Metab 1983;56:1139–44.

59. Marcocci C, Bartalena L, Bogazzi F, et al. Orbital radiotherapy combined with high dose systemic glucocorticoids for Graves' ophthalmopathy is more effective than radiotherapy alone: results of a prospective randomized study. J Endocrinol Invest 1991;14:853–60.

60. Chang TC, Liao SL. Slow-release lanreotide in Graves' ophthalmopathy: a double-blind randomized, placebo-controlled clinical trial. J Endocrinol Invest 2006;29(5):413–22.

61. Stan MN, Garrity JA, Bradley EA, et al. Randomized, double-blind, placebo-controlled trial of long-acting release octreotide for treatment of Graves' ophthalmopathy. J Clin Endocrinol Metab 2006;91(12):4817–24.

62. Kahaly G, Schrezenmeir J, Krause U, et al. Ciclosporin and prednisone v. prednisone in treatment of Graves' ophthalmopathy: a controlled, randomized and prospective study. Eur J Clin Invest 1986;16:415–22.

63. Wiersinga WM, Prummel MF, Mourits MP, et al. Classification of the eye changes of Graves' disease. Thyroid 1991;1:357–60.

64. Paridaens D, van den Bosch WA, van der Loos TL, et al. The effect of etanercept on Graves' ophthalmopathy: a pilot study. Eye 2005;19:1286–9.

65. Nielsen CH, El Fassi D, Hasselbalch HC, et al. B-cell depletion with rituximab in the treatment of autoimmune diseases. Graves' ophthalmopathy: the latest addition to an expanding family. Expert Opin Biol Ther 2007;7(7):1061–78.

66. Vannucchi G, Campi I, Bonomi M, et al. Rituximab treatment in patients with active Graves' orbitopathy: effects on proinflammatory and humoral immune reactions. Clin Exp Immunol 2010;161(3):436–43.

67. Salvi M, Vannucchi G, Campi I, et al. Rituximab treatment in a patient with severe thyroid-associated ophthalmopathy: effects on orbital lymphocytic infiltrates. Clin Immunol 2009;131(2):360.

68. El Fassi D, Banga JP, Gilbert JA, et al. Treatment of Graves' disease with rituximab specifically reduces the production of thyroid stimulating autoantibodies. Clin Immunol 2009;130(3):252.

69. Silkiss RZ, Reier A, Coleman M, et al. Rituximab for thyroid eye disease. Ophthal Plast Reconstr Surg 2010;26(5):310–4.

70. Salvi M, Vannucchi G, Campi I, et al. Efficacy of rituximab treatment for thyroid-associated ophthalmopathy as a result of intraorbital B-cell depletion in one patient unresponsive to steroid immunosuppression. Eur J Endocrinol 2006; 154(4):511.

71. Salvi M, Vannucchi G, Campi I, et al. Treatment of Graves' disease and associated ophthalmopathy with the anti-CD20 monoclonal antibody rituximab: an open study. Eur J Endocrinol 2007;156:33–40.

72. El Fassi D, Nielsen CH, Hasselbalch HC, et al. Treatment-resistant severe, active Graves' ophthalmopathy successfully treated with B lymphocyte depletion. Thyroid 2006;16:709–10.

73. Khanna D, Chong KK, Afifiyan NF, et al. Rituximab treatment of patients with severe, corticosteroid-resistant thyroid-associated ophthalmopathy. Ophthalmology 2010;117:133–9. e2.

74. Krassas GE, Stafilidou A, Boboridis KG. Failure of rituximab treatment in a case of severe thyroid ophthalmopathy unresponsive to steroids. Clin Endocrinol (Oxf) 2010;72:853–5.

75. El Fassi D, Nielsen CH, Kjeldsen J, et al. Ulcerative colitis following B lymphocyte depletion with rituximab in a patient with Graves' disease. Gut 2008;57: 714–5.

76. Marcocci C, Kahaly GJ, Krassas GE, et al. European Group on Graves' Orbitopathy. Selenium and the course of mild Graves' orbitopathy. N Engl J Med 2011; 364(20):1920.
77. van Steensel L, van Hagen PM, Paridaens D, et al. Whole orbital tissue culture identifies imatinib mesylate and adalimumab as potential therapeutics for Graves' ophthalmopathy. Br J Ophthalmol 2011;95(5):735–8.
78. Tian XL, Yao W, Guo ZJ, et al. Low dose pirfenidone suppresses transforming growth factor beta-1 and tissue inhibitor of metalloproteinase-1, and protects rats from lung fibrosis induced by bleomycin. Chin Med Sci J 2006;21(3): 145–51.
79. Kim H, Choi YH, Park SJ, et al. Antifibrotic effect of Pirfenidone on orbital fibroblasts of patients with thyroid-associated ophthalmopathy by decreasing TIMP-1 and collagen levels. Invest Ophthalmol Vis Sci 2010;51(6):3061–6.
80. Sakula A. Henry Hyde Salter (1823-71): a biographic sketch. Thorax 1985;40: 887–8.
81. Asthma Facts and Figures. Available at: http://www.aafa.org. Accessed March 20, 2012.
82. Mutius EC, Drazen JM. A patient with asthma seeks medical advice: 1828, 1928 and 2012. N Engl J Med 2012;366:827–34.
83. Shalev I, Schmelze M, Robson SC, et al. Making sense of regulatory T-cell suppressive function. Semin Immunol 2011;23:282–92.
84. Holgate ST. Pathophysiology of asthma: what has our current understanding taught us about new therapeutic approaches. J Allergy Clin Immunol 2011;128: 495–505.
85. Kim H, Mazza J. Asthma. Allergy Asthma Clin Immunol 2011;7(Suppl 1):S2.
86. Noon L. Prophylactic inoculation against hay fever. Lancet 1911;1:1572.
87. Abramson MJ, Puy RM, Weiner JM. Allergen immunotherapy for asthma. Cochrane Database Syst Rev 2003;4:CD001186.
88. Calamita Z, Saconato H, Pela AB, et al. Efficacy of sublingual immunotherapy in asthma: systematic review of randomized clinical trials using the Cochrane collaboration method. Allergy 2006;61:1162–72.
89. Calderon MA, Casale TB, Togias A, et al. Allergen specific immunotherapy for respiratory allergies: from meta-analysis to registration and beyond [Erratum appears in J Allergy Clin Immunol 2011;127(4):859]. J Allergy Clin Immunol 2011;127:30–8.
90. Cox L, Nelson H, Lockey R, et al. Allergen immunotherapy: a practice parameter third update [Erratum appears in J Allergy Clin Immunol 2011;127(3):840]. J Allergy Clin Immunol 2011;127(Suppl 1):S1–55.
91. Akdis CA, Akdis M. Mechanisms of allergen-specific immunotherapy. J Allergy Clin Immunol 2011;127:18–27.
92. Cox L, Larenas-Linnemann D, Lockey RF, et al. Speaking the same language: the World Allergy Organization subcutaneous immunotherapy systemic reaction grading system. J Allergy Clin Immunol 2010;125:569–74.
93. Smith SL. Ten years of Orthoclone OKT3 (muromonab- CD3): a review. J Transpl Coord 1996;6(3):109–19.
94. Hanania NA, Alpan O, Hamilos DL, et al. Omalizumab in severe allergic asthma inadequately controlled with standard therapy: a randomized trial. Ann Intern Med 2011;154:573–82.
95. Clienti S, Moijaria JB, Basile E, et al. Monoclonal antibodies for treatment of severe asthma. Curr Allergy Asthma Rep 2011;11:253–60.

96. de Mos M, de Bruijn AG, Huygen FJ, et al. The incidence of complex regional pain syndrome: a population based study. Pain 2007;129:12–20.
97. Huygen FJ, de Bruijn AG, de Bruin MT, et al. Evidence for local inflammation in complex regional pain syndrome type 1. Mediators Inflamm 2002;11:47–51.
98. Uceyler N, Eberle T, Rolke R, et al. Differential expression patterns of cytokines in complex regional pain syndrome. Pain 2007;132:195–205.
99. Goebel A, Baranowski A, Maurer K, et al. Intravenous immunoglobulin treatment of the complex regional pain syndrome. Ann Intern Med 2010;152:152–8.

Index

Note: Page numbers of article titles are in **boldface** type.

A

A Crohn's Disease Clinical Trial Evaluating Infliximab in a New Long-Term Treatment
  Regimen (ACCENT) studies, 528–529, 533–534, 536
Abatacept
  for diabetes mellitus prevention, 626
  for rheumatologic disorders, 487, 489–490
Abciximab, historical view of, 426
ABX-CBL, for hematologic disorders, 586, 600–601
ACCENT (A Crohn's Disease Clinical Trial Evaluating Infliximab in a New Long-Term
  Treatment Regimen) studies, 528–529, 533–534, 536
Acquired inhibitors of coagulation, 603–607
ACT (Active Ulcerative Colitis Trials), 529, 533–534
Activated protein C, for infections, 466–467
Active immunotherapy, historical view of, 422–424
Active Ulcerative Colitis Trials (ACT-1 and ACT-2), 529
Acute inflammatory demyelinating polyradiculopathy, 513–514
Adalimumab
  antibodies against, 536
  for dermatologic disorders, 569–570
  for IBD, 527, 529–532, 534, 536–538
  for kidney diseases, 557
  for rheumatologic disorders, 484–486, 490
  side effects of, 537–538
ADAMTS13 deficiency, 596–598
Adipocytes, in Graves ophthalmopathy, 637–638
AFFIRM trial, for multiple sclerosis, 501, 502
Agammaglobulinemia, X-linked, 434, 436, 441–443
Alefacept, for dermatologic disorders, 570
Alemtuzumab
  for dermatologic disorders, 570
  for hematologic disorders, 586, 592–594, 601, 608
Allergen-specific immunotherapy
  for asthma, 646–647
  for dermatologic disorders, 567–568
  historical view of, 427–428
ALMS trial, for glomerulosclerosis, 552
Anakinra
  for diabetes mellitus prevention, 628
  for rheumatologic disorders, 488–490
Anaphylaxis, to immunoglobulin therapy, 440

Med Clin N Am 96 (2012) 655–670
doi:10.1016/S0025-7125(12)00100-9
0025-7125/12/$ – see front matter © 2012 Elsevier Inc. All rights reserved.

medical.theclinics.com

Metabolism
Fast and Free Publication

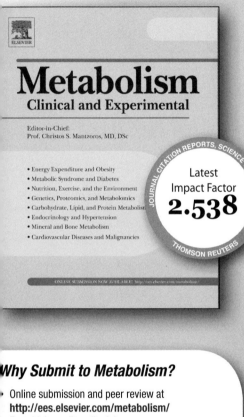
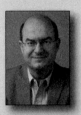

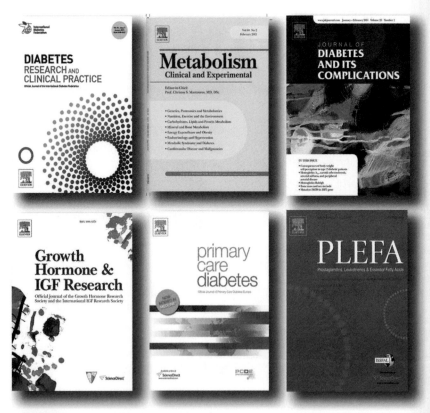

Moving?

Make sure your subscription moves with you!

To notify us of your new address, find your **Clinics Account Number** (located on your mailing label above your name), and contact customer service at:

Email: journalscustomerservice-usa@elsevier.com

800-654-2452 (subscribers in the U.S. & Canada)
314-447-8871 (subscribers outside of the U.S. & Canada)

Fax number: 314-447-8029

Elsevier Health Sciences Division
Subscription Customer Service
3251 Riverport Lane
Maryland Heights, MO 63043

*To ensure uninterrupted delivery of your subscription, please notify us at least 4 weeks in advance of move.